THE LONG QUIET

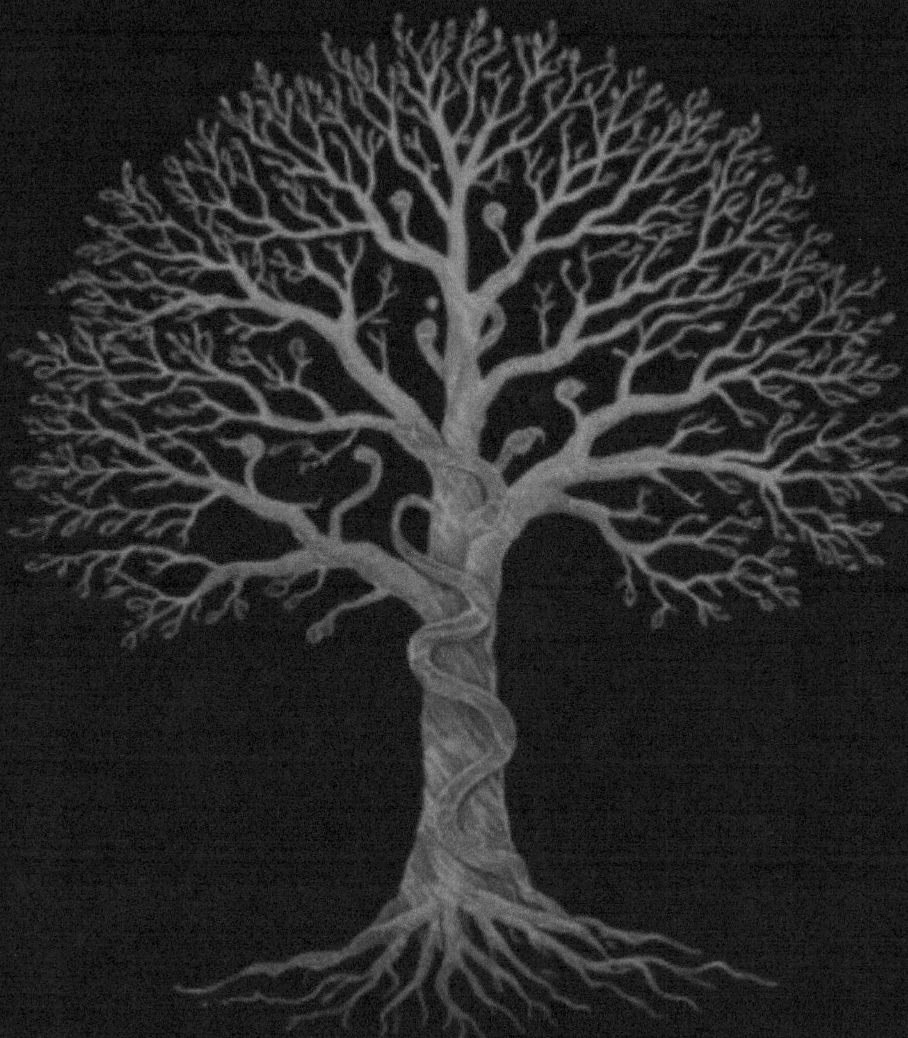

MARK W. BOUTWELL II

The Long Quiet

A Complete Guide to Prolonged Water Fasting,

Biological Renewal, Gut and Parasite Cleansing

Mark W. Boutwell II

The Long Quiet

Excerpts from The Essene Gospel of Peace, translated by Edmond Bordeaux Szekely, are drawn from a work in the public domain.

Published by Eight Hours, an imprint of Lism, LLC
Denver, Colorado, USA
eighthrs.com
First edition · 2026
ISBN (paperback): 978-0-9998990-4-5
ISBN (ebook): 978-0-9998990-3-8
Library of Congress Control Number: 2026917418

Medical Disclaimer

This book describes the author's personal experience with prolonged water fasting and related practices, together with the research that informed it. It is offered for educational purposes only. It is not medical advice, and it is not a substitute for the care of a qualified health professional.

Prolonged fasting, gut-cleansing, and the other practices described in these pages carry real risks and are not appropriate for everyone. What one body can do, another cannot. Before beginning any fast, cleanse, or protocol in this book, consult a licensed physician who knows your history — especially if you are pregnant or nursing, under eighteen, taking medication, or living with any medical condition, including diabetes or any heart, kidney, or liver condition, or any history of disordered eating.

This book is not for anyone with a current or past eating disorder, or with a disordered relationship to food or to the body. Fasting is not a tool for weight loss or control, and it should never be used as one. If any part of this book stirs that kind of impulse, set it down and reach out for support. In the United States, the National Alliance for Eating Disorders offers a helpline staffed by licensed therapists at 1-866-662-1235 (Monday through Friday). It is not a 24-hour crisis line; in a crisis, call or text 988.

The author and publisher accept no responsibility or liability for any loss, injury, or harm claimed to arise, directly or indirectly, from the use or application of any information in this book. By continuing to read, you accept full responsibility for your own choices and your own care.

For Little Marky

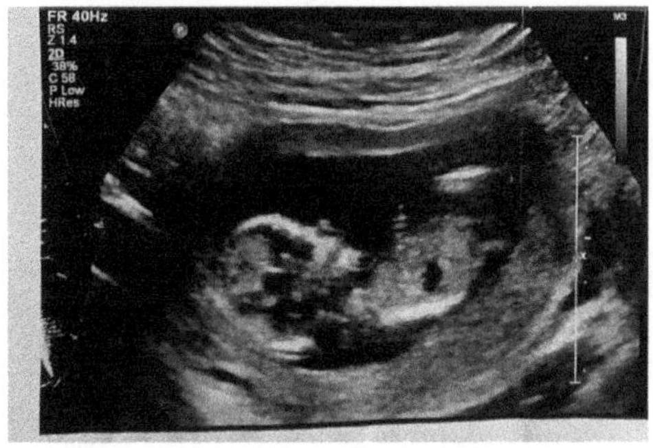

You were smaller than the size of a closed hand.
I held you against my chest
on a hard plastic couch
and for eight hours fell asleep against you
in the gratitude
I have only ever known
next to your sister,
knowing it was the only sleeping
we would ever do together.
Your mother and I drove you home,
determined not to let you miss a moment.
You were touched and loved by your family.
You were laid in soil
cultivated by the lineage you came from,
and we decided to bring you with us,
season after season.
It is still growing.
Everything I have learned to do
since the day I held you,
I learned because I held you.
This book is one of the things that grew.
— your father

For my daughter

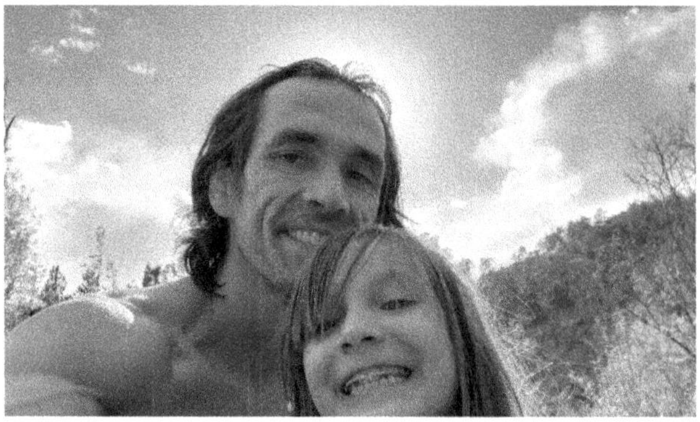

The moment you were made,
I felt something leave me
and arrive in the woman I loved
and I looked her in the eyes
and said her name
and told her we had become three.
She had been preparing her body
for months before that moment.
Fasting. Cleansing. Walking long.
Making herself a place
that you could come into
without the weight of what we had carried before.
I had been preparing for longer.
Years longer.
Without knowing
that what I was preparing for
was you.
Every page of this book
is what I learned
on the way to becoming someone
who could be your father.
— your father

For Sarah

Thank you for being willing to bring two lives into the circle.

A sacred contract — December 20, 2014

This is a sacred contract bonding my commitment to Mark Boutwell. I will walk in line with these values as we create our lives together. I will speak with honesty, be true to myself, to you, living in truth. I will come from a place of understanding and operate with compassion, knowing my source is love. I will do my best to apply non-violent communication, speak with integrity, driven by passion to apply our knowledge that creates growth, stability, and partnership — creating an environment which allows a safe container to express ourselves freely with respect, confidence, and harmony, joining our creative forces to live authentic lives co-creatively in partnership.

— Sarah

For Elizabeth

Thank you for being the spoke that ignited the spark that relit my flame.

Table of Contents

Before You Read This Book

This book was born from personal experience — not a medical degree.

What you are about to read is one person's journey — documented honestly, shared openly and offered with the deepest respect for your individual path.

Please read what follows carefully before going any further.

Medical Disclaimer

The information contained in this book is based entirely on the author's personal experience with prolonged water fasting and gut cleansing protocols. It is shared for educational and informational purposes only.

This book is not medical advice.

The author is not a licensed physician, registered dietitian or certified medical professional. Nothing written in these pages should be interpreted as a diagnosis, treatment recommendation or substitute for professional medical guidance.

Before attempting any prolonged fast or cleansing protocol you should:

• Consult your physician or qualified healthcare provider

• Disclose all existing medical conditions

• Disclose all medications and supplements you are currently taking

• Obtain medical supervision for any fast exceeding 24 hours

• Undergo baseline blood work and health assessment

• Have a qualified medical professional monitor your progress throughout

Prolonged fasting carries serious medical risks including but not limited to:

• Severe electrolyte imbalances

• Cardiac arrhythmias

• Refeeding syndrome — which can be fatal if managed incorrectly

• Muscle wasting including cardiac muscle

• Immune suppression

• Psychological complications

These risks are real. They are serious. They require medical oversight.

The author and publisher accept no liability whatsoever for any harm, injury or adverse outcome resulting from the application of information contained in this book. By continuing to read you acknowledge that you do so entirely at your own risk and with full personal responsibility for your choices.

A Note on Who This Book Is For

This protocol is powerful.

Precisely because it is powerful — it is not for everyone.

This book is written for adults who are:

• In generally good health with no serious underlying medical conditions

• Working with or intending to work with qualified medical supervision

• Approaching fasting from a place of genuine health seeking

• Psychologically stable and in a healthy relationship with their body and food

• Fully informed of the risks and proceeding with clear conscious intention

---

An Important Message About Eating Disorders

This section matters deeply. Please do not skip it.

Prolonged fasting — when approached from the wrong place — can cause profound harm to people struggling with disordered eating or difficult relationships with food and body image.

The language of cleansing, purification and gut health can sometimes become a way of justifying patterns that are not about health at all — but about control, punishment or fear.

If any part of you recognizes that pattern — this book is not your next step.

Your next step is support.

If you or someone you know is struggling with disordered eating please reach out to:

Alliance for Eating Disorders Helpline 📞 1-866-662-1235 *Free support and connection to specialized care*

There is no shame in recognizing that something deeper needs attention first. In fact — recognizing it is an act of profound courage and self awareness.

Healing the gut means nothing if the relationship with the body remains broken.

True healing begins from the inside out — in every sense of those words.

How to Use This Book

This book is designed to be read in order.

Each chapter builds on the last — creating a complete understanding before moving to the next layer of the protocol. Jumping ahead without the foundation is like building a house from the roof down.

Read it once fully before attempting anything described within it.

Then read it again with a pen in your hand.

Knowledge without understanding is just information.

This book is designed to give you both.

A Personal Note From the Author

I almost did not write this book.

The experiences contained in these pages are deeply personal. The protocol described here has transformed my life and the lives of hundreds of people I have had the privilege of guiding through it.

But I am aware that information this specific — this detailed — carries responsibility.

I wrote it anyway — because the alternative is that people attempt these protocols without guidance, without context and without the understanding that makes the difference between transformation and harm.

My intention is your safety as much as your healing.

Please honor that intention by proceeding with care, with medical support and with deep respect for your own body.

It has carried you this far.

Treat it accordingly.

Now — if you are ready — let us begin.

Who This Book Is Not For

A Necessary Conversation Before We Go Further

This section exists because the author cares more about your wellbeing than about selling a protocol.

Please read it carefully.

Please read it honestly.

The Most Important Pages in This Book

Every protocol has boundaries. Every intervention has contraindications. Every powerful tool can cause harm in the wrong hands — or at the wrong time — or for the wrong reasons.

Prolonged water fasting is no exception.

What follows is not a disclaimer written by a lawyer. It is a genuine and direct conversation about who should not undertake this protocol — and why.

If you find yourself in any of the categories below — this book is not your next step.

Something else is.

And that something else is equally worthy of your attention and care.

Absolute Medical Contraindications

The following conditions make prolonged water fasting **medically dangerous** regardless of supervision:

Cardiac conditions:

- Any history of cardiac arrhythmia
- Heart failure or cardiomyopathy
- Recent cardiac event or procedure
- Prolonged QT syndrome
- Electrolyte sensitive cardiac conditions of any kind

Metabolic conditions:

• Type 1 diabetes — insulin dependent

• Severe Type 2 diabetes with complications

• Any history of diabetic ketoacidosis

• Adrenal insufficiency or Addison's disease

• Thyroid disorders that are uncontrolled

Nutritional status:

• Current malnutrition or underweight status

• Any history of significant nutritional deficiency

• Active eating disorder — see dedicated section below

• Recent significant unintentional weight loss

Organ function:

• Kidney disease — any stage of chronic kidney disease

• Liver disease — cirrhosis, hepatitis, liver failure

• Pancreatic conditions

• Severe gastrointestinal disease — Crohn's disease, severe IBD, recent bowel surgery

Other absolute contraindications:

• Pregnancy or breastfeeding

• Active cancer — particularly any involving the digestive tract

• Any condition requiring daily medication that cannot be safely paused

• Recent major surgery — within 6 months

• Active infection or acute illness

• Children and adolescents — under any circumstances

(Figure C.1 — see the online Figure Guide)

Conditions Requiring Exceptional Medical Oversight

The following conditions do not absolutely prohibit prolonged fasting — but require direct ongoing medical supervision throughout:

• Controlled Type 2 diabetes — medication adjustment essential

• History of cardiac conditions — currently stable

• History of kidney stones

• Autoimmune conditions — fasting affects immune function significantly

• Any psychiatric condition — including anxiety and depression

• History of substance use — fasting can trigger relapse vulnerability

• Older adults — over 65 — physiological reserves require careful monitoring

• Anyone on prescription medications of any kind

If you fall into any of these categories and still wish to undertake this protocol — the conversation begins with your physician.

Not with this book.

A Dedicated Section on Eating Disorders

This requires its own space.

Because it is the most important contraindication in this entire book.

Prolonged fasting — undertaken from a place of genuine health — is a powerful therapeutic tool.

Prolonged fasting — undertaken from a place of disordered relationship with food and body — is not fasting.

It is restriction with a protocol wrapped around it.

The difference matters enormously. And the most dangerous thing about that difference is that it is often invisible from the inside.

You should not undertake this protocol if:

• Food restriction brings a sense of **control, safety or relief** that feels disproportionate to its physical effects

• The idea of eating feels threatening, frightening or morally significant

• You have a history of **anorexia, bulimia, binge eating disorder or any restrictive eating pattern**

• You have previously used fasting, cleanses or detox protocols as a way of **compensating for eating**

• The language of **purity, contamination or control** in relation to food resonates strongly with you

• Weight loss is a primary motivation — even if framed as a secondary one

• You have been told by a doctor, therapist or person close to you that your relationship with food concerns them

• Reading this book produces a sense of **excitement or relief** that feels more emotional than intellectual

None of these things make you broken.

None of them are shameful.

All of them are signals that a different kind of support is what is actually needed right now.

The honest truth:

A prolonged fast will not heal a difficult relationship with food and body.

It will intensify it.

The restriction, the control, the sense of purity — these things feel like healing when they are not. They feel like progress when they are circling. They feel like strength when they are a symptom.

Real healing of this kind of difficulty requires specialized support.

Not a longer fast.

Not a stricter protocol.

Human connection with someone trained to help.

If any of this resonates — please reach out:

Alliance for Eating Disorders Helpline 📞 1-866-662-1235 *Free support and connection to specialized care Available to anyone — not just those with a formal diagnosis*

You do not need to be certain something is wrong to call.

Uncertainty itself is enough of a reason.

A Note on Using This Protocol for Weight Loss

This needs to be said directly.

The protocol in this book is designed for **gut cleansing, parasite elimination and biological renewal.**

It is not a weight loss protocol.

Weight loss will occur during a prolonged fast — this is unavoidable and not the point. Using this protocol primarily or significantly as a weight loss tool:

• Misses the actual purpose entirely

• Creates a relationship with the protocol that is psychologically risky

• Is not what this book is designed to support

If weight management is your primary goal — this is not the right tool.

There are better, safer and more sustainable approaches.

Please seek guidance from a qualified healthcare provider.

The Question Worth Sitting With

Before you go further in this book — sit with this question honestly:

Why do I want to do this?

Not the answer that sounds best. Not the answer that feels most defensible.

The real answer. The one underneath the first answer.

If that answer — honestly examined — is about health, healing, spiritual practice or biological renewal — then continue.

If that answer — honestly examined — carries something else alongside it — fear of food, desire for control, punishment, a need to feel small or pure or empty —

Then the most courageous thing you can do is set this book down.

And pick up the phone instead.

Alliance for Eating Disorders Helpline: 1-866-662-1235

This section was written with care.

It was written because the author has sat with enough people through enough difficult moments to know that the most important thing is not the protocol.

It is you.

Your health.

Your wholeness.

Your life beyond this fast.

That matters more than any chapter that follows.

If you have read this section honestly — and you are in the right place to continue — then let us proceed.

*Chapter 26** is waiting.*

A Self-Reflection Before You Begin

The 15 Questions

This is one of the most important sections in this book.

Please do not skip it.

Please do not rush it.

Please answer honestly — even if the honest answer is uncomfortable.

Why This Assessment Exists

This protocol is powerful. That power can serve you — or it can harm you — depending on what you bring to it.

The questions that follow are not designed to test you. They are designed to help you see yourself clearly.

The author has guided enough people through this work to know that the difference between a healing fast and a harmful one is rarely about the protocol itself.

It is about who is doing it — and why.

How to Use This Tool

• Find a quiet moment when you can be honest with yourself

• Read each question carefully

• Answer based on your actual experience — not the answer you think is correct

• Score each question

• Add your total at the end

• Read the score interpretation honestly

This is not a test you can pass or fail by giving the right answers.

It is a mirror.

Look into it honestly.

Scoring Each Question

For each question — assign a number based on how true the statement is for you:

0 — Never or rarely true **1** — Sometimes true **2** — Often or always true

---

The Questions

---

1. I think about food, calories, weight or my body for significant portions of each day.

Score: ___

---

2. When I restrict my food intake or fast — I feel a sense of accomplishment, control or relief that goes beyond the physical effects.

Score: ___

---

3. I have used or considered using fasting, cleanses or detox protocols specifically as a way to compensate for eating, drinking or weight gain.

Score: ___

---

4. The thought of eating a normal meal — particularly if it includes foods I consider impure or unhealthy — produces anxiety, guilt or fear in me.

Score: ___

---

5. I have a history of restrictive eating, binge eating, purging, excessive exercise or other behaviors that someone else might describe as disordered.

Score: ___

6. Someone close to me — a family member, friend, doctor, therapist or partner — has expressed concern about my relationship with food, exercise or my body.

Score: ___

7. The idea of completing a 28 to 40 day fast produces excitement, pride or relief that feels disproportionate to its medical purpose.

Score: ___

8. I weigh myself frequently or check my body in the mirror multiple times a day to monitor changes.

Score: ___

9. I find it difficult to eat in front of others — or I feel anxious about meals I do not control.

Score: ___

10. Weight loss is one of my motivations for this protocol — even if I tell myself it is a secondary or unimportant one.

Score: ___

11. The language of purity, contamination, cleanness or detoxification in relation to food strongly resonates with me.

Score: ___

12. I have felt that I deserve to be hungry — or that hunger is a form of strength, virtue or moral cleanliness.

Score: ___

13. My self worth fluctuates significantly based on what I have eaten, my weight or how my body looks.

Score: ___

---

14. I have used food restriction or fasting in the past to manage difficult emotions, stress or trauma rather than for clear health reasons.

Score: ___

---

15. Reading this book — or thinking about this protocol — has produced an emotional excitement that feels more intense than my excitement about other health practices.

Score: ___

Calculating Your Score

Add up the numbers from all 15 questions.

Your total score: ___

What Your Score Means

Score of 0 to 5 — Low Concern

Your answers suggest a relatively healthy relationship with food, your body and your motivations.

This protocol — undertaken with proper medical supervision and full understanding of the contraindications in the previous section — appears to be appropriate for you.

Continue reading.

Proceed thoughtfully.

The intention behind your interest appears to come from a place of genuine health seeking.

Score of 6 to 12 — Moderate Concern

Your answers suggest some areas of complexity in your relationship with food and body.

This score does not necessarily mean you have an eating disorder. It does mean that some of your motivations and experiences around food may benefit from examination before undertaking a protocol this powerful.

Recommended actions:

- **Speak with a qualified mental health professional** — particularly one with experience in eating behaviors — before beginning this protocol
- Discuss your interest in this fast openly with them
- Examine specifically the questions where you scored 1 or 2 — what is underneath those answers?
- Consider whether less intensive interventions might serve your actual goals

A score in this range is not a verdict.

It is an invitation to deeper self examination before proceeding.

Score of 13 to 30 — Significant Concern

Your answers strongly suggest patterns that this protocol could intensify rather than heal.

The features described in the questions you scored higher on are not character flaws. They are not signs of weakness. They are signs that something deeper is asking for attention — and this protocol is unlikely to be the kind of attention that helps.

Please consider this strongly:

- This protocol — undertaken at this score range — carries significant risk of exacerbating disordered eating patterns
- The structure and discipline of fasting can feel like healing while reinforcing patterns that are quietly harmful
- The clarity and control that prolonged fasting produces can become reinforcing in ways that are not in your best interest

What this book recommends — directly and with care:

- Set this book aside for now
- Reach out for professional support — a therapist or specialist in eating disorders
- Begin with healing the relationship — not with restriction
- The fast will still be available to you in the future if it ever becomes appropriate

Alliance for Eating Disorders Helpline 📞 1-866-662-1235

Free support — available to anyone — no formal diagnosis required

---

A Direct Word From the Author

If you scored in the higher ranges — please hear this carefully.

The author has guided hundreds of people through prolonged fasting.

The people who came to it from a place of genuine health seeking found healing.

The people who came to it from a place of disordered relationship with food — even when they passionately believed they were seeking health — almost universally caused themselves harm.

That harm was rarely visible to them in the moment. It looked like progress. It felt like discipline. It seemed like exactly what they needed.

Until it wasn't.

Some of those people sought help months or years later — having compounded the difficulty rather than healed it.

This assessment exists because the author would have given anything to put a tool like this in those people's hands before they started.

If you are reading this and you scored in a concerning range — you are being given that tool.

Please use it.

The protocol in this book will exist whenever you genuinely need it. It is not going anywhere. You are not missing your only chance by waiting.

What may be missing — and what professional support can help you find — is the foundation of self-relationship that would let any healing protocol actually heal.

That foundation is more important than this fast.

It is more important than any fast.

It is what makes everything else possible.

Before You Continue Reading

If your score was in the **low concern range** — proceed with the book.

If your score was in the **moderate concern range** — please pause until you have spoken with a qualified mental health professional. They can help you understand whether and when this protocol is appropriate for you.

If your score was in the **significant concern range** — please set this book aside. Reach out for support. The path forward begins somewhere different than these pages.

Your wellbeing matters more than completing this book.

With genuine respect for whatever brought you here — and genuine care for what comes next — let us continue only if continuing serves your actual healing.

The Ancient Practice

A History of Fasting Across Human Civilization

Before any of the science in this book existed, before the word *fasting* could be uttered in any language a modern reader would recognize, before there were physicians or universities or printed books, human beings were doing this. They were setting down food on purpose. They were going without, for stretches of days and weeks, and emerging from the experience changed.

We know this because they wrote about it. They painted it on temple walls. They built rituals around it that have survived, in some cases, for five thousand years and continue, this morning, in cities across the world. Whatever else has divided human beings across continents and centuries — language, religion, climate, technology — the practice of voluntary fasting has run beneath the surface of nearly every culture we have records of. It is one of the oldest things our species does.

This protocol is new. The practice it serves is older than recorded history. This preface places you in that lineage.

The Universal Practice

The fact that humans fast is not in itself unusual. Many animals fast — bears in winter, snakes between meals, salmon during the long swim home. What makes human fasting unusual is that we do it deliberately, for reasons we can articulate, in patterns we have refined across thousands of years.

What is more striking is that we have refined those patterns independently. The Egyptian priest of three thousand years ago did not consult the Hindu sage. The Hindu sage did not exchange notes with the Christian mystic. The indigenous shaman of the American plains had never heard of the Sufi practitioner of the Persian desert. And yet, across continents and centuries that had no contact with one another, they all arrived at the same essential observation. That to set food down for a period of days does something to the human body and the human mind that nothing else does. That the experience produces clarity. That it produces healing. That it produces, sometimes, a kind of contact with something larger than the self that the practitioner never afterward forgets.

When unrelated cultures arrive independently at the same conclusion, what we are seeing is not coincidence. We are seeing something true about human biology. About human consciousness. About the relationship between the two.

The protocol in this book draws on that long observation. It does not invent. It refines. The fasting itself is the inheritance.

Ancient Egypt

The oldest documented therapeutic fasting we have records of comes from Egypt, around three thousand years before the common era. The papyri describe specific protocols — fasts of three days, of seven, of longer — prescribed for digestive complaint, for spiritual purification, for preparation before sacred ceremony. The Egyptians had observed that withholding food produced effects that food itself could not produce. They had no theory of autophagy. They had no understanding of ketones or the migrating motor complex. What they had was five centuries of accumulated observation, passed from priest to priest and physician to physician, and recorded with a precision that startles modern readers when they encounter it.

The healing god Imhotep — later worshipped as a deity, originally a physician who lived around 2600 BCE — was associated with fasting protocols that the temples maintained for centuries after his death. The priestly classes fasted regularly, both as health practice and as spiritual discipline. The temple kitchens were sometimes idle for days at a time while preparation rituals proceeded.

The earliest written records of human medicine, in other words, include fasting at their center. Whatever else medicine has become in the four thousand years since, this is where it began.

Ancient India

In India, fasting reached a degree of sophistication that has not been matched anywhere else in the world. The Ayurvedic tradition, which developed over thousands of years on the Indian subcontinent, recognized fasting as one of the primary therapeutic modalities — to be applied in different ways for different body constitutions, in different patterns for different ailments, with detailed guidance on how to prepare for the fast, conduct it, and break it.

The Hindu spiritual traditions added layers of meaning the medical traditions had not articulated. *Ekadashi*, the fast on the eleventh day of each lunar fortnight, has been observed continuously for thousands of years. *Navratri*, nine days of fasting and worship, marks the seasonal transitions. *Maha Shivaratri*, the great night of Shiva, is accompanied by a fast that lasts from sunrise to sunrise the following day. Each fast is woven into a calendar of remembrance and devotion that does not separate the bodily practice from the spiritual one.

The Jain tradition went further than any other. Jain practitioners — including monks who took vows for life and laypeople who maintained the practice alongside ordinary work and family — undertook fasts that astonish modern medicine. *Paryushana*, an annual fasting festival, asks practitioners for eight days of strict abstention. *Maskhaman*, a one-month water fast, is undertaken by some advanced practitioners. There are recorded cases of Jain practitioners undertaking fasts of sixty days, ninety days, even a hundred days for spiritual purification, with the support of the community and under the guidance of teachers who themselves had passed through similar experiences.

Buddhist practice, which arose in this same cultural soil, inherited and modified these traditions. The Buddha himself fasted for extended periods before his enlightenment under the Bodhi tree. Theravada Buddhist monks, to this day, do not eat after noon. The morning meal is the only meal, and the long afternoon and evening are spent in meditation, study, and the work of the monastery.

What we are seeing in India is not occasional fasting. It is a civilization in which the practice of voluntary fasting has been continuously maintained, taught, and refined for as long as the civilization has existed.

Ancient China

In China, fasting was woven into both the medical tradition and the spiritual one, and the line between them was rarely sharp. Traditional Chinese Medicine, which emerged over thousands of years of clinical observation, recognized fasting as a means of restoring qi — the life force whose smooth circulation through the body was understood to be the foundation of health. The TCM physician prescribed fasting for stagnation, for excess, for conditions that required not the addition of something but the subtraction of it. The body, the tradition held, required periodic rest from the work of digestion as much as the muscles required rest from labor.

The Taoist tradition, which intersected with TCM at many points, developed its own fasting practices in the service of internal alchemy. *Bigu*, the practice of grain abstention, sometimes lasted weeks or months. Some advanced practitioners abstained from food entirely for periods that stretched the limits of what modern physiology would consider possible — and there are credible historical accounts, from observers who had no reason to exaggerate, of practitioners maintaining fasts that should not have been survivable. Whether these accounts are accurate in every detail or contain the embellishment that often accompanies religious narratives, what they tell us is that the upper limits of human fasting were being explored, in a disciplined and intentional way, in monasteries across China for many centuries before modern medicine took notice.

When Buddhism arrived from India, it brought additional fasting practices that integrated with the existing Taoist framework. Chan Buddhism, which would later be transmitted to Japan as Zen, incorporated fasting into the rhythm of monastic life. The combined traditions produced sophisticated fasting protocols that influenced not only Chinese culture but every culture that encountered Chinese thought.

The medical texts that survive from this period describe fasting practices that are remarkably similar to what is taught in this book. The wisdom is not new. It is being recovered.

The Hebrew and Jewish Tradition

The Hebrew scriptures are saturated with fasting. Moses fasted forty days on Mount Sinai before receiving the Torah. Elijah fasted forty days journeying to Mount Horeb. David fasted in mourning. Esther called for a three-day fast before approaching the king on behalf of her people. The prophet Daniel undertook multiple extended fasts, recorded in such detail that modern readers can reconstruct the protocols he followed.

The forty-day fast — which appears in the Mosaic narrative and which has shaped much of what Western culture associates with prolonged fasting — finds its roots here. Every person who has undertaken a forty-day water fast in the centuries since, regardless of their tradition, is walking in a path traced thousands of years ago in the deserts of the Near East.

The Jewish tradition has maintained these practices continuously, without break, for more than three thousand years. *Yom Kippur*, the Day of Atonement, asks observant Jews for a complete fast lasting twenty-five hours — no food, no water, no comfort. *Tisha B'Av*, mourning the destruction of the temples, asks the same. There are several other fast days in the Jewish calendar, each tied to a moment of historical or spiritual weight, each observed by communities scattered now across every continent on earth.

The scale of this is difficult to grasp at first. Tens of millions of people, year after year, century after century, have set food down on the same days, for the same reasons, in continuity with their ancestors who did the same. Whatever fasting is — and the practitioners themselves have offered many answers across the millennia — it is something that this tradition has held onto with rare tenacity, through diaspora and persecution and the loss of nearly everything else.

The Christian Tradition

Christianity inherited the fasting practices of Judaism and expanded them. Christ's forty days in the wilderness — itself an echo of the Mosaic forty days — became the foundational fast of Christian tradition, and the season of Lent, observed by hundreds of millions of Christians today across the world, is its long shadow.

In the Eastern Orthodox tradition, the fasting practice has remained particularly strong. Orthodox Christians fast on Wednesdays and Fridays year-round, in remembrance of the betrayal and the crucifixion. They fast through Lent before Easter. They fast through Advent before Christmas. They fast at other points in the liturgical year that the Western churches have largely forgotten. The Ethiopian Orthodox Christians fast more days than any other Christian community — over two hundred days a year for the most observant — in a continuous tradition that stretches back nearly two thousand years.

The Christian mystical tradition produced practitioners who took the fast further than the liturgical calendar required. Saint Catherine of Siena, in the fourteenth century, was reported to have lived for years on minimal food. Saint Teresa of Avila practiced regular extended fasts. The Desert Fathers, the early Christian monastics who withdrew into the deserts of Egypt and Syria in the third and fourth centuries, developed protocols of fasting and meditation that are still studied for what they reveal about the limits of human asceticism.

The Lenten fast remains, today, the most widely observed prolonged fast in the Western world. Forty days, in shadowed echo of the desert that began it.

Islam

Of all the fasting traditions on earth, none is currently practiced at the scale of Ramadan. Each year, for one lunar month, an estimated 1.8 billion Muslims across the world fast from dawn to sunset — no food, no water, no smoking, no marital intimacy during the daylight hours. They have done this every year for nearly fifteen hundred years, since the Prophet Muhammad first received the verses of the Quran that established the practice as the fourth pillar of the faith.

Beyond Ramadan, Islamic tradition includes voluntary fasting practices that observant Muslims maintain throughout the year. Mondays and Thursdays are recommended fast days. The middle three days of each lunar month are recommended fast days — the so-called White Days, when the moon is full. Six days of Shawwal, the month following Ramadan, are observed by many. The Day of Ashura is fasted by Sunni and Shia alike, in remembrance of different but overlapping events.

The cumulative effect is that observant Muslims spend a substantial fraction of every year in some form of fasting practice. The Prophet himself emphasized the health benefits of the fast alongside the spiritual ones, and modern research has confirmed many of the physiological effects he described. The annual Ramadan fast represents the largest coordinated fasting practice in human history, performed by more people than any other voluntary practice on earth.

It has continued, without interruption, for nearly fifteen centuries.

Native American and Indigenous Traditions

Across the Americas, before any European contact, indigenous peoples maintained fasting traditions of their own. The vision quest — a multi-day fast undertaken in solitude, often in a high or remote place — was practiced across many tribal traditions and continues today among many indigenous peoples who have preserved their ceremonial life. The fast was sought for guidance. For passage from youth to adulthood. For contact with whatever the tradition recognized as sacred. For healing of body and spirit at moments when ordinary medicine could not reach.

The traditional healers — the medicine people of various tribes — used fasting as part of their treatment protocols, often combined with sweat lodge ceremonies and specific herbal preparations. The knowledge was passed from teacher to student through long apprenticeship. Much of it was nearly lost during the centuries of colonization, suppression, and forced assimilation that followed European contact, and what remains exists today in the keeping of practitioners who have worked, often at great cost, to preserve their inheritance.

What these traditions emphasize, with particular clarity, is the spiritual dimension of fasting. The body's surrender becomes the gateway to vision and connection. The hungry body, properly supported, opens to something the fed body cannot perceive. This is observation, not belief — repeated across many tribes who never met one another, and consistent enough that the modern Western practitioner who undertakes a prolonged fast often experiences, with surprise, what indigenous traditions described long ago.

Ancient Greece

The Greek tradition gave us the foundations of Western medicine, and from the beginning, fasting was central to it. Hippocrates, in the fifth century before the common era, prescribed fasting for many of the conditions his patients brought to him. His most famous remark on the subject — *to eat when you are sick is to feed your sickness* — has echoed through Western medicine for two and a half thousand years. He had observed, as physicians before him had observed, that the body in illness required not the addition of nourishment but the lifting of the burden of digestion.

Plutarch, four centuries later, would write that one should *use medicine, only as a last resort, and rather fast a day*. The Greek understanding of fasting was practical and clinical, rooted in observation of what worked and what did not. It was passed forward into Roman medicine through Galen, who served as physician to the Roman emperors and whose writings shaped European medicine through the medieval period.

When Western medicine, in the modern era, began to lose its fasting traditions, what was being lost was not a fad of the moment. It was a thread of practice continuous for two thousand years.

Medieval Europe

Through the medieval period, fasting remained central to European life. The Christian monastic orders — Benedictines, Cistercians, Carthusians, and many others — maintained fasting protocols that varied by order and by season but together meant that some monks fasted half the days of every year. The fasting was woven into the rhythm of liturgical time, marking the seasons, preparing the body and spirit for the great feasts that punctuated the calendar.

The medieval physicians prescribed fasting as routinely as their predecessors had. Therapeutic fasting was considered standard practice for many conditions and was applied in protocols that continued the Hippocratic tradition with little modification.

The mystical tradition, which had been quietly present in Christianity from the beginning, produced women in particular — and the historical record is unusually full of them — who practiced extended fasts in pursuit of spiritual experience. Some of them lived for years on minimal food, by the testimony of contemporaries who observed them and had no reason to embellish. Modern medicine, when it considers these accounts, generally concludes either that the accounts contain exaggeration or that the practitioners had access to small amounts of food we would consider substantial. Either way, what we are seeing is a culture in which prolonged fasting was not unusual. It was simply part of the spiritual landscape.

The cultural memory of how to fast — passed down generation after generation in monasteries, in households, in the rhythm of village life — was widespread in Europe until comparatively recently. It has only been in the past century or so that most Europeans have lost the practice. The recovery of the practice, in our own time, is the recovery of something that was once universal.

Africa

African fasting traditions have not received the attention given to those of other continents, but they are deep and varied. Ethiopian Orthodox Christianity maintains some of the most extensive fasting traditions in any branch of Christianity, with practitioners observing more than two hundred fast days in a typical year. The tradition is continuous and has been since the conversion of the Ethiopian kingdom to Christianity in the fourth century, making it one of the longest unbroken Christian fasting practices on earth.

Beyond the Christian tradition, various African cultures have incorporated fasting into their healing and spiritual practices for as long as anyone can remember. Initiation rituals across many tribes have used fasting as part of the passage from one life stage to the next. Traditional healers have used fasting protocols alongside herbal treatments. The Islamic presence across much of the continent, combined with these older traditions, produces in many regions a layered fasting culture in which Ramadan is observed alongside practices that predate Islam by centuries.

What the African traditions remind us is that fasting wisdom is not the property of any single culture. It is part of the human heritage. Wherever humans have lived in community, in continuity with their ancestors, they have eventually arrived at the practice — usually without instruction from anyone outside their own tradition.

The Modern Revival

By the nineteenth and twentieth centuries, much of the traditional fasting wisdom had been forgotten in mainstream Western culture. The rise of industrial agriculture had made food abundant in a way it had never been before. The rise of pharmaceutical medicine had given physicians tools that did not require their patients to do anything difficult. The cultural conditions that had supported fasting — religious calendars observed by communities, knowledge passed from teacher to student, sufficient cultural patience to wait while a body did its slow work — were eroding.

But the practice did not die. It persisted in pockets — in monasteries, in immigrant communities, in the homes of people who remembered what their grandparents had taught them — and in the late nineteenth century, it began to return.

Edward Hooker Dewey, an American physician of the late 1800s, wrote extensively on therapeutic fasting at a time when the medical establishment had largely abandoned the practice. His book, *The No-Breakfast Plan and the Fasting Cure*, documented numerous successful prolonged fasts and influenced generations of practitioners who followed.

Herbert Shelton, in the early twentieth century, founded the natural hygiene movement and operated fasting clinics for decades. He supervised thousands of prolonged fasts personally. His foundational text, *The Hygienic System: Fasting and Sun Bathing*, remains in print and continues to influence modern protocols, including this one.

Otto Buchinger, in Germany, founded clinics that still operate today and that have offered medically supervised multi-week fasts for nearly a century. The Buchinger clinics established standards of medical supervision that have allowed prolonged therapeutic fasting to be practiced safely on a scale that would not otherwise have been possible.

Arnold Ehret, working in the early twentieth century, developed the *mucusless diet* theory and wrote *The Mucusless Diet Healing System*, which remains a foundational text for many modern fasting protocols. His understanding of accumulated layers in the gut prefigured much of what later research would confirm.

In our own time, Joel Fuhrman has supervised prolonged therapeutic fasts and brought medical credibility to the practice in a way that made it accessible to mainstream patients. Valter Longo, at the University of Southern California, has produced research on the cellular effects of prolonged fasting that has shaped current understanding. And in 2016, the Nobel Committee awarded the Prize in Physiology or Medicine to Yoshinori Ohsumi for his discoveries about autophagy — the cellular self-cleaning process that prolonged fasting activates more powerfully than any other intervention. The Nobel Prize, in effect, vindicated thousands of years of practice with the language of molecular biology. What the Egyptian priests had observed without instruments, the Indian sages had refined without theory, the Christian mystics had pursued without medical sanction — twenty-first-century cell biology had now confirmed.

The wisdom never disappeared. It simply waited for the right moment to be rediscovered.

What This Lineage Means for You

When you undertake the protocol in this book, you join a lineage. Not metaphorically. Practically. The lineage extends back through the modern researchers who recovered the practice, through the natural hygienists of the nineteenth century, through the medieval monks and the desert mystics, through the Sufi practitioners and the Buddhist nuns, through the Christian saints and the Hindu sages, through the Egyptian priests and the indigenous shamans, all the way back to the earliest humans who, for reasons we will probably never fully recover, set food down on purpose and discovered what happened.

You are not the first to do this. You will not be the last. You are one in an unbroken chain that stretches back to the earliest days of recorded history and probably much further than that.

When you struggle in the first three days of the fast, remember that millions of others have struggled in those same days for thousands of years. When you experience the lightness and clarity that emerges in deep ketosis, remember that Egyptian priests and Hindu sages and Christian mystics and indigenous shamans have all known that exact state. When emotional content surfaces unexpectedly during the fast, remember that this is what fasting has always done across every culture that has practiced it seriously. When you reach the deeper insights of prolonged fasting in the second and third weeks, remember that you are accessing something humans have accessed forever.

You are not alone in this practice. You have never been alone in this practice. The companions of your fast are everyone who has ever undertaken what you are undertaking — across every culture, every century, every continent. Some left records. Some did not. All of them did the work. Now it is your turn.

This book teaches a specific modern protocol. The herbs are particular. The enemas are detailed. The supplements are precise. The science is current. But what underlies it all is ancient. The setting down of food. The allowing of the body to do what only fasting allows it to do. The trusting of a process that has worked for thousands of years.

Welcome to the practice. You are exactly where countless humans have been before you. Now begin.

Journal Entry — Day Zero

Twelve years ago I read four passages, in four small books, and walked into a forest because of them.

The books were the four Gospels of Peace, translated by Edmond Bordeaux Szekely from a manuscript he said he had found in the Vatican. Across the four volumes there were perhaps four hundred pages. I read them and four passages held. The rest passed through me. The four that held described worms that lived in the bowels of men, and an apparatus made of a hollow tree-trunk and a vessel of water that the sick were instructed to use to wash the inside of themselves clean. I had never read anything that named what I had been feeling for most of my life. I read those four passages and a question opened in me that I could not close again.

I did not know whether to believe the man who translated them. The scholars who have read him since say the manuscript cannot be traced to where he claimed to find it — that he was, perhaps, a man who knew how to tell a story. I cannot answer that question and I have stopped trying. What I can say is that something in those four passages was old, and something in them was true, and the part that was true was enough to make me walk into a forest at twenty-eight years old and stay there until my body had answered me.

This is the book I wish I had been handed at twenty-eight, in place of those four passages. The four passages set me walking. They were not enough to walk me through. The technical instructions a reader actually needs to do this work were not in them anymore. They had been pulled out, or eroded, or lost in translation between languages that did not have the words. What remained was enough for me, because of who I am. It would not be enough for most people. That is what this book is for.

— M.W.B. II

Journal Entry No. 1

Day 25 of the Second Fast

My daughter walked me into the forest tonight, the way she has been doing all month, and the trees gave back something I did not know I had lost.

Twelve years ago I went into a forest in the Upper Peninsula and stayed there for forty days. The forest from that fast has lived in me as a place I could return to with my eyes closed. It has been the room I went to when I needed to remember what I was doing. Some time in the last few years — I cannot say when, exactly — the room had begun to dim. I did not notice it dimming. I only noticed, tonight, that the light came back.

My daughter is eight. She has been carrying me through this fast more steadily than any adult in my life has carried me through anything. She does not know she is doing it. She *thinks* she is finding a place by the water for me to break the fast. She *is* finding a place by the water for me to break the fast. She is also, in the doing of it, handing me back a forest I had walked away from without realizing.

The body in the chapter that follows is the body that walked into that first forest. The man writing this entry is the body that walked back out, and walked in again, twelve years later, holding a small hand.

— M.W.B. II

Chapter 1

My Story

* * *

The body that began this story was assembled in the early nineteen-eighties, in a household where my mother and father had been working at a high level in industrial agriculture for more than a decade by then. The chemicals they handled in their work had moved through their lives — on their hands and clothes when they came home, in the air of the rooms I would later be brought into, in the food and the water and the soil of a childhood the broader culture would not yet understand was being conducted in a chemical bath. My body was assembled inside my mother's body during those months, and what was around her was around me. I have come, over the decades since, to think of this as the first inheritance — the body I would later spend twenty-eight days trying to clean was, in some measure, the body I had been given before I was born.

I was the youngest of six. The household I came into was a complicated one. My oldest brother was Spanish. My oldest sister was Korean. My next brother was Spanish. The next sister came after that. The youngest sister before me was Black. I was the baby. By the time I was old enough to look around at my family, the household had its own internal weather — the loyalties, the rivalries, the small daily violences and large occasional ones that circulated among my siblings, in the way that they circulate in any house where many children have been gathered. I will not dwell on what was done to me by my brothers and sisters across those years. It is enough to say that I learned, before I had words for it, that what was happening in the rooms around a child could reach all the way down into him — into the body, into the cells, into the smallest places a child does not yet know he has. The surroundings of a person, when they are unsafe enough, become the person.

What ran underneath all of it, holding everything together, was the example of my parents.

My mother and father were not perfect. They had their own difficulties, their own susceptibilities, their own places where the discipline they brought to their work did not extend into the rest of their lives. But what they offered me, and what shaped me more than anything else in those years, was a kind of contrast I could see clearly even as a child. My siblings, in their various ways, were getting into the kinds of trouble that follow from absent attention — to the body, to the consequences, to the future. My parents were not. My parents got up early. They worked hard. They put their bodies into a long stretch of useful labor every day of every week, and the bodies that emerged from that labor were strong bodies, capable of more years of useful work, that had been kept alive by the practice of being used well.

I watched both. I watched my siblings, and I watched my parents, and I made a decision that I did not at the time recognize as a decision. I decided to follow the parents.

It was not a moral decision. It was not a decision I formed in any kind of conscious way at eight or ten or twelve. It was a decision the body made, watching the two paths in front of it, and recognizing that one of them led somewhere that looked like a life and the other one did not. I gravitated toward my parents the way a plant gravitates toward light. I did the work they asked. I learned to wake early. I learned to put a body into a job and let the job do what jobs do to a body. I did not yet have a vocabulary for any of this. I had only the seeing, repeated daily, of what discipline produced in a person and what its absence produced.

I was given a body that had been chemically loaded before I was born, into a household where the patterns of harm were close at hand and the patterns of discipline were also close at hand. I was given the chance, by accident of birth order and temperament, to choose between them. I chose, mostly without knowing I was choosing, the patterns that were keeping my parents alive.

That choice is the seed of everything that follows.

* * *

Construction was the first place I learned that work produced response.

I was eight the year my father began picking me up after school and bringing me along to his job sites. The work he gave me was small. I swept. I picked up nails the men had dropped. I carried things from one part of a site to another. I rode in the truck with him, watching the way the older men moved around the site. I came back on the weekends and did more of the same. I was eight years old and was being trusted, in the small ways an eight-year-old can be trusted, with the work of being part of a crew. None of it was forced. My father needed someone to bring along, and I wanted to go.

By the time I was thirteen, the work had grown into something larger. I was small still, and the work was not made for me. But by then I had been on enough sites to know how to hold the dumb end of a measuring tape, how to fetch what an older man asked for and bring it back without complaint, how to be useful without being in the way. The men around me were larger and louder than I was. They had been doing this for years. They knew what they were doing in a way I did not. What I learned, across those summers, was that a body that showed up early, that did not complain, that picked up what needed picking up before being asked, became, slowly, a body the older men trusted. The trust was not stated. It arrived in small ways. The keys to the truck. The harder job. The quiet word at the end of the day that said the work had been seen.

Something began to register, across those years, that I would not have words for until much later. The body, used carefully, gave back what was put into it. Not the body in any abstract sense. The actual body, on a job site, in heat, doing useful work for ten or twelve hours, would respond by becoming a body that could do useful work for ten or twelve hours. The strength came from the doing. The capacity came from the being asked. The body that was used carefully became a body that could carry more.

Wrestling came next. I was fourteen the year I joined the team, and the discipline of the sport went deeper into the body than the construction work had. Wrestling did not only ask the body to work; it asked the body to weigh a certain amount on a Friday afternoon, three days after a Tuesday weigh-in, in conditions that were not always conducive to the careful loss of ten or fifteen pounds. The methods I learned for making weight, in those years, were the crude methods of a high school sport on the West Coast in the late nineties. Plastic sweat suits. Spitting into cups. Sitting in saunas with friends, watching the dial on the scale come down. None of this was wisdom. All of it was the body learning a particular thing about itself — that it could be asked to do without, and that it would respond, and that the response would be controllable if you paid enough attention to it.

The Jay Robinson camps were the next layer, and the layer that did the deepest work. Three summers running, twenty-eight days at a time. Three of those camps, each one twenty-eight days, in conditions designed to break a wrestler down to where he could be rebuilt. The number meant nothing to me at the time. The structure was simply the structure. Years later, when I walked into the forest at twenty-eight to fast for twenty-eight days, the rhythm I was stepping into was a rhythm I had already, without knowing it, lived inside. The training was harder than anything I had encountered. Five practices a day. The first one started at six in the morning. The last one finished at nine at night. Long runs between practices, when there were any gaps. The kind of fatigue that does not lift between sessions, that accumulates across the days, until by the end of the camp the body has been remade into a different body. I came home each summer as a slightly different person.

What J Robinson gave me, beyond the training itself, was the first real teaching about food. Until I joined wrestling, food in my house had been whatever I wanted. My parents would let me eat anything I reached for, in the kind of household where the question of what a child put in his body had not, in any structured way, been a question. For a long stretch of my childhood, the only thing I would eat was frozen bean burritos. My mother would ask my father, on more than one occasion, whether they ought to be giving me something different. My father would say, he'll grow out of it. He was, eventually, right. I did grow out of it. But what I grew into was not a structured eating; it was simply a wider variety of whatever I wanted. The crude methods of high school weight-cutting that I had been picking up around the team — the plastic suits, the spitting cups, the saunas — were the first time food had registered as a thing that mattered, and they were not wisdom. What J Robinson taught was different. They taught what real food was. They taught what real rest was. They taught the timing, the proportions, the rhythm of meals across a day. They taught that the food itself was the support, and that the structure of the eating was part of the support. I had not, before those camps, had any vocabulary for any of this. They gave me the vocabulary. The body, given the vocabulary, began to learn what it could become when it was being properly supported.

This is also where the first crack in the wall appeared. I had been raised on the food of a household where industrial agriculture was the family business, and where the food in the house was, accordingly, the food the industry was producing. I had not, until those camps, had reason to question any of it. What I learned there opened a small door I would not be able to close again. The door did not open all at once. It cracked. Through the crack came the first thought that the food in the house I had grown up in might not have been the food my body was best served by. It was a small thought. It would become, over the years that followed, a much larger one.

What I did with what they had given me, after the camps ended each summer, was take it home and keep going. I built my own program around what I had learned. I refined it. I added to it. The teaching had been the seed. The years that followed were what I made of the seed on my own.

What I had been given by the end of those summers was a body that knew it could be worked, a body that knew it could be restricted, and a body that had been told, by men who had been paying attention, that food itself had structure that mattered. That is most of what I had when I left for college, and most of what I would take with me into the years that followed.

* * *

By the time I was eighteen I had been asking the same question of nearly everyone I met. I had asked it of friends and of strangers, of girlfriends and of their mothers, of teachers and of the older men who showed up at the wrestling tournaments to watch their sons and grandsons. I had asked it, by my own rough count, of more than a thousand people. The question was what is love.

The answers I had been given were not bad answers. They were the answers a thousand ordinary people give. Love is a feeling. Love is when you cannot stop thinking about someone. Love is the chemistry. Love is what you fall into. Love is the first year and then it changes into something else. Love is what your parents had if they were lucky and what your parents did not have if they were not. I had collected the answers carefully, the way some people collect coins. I had laid them out next to each other and looked at them. None of them had ever quite settled the question for me. The thousand answers had begun to feel, taken together, like the absence of an answer.

I was a college pilot then, in ROTC, training for a slot in the air. The flying was new and was teaching me a kind of attention I had not had before. The plane did not care what you felt. It cared what you did. The instruments told the truth. The weather told the truth. The engine told the truth. A pilot who confused his feelings about any of those things with the things themselves did not become an old pilot. I did not yet know what to do with that lesson outside the cockpit. But I had begun to suspect that whatever love was, it was probably more like the engine than like the weather of the heart.

On a clear afternoon I landed at a small airfield in Prescott, Arizona, to refuel. I taxied in, shut the engine down, climbed out, and walked into the office to pay for the gas. There was a woman behind the counter. She was older, in her seventies maybe. Silvery hair down past her shoulders. About five foot two. She moved swiftly behind the counter in the way that people move when they have kept their bodies well, and she had the kind of quiet glow on her that people sometimes have when they have lived a careful life all the way through. I handed her my card. She took it.

I had asked the question of nearly everyone I had met since I was a boy. I asked her too.

She did not answer right away. She set the card down. She looked at me for a moment, the way a person looks when they are deciding whether to give a small answer or a true one. Then she gave me the true one.

She said love is not a feeling. It is a decision.

She let that sit for a beat. Then she said: every time I told my husband I loved him, I had already decided. Whatever he did, I had already accepted him for who he was.

She handed the card back. She said something else, probably, about the gas or the weather or the sky I was about to go back into. I do not remember it. I remember walking out of the office with her two sentences in me and standing on the apron next to the plane and feeling something rearrange itself inside my chest.

Love was not a feeling. It was a decision. It was a thing a person made, ahead of time, and then kept making, every morning, for as long as they were going to keep making it. The feeling came and went. The decision stayed. That was the difference between the marriages that lasted and the marriages that did not. That was, possibly, the difference between every relationship a person was going to have in their life with anything that mattered to them.

I did not, at eighteen, understand all of what she had said. I am not sure I understand all of it now. But the shape of it has stayed with me for more than twenty years, and the longer I have lived the more I have found that almost every relationship worth having turns out to obey the same law she named at that counter. Including, as I would learn much later, the relationship a person has with their own body.

* * *

By the time I was in my last semester of college, I had begun to surrender to the seven sins.

I do not mean this as theology. I mean it as honest self-report. I had carried, since childhood, a body that had not been safe inside a household. What had been done to me by my brothers and sisters in those years had laid something down in me that wanted out, and that had not yet found a place to go. Wrestling had been the first place. The sport had given me a body that could hold its own, that could not be made to absorb what it did not want to absorb. I had joined the team in part because I wanted to be able to defend myself, in the simplest sense — to be a body that other bodies could not, any longer, do as they pleased with. The discipline of the sport was real. So was the other thing the sport was teaching me, which was how to put a man on the ground.

By twenty I had a 3.9 grade point average, the dean's list, and a clean trajectory toward a degree in applied meteorology. I had also, across the previous year, begun to feel something inside me arriving at a place I did not have a name for. The aggression I had been carrying since I was a boy was no longer staying in the corners of the body where I had been keeping it. It was leaking. Into the choices of an ordinary week. Into the way I moved through rooms. Into the kinds of decisions a young man makes when he is trying to make himself feel something other than what he is feeling. I will not catalogue the surrender. I will only say that I knew, by the last semester, that I was inside a slope I could not climb out of by continuing the life I was in. I was about to graduate into a future that would not know what to do with what I was carrying.

I dropped out.

I had been thinking, for some time, about the military. Specifically about Pararescue. The career field's job was to go into the worst places a person could go — combat zones, downed aircraft, ocean rescues, mountain extractions — and bring people back alive. The motto of the career field was four words: That Others May Live. The second guiding line, the one that ran beneath the daily work, was that the team came before personal desires and comforts. I had read about the work and known, in the way a young man knows certain things before he can argue for them, that this was where what I was carrying needed to go. I would not be an officer. If I was going to serve men, I would serve them from the bottom up, the way the men I had worked with on construction sites had taught me a body could be useful — by being used, in the same place, alongside the same people, until the people on either side of you could trust you with what mattered.

I called the unit. They told me I could come up to Anchorage in a few months, and they would schedule something. I said no. I hung up the phone, packed what would fit in my car, and started driving from Daytona Beach to Anchorage that afternoon.

The drive took six and a half days. Some of the days I drove the full twenty-four hours straight through. Most of the days I drove twenty hours and slept for four. I did not stop for things that did not have to be stopped for. The country went past in a single long unbroken stretch — the Florida flatness, the Mississippi crossing, the plains opening up in Kansas, the Rockies, the high western roads going north, then the Yukon, then the long final descent into Alaska. I arrived less than ten days from the phone call.

The fastest the unit had ever gotten a recruit through the initial selection process to basic training was ten months. I did it in four and a half. I was not, in any technical sense, a better candidate than the men who had taken ten months. I was just a man who would not leave.

What I did, when I arrived, was sleep in their parking lot. In my car. Every night. I would show up at the unit in the mornings, do whatever they asked of me, and at the end of the day I would walk back to the car and sleep in it. I was twenty years old and I had come from California and I did not, at that point in my life, have a working understanding of what an Alaskan winter actually was. The summer thinned. The light began to go earlier. The first cold nights arrived. I kept sleeping in the car. One morning a man from the unit came out into the lot as I was climbing out of the back seat. There was snow on the ground. He looked at me, then at the car, then back at me, and he said, you cannot sleep out here, you are going to die. After that they let me sleep inside the unit, even before I was officially in the military. They let me in for two reasons. The first was that they had realized I was not going to leave. The second was, I think, that I had probably annoyed some of them just enough that finding me a cot was easier than finding another way to make me go away. But underneath both of those reasons was the thing that actually mattered. They had seen, across those weeks in the parking lot, that I was going to put my life on the line to be there. That, more than anything else, was what the career field was looking for.

I served six years.

Some of what was done in those six years is not mine to set down on a page. Some of it is, but does not belong here. The work of Pararescue is the work of going, on a regular basis, into situations in which the daily question is not whether someone will live or die. It is who will live, and how, and at what cost, and what a man who has been trained for this will be asked to do in the next several minutes to bring it about. Every day in that work, in some form, was the day a man had to decide between saving someone's life and taking someone's life. Sometimes both, in sequence, in the same hour. The polarity of the work was not metaphysical. It was the daily medium.

That Others May Live. Before personal desires and comforts. Those two phrases were the air the career field breathed. They have been the air I have breathed, in some form, for the twenty years since.

What I carried out of those six years, when I left the military, was something I did not have a clean name for. The aggression that had leaked out of me in college had been put back into a container — the work had given it somewhere to go, and the container had held while I was inside it. But the aggression had not gone away. It had only been redirected. The violence I had absorbed as a child had been transformed, across two decades, first into the body of a wrestler who could defend himself, then into the body of a Pararescueman who could enter situations of life and death, and then, when I came home, into the body of a man in his late twenties who was no longer in either of those structures, and who was carrying inside him the residue of all of it.

I tried, for a stretch of months, to put it down through ordinary means. The means did not work. The body that had been in that container for six years did not unwind on its own, and the things I had seen and done while I was inside the container did not, on their own, find a way out. They stayed.

By the time I was twenty-eight, I had arrived at a level of conviction that what I was carrying was going to require something more than ordinary means to put down. I had also arrived at a kind of certainty, which I did not entirely articulate to myself even then, that if I could not get this done — if whatever I was about to attempt did not work, or if I could not finish it, or if the body could not survive what I was going to ask of it — my life, in some real sense, was going to end. Not by the body's death. By the slow extension of what I was already inside, into a future I could not picture and did not want.

* * *

Four of us drove north into the Upper Peninsula of Michigan in the late summer of my twenty-eighth year, intending to fast for twenty-eight days in the woods. The leaves had not yet turned. The afternoons were warm. The air, where it moved through the trees, still carried the soft weight of late summer. We walked into the forest with what we had brought, made camp, and began.

The four men with me had each come to the fast in their own way. I had come carrying a book a friend had given me the year before — the Essene Gospel of Peace — and a reading of that book that was my own. I had read it and pulled an interpretation out of it that no one had taught me and that I had not heard anyone else describe. The interpretation was that the tree of life inside a person is the gut. The seven sins are the origin point — the lower-level energies that begin as bad habits, as small daily compromises, as the choices a person makes when no one is watching. Left in the body across enough time, those energies do not stay abstract. They take form. They become the diseases that follow from them, and eventually they take physical shape as the organisms that live inside the gut. The snakes on the tree of life are what the seven sins finally manifest as. The long energy of the body, moving from the base of the spine to the place behind the eyes, passes through these snakes on its way upward, shaped by what they are. Christ was a man who had cleared his own snakes. The fast was the way the snakes were cleared. I did not know whether the reading was true. I knew it was the reading I had. I knew I had carried it with me into the forest, and I was about to find out what the next twenty-eight days would do with it.

The first weeks were spent on the work of being there. Building a small shelter, gathering wood, hauling water. The body that has stopped eating is not the body that should be lifting logs in country that turns cold without warning, but we did the work because the work was what was in front of us. There is a kind of clarity that arrives in a body that has both no food and no choice but to keep moving. The afternoons were still warm. The evenings cooled a little more each night than they had cooled the night before. None of us, I think, quite registered the slope.

On the fourth day, my first friend walked out.

He had been quiet for a day before he said anything. Then he said it plainly. He had looked at the cold beginning to arrive earlier in the evenings than it had the week before, at the four of us still building a shelter that none of us could honestly have called finished, at the work of survival a fasting body was about to be asked to do across the next three weeks in country that was already turning, and he had concluded that one of us could realistically die out there. He did not want to be present for that. He left.

I have thought about my first friend many times in the years since. He is still in my life, more than a decade on, and one of the people I trust most in this world. What I have come to understand about his leaving on the fourth day is that he was operating from the highest level of safety, and that what looked like worry from inside the fast was, in fact, careful seeing from outside it. In a moment of that kind of intensity, it is hard to tell concern apart from worry. It is harder still to grant the difference to the person naming the danger. My first friend was right. He was the one of us who saw the actual situation most clearly. I did not know that then; I know it now.

In the years before the forest, my life had been moving at a speed I did not yet know was a speed. I had been pushed, by what I had been carrying and by what I had been chasing, to a kind of breaking point in which the days no longer registered as days. They registered as a single rushing forward that ate one morning and produced the next without my ever quite looking at either. I had not known this was the shape of the life I was inside. A person inside that kind of speed does not, as a rule, know they are inside it. The speed becomes the air, and the air is invisible.

The forest began to slow the air down. By the end of the first week, the day was no longer a thing I was rushing through. It was a thing I was inside. By the second week, the slowing had gone deeper than I had thought possible. I would sit at the edge of the camp in the morning and watch a single ant carry something across the surface of a leaf. The watching would take an hour. The hour would not feel long. I noticed a squirrel moving through the upper branches of a tree above me and registered, for the first time in my life, that the squirrel was a creature with its own concerns, conducting its own day, in a world that overlapped mine without having anything to do with me. The sound of the wood the wind moved through the canopy, the small rustlings of things I could not see, the call of a bird I would not have been able to hear three weeks before because the inner noise of the life I had stepped out of would have drowned it. All of it began to arrive. None of it had not been there before. I had simply been moving too fast to receive any of it.

This is part of why I stayed when the others left. The framework held me. The determination held me. But underneath both of those, something quieter was holding me. The forest had begun to give me back a register of attention I had not known I had lost. To leave on the fourth day, or the tenth, or the fourteenth, would have been to leave that too. I was twenty-eight years old, and the forest was teaching me, for the first time, what it meant to be inside a day rather than to be running through one. I was not going to give that back to the cold or to the framework's predicted temptations or to anything else. I was going to stay until the fast itself said the staying was done.

On the tenth day, my second friend walked out.

My first friend came back to camp that morning. During his days down in town he had been thinking about who else among us might also be needed at home, and he had concluded that my second friend was needed. He brought the word kindly. My second friend received it. The two of them left together. The arrival and the departure were the same moment.

I noticed something then that I have not stopped noticing since. The thing that called my second friend out of the forest did not arrive as the voice of his own hunger or his own cold or his own doubt. It arrived in person, in the form of a friend who had already left, carrying a true and loving message that happened to be the exact thing that would pull the next man out. The framework I had carried in with me had a name for what I was watching. The snake does not speak in its own voice; it speaks in the voices of the people you love. That is what makes it a temptation rather than a threat. That is what makes it work.

By the fourteenth day, the cold that my first friend had seen arriving on the fourth day was no longer arriving slowly. It was arriving fast. The shelter was not enough. The bodies of two men who had been fasting for fourteen days were not the bodies that were going to survive what was coming. My third friend had been holding the fast cleanly until then, but by the fourteenth day a cell phone had appeared in camp — my first friend had brought it on the day he came back for my second friend — and my third friend had been carrying it for the four days since. There was no signal in that part of the woods. He could not call his girlfriend on it. He could not text her. He could only hold it and know that she existed at the other end of the device, somewhere four days' walk away, in a world the phone reminded him of without delivering. The wanting built across those four days. The cold built alongside it. By the fourteenth day, the wanting in his pocket and the cold in the air had together become a steady pressure neither of us could set aside.

My third friend and I walked out together.

I saw, in his leaving, the same shape I had seen in my second friend's. The phone in my third friend's pocket had not asked him to leave the fast. It had only shown him what he could not have inside the forest. The cold had not asked him to leave either. It had only made staying harder. Neither had spoken in its own voice. Together they had spoken in the voice of the life my third friend had stepped out of, calling him back to it. That was the third time, in fourteen days, that I had watched the framework I had brought into the forest predict precisely what was happening in front of me. I was a man at twenty-eight watching the Gospels become literal. The temptations did not arrive as voices in the wilderness. They arrived as departing friends, as a true and loving message, as a phone in a pocket with no signal. They arrived in the ordinary forms of a life that wanted its men back.

My own leaving was simpler. The cold had finished what it had started. The fast was not over — twenty-eight days had been the intended length, and I was only halfway there — but the forest was no longer a place a fasting body could continue. I flew home to California with the fast still continuing, intending to finish the twenty-eight days indoors, in a body that was no longer being asked to chop wood in the dropping temperatures of country that had turned without warning.

The purging had begun in earnest by then. It had started in the first week and had grown stronger as the second week progressed. Around day nine the parasites began to come out, and they continued to come out, day after day, in different forms and at different sizes, all the way through to the end of what I would do. I had never seen anything like what was leaving my body. The framework had told me what I would see. The body confirmed it. There was a moment somewhere around day ten or eleven when the framework I had brought into the forest stopped being a framework I was holding and became, simply, what was happening. I was no longer a man interpreting his fast through a book. I was a body in a forest, doing what the book had said the body would do, watching the things the book had said would leave me leave me.

As the days went on, the sevens kept surfacing. They did not surface in the parasites themselves; they surfaced in the corners of ordinary days. A calculation I had to work out for some practical reason during the second week came out to seven thousand seven hundred and seventy-seven. A number on a page in a notebook would be seven, and then the next number I needed would also be seven, and then the next. None of these on its own would have meant anything. Taken across the long quiet weeks of a fast, with the framework I had carried in already running underneath everything, the accumulation of small sevens stopped looking like coincidence and started looking like something the fast was telling me. By the time I reached the third week, the structural rightness of finishing on the twenty-eighth day was no longer something I was holding as an intention. It was something the days themselves were confirming. Four sevens. The fast had been built around that number from the beginning, and as I approached it, the number kept returning to me in the small ordinary places a person might not otherwise have noticed it.

On the twenty-eighth day I was invited to a small gathering in Monterey. I went. I do not now remember why I went; the body that goes to a party on the twenty-eighth day of a water fast is not the body of a person making decisions in any ordinary way. At some point in the evening I separated myself from the gathering and walked down to the water alone. The sun was setting. It was the sky a person sees once or twice in a life, if they are lucky. The light was crystallizing on the water in a way I did not know light could. The reds were going deeper than I had ever seen reds go in a sky. The whole western horizon had become a thing the body was being permitted to witness. I broke the fast there. A piece of bread. A few apples. A little goat's milk. The breaking was, in its moment, one of the most joyful things I have ever felt. I did not know, then, that it was also the moment the danger of the whole undertaking actually arrived.

The bowel movement came a few days later.

It is hard to write plainly about what happened in that bathroom, but I will try. The first movement was larger than a body is built to pass. It was, in size, more than the body had been carrying when the fast began — a thing that had been compacting and accumulating across the days since the breaking, around four days in all, in a gut no longer moving anything through, drying and consolidating in the dark. It did not move easily. It took its time. When it finally began to move, the pain was beyond what I had ever known a body to be capable of producing. I was alone in the house. There was no one in the next room, no one I could have called who would have understood what I was doing or why. The movement took, in real time, longer than I want to remember. Halfway through it I understood, with a clarity I had not had at any point inside the forest or at any point during the meal at the water, exactly how badly I had just hurt myself, and exactly how much worse than this it could have gone. I was not, in that bathroom, dying. I was, in that bathroom, finally seeing the place a person can bring themselves to by breaking a long fast on bread and apples and goat's milk in a moment of joy on a cliff over the Pacific.

The fast had worked, in its primary purpose. The parasites had come out. The framework I had gone in with had borne, in its own way, the weight I had asked it to bear. Something fundamental had shifted in me, in the forest, that I did not have words for at twenty-eight and do not entirely have words for now. The body that came back from those four sevens of days was not the body that had gone in. The breaking of the fast — the wrong food, the wrong order, the wrong amount, in a body that no longer had the lining or the enzymes or the gut motility to handle any of it — was the part that almost cost me everything I had just gained. The fast did not nearly kill me. The refeeding nearly did. What I did in the forest at twenty-eight was the easier half. The harder half was the one I did wrong.

This book is what I wrote so that no one else would have to learn that the way I did.

* * *

Twelve years passed.

I came back from that first fast a different man, and the years that followed were the years I built a life on what the forest had given me. I taught what I had learned. I sat on the phone with people who were on day six, on day eleven, on day nineteen, walking them through what their bodies were doing and why. I guided men and women through the liver-gallbladder flush, in their own kitchens, in their own bathrooms, hundreds at first and then thousands across the years. By the time the years had run their course, I had reached, in one way or another, somewhere near twenty thousand people about prolonged fasting. I had taken roughly five hundred phone calls. I had walked over ten thousand people through a flush. None of these numbers had been a goal. They were the slow accumulation of one man being present, again and again, for someone else's first time.

There was a wider reach, too, that built itself almost without my doing anything. In the months after I came out of the forest, I had begun posting videos to a YouTube channel — small pieces about what I had learned, made without much thought beyond the wanting to set the work down somewhere it could be found. The videos found people. The channel grew on its own. Across the next stretch of years it gathered something near two million views before it slowed down. A Facebook community I started about parasites grew, in the same way, to twenty-one thousand followers. A second one I started about the liver-gallbladder flush grew to twenty thousand. None of this was the result of any plan I had made. After the forest, things lined up. I would do something. It would work. The working would draw more people in. The next thing would also work. The years after the fast were a stretch in which the world seemed, for a while, to be agreeing with what I was doing.

Inside those years, I was also doing the slower work of trying to understand what kind of value system was now mine. I had come out of the military with a body that had spent six years inside the polarity of saving and taking. I had walked into the forest carrying what was left of that polarity. I had come back from the forest with much of it dissolved. What I was now trying to understand was what to put in its place. A man who has known harm primarily as a thing the body does to other bodies — who has been trained for that work, who has done that work, who has been paid to do that work — has a particular kind of recalibration to do when he comes home. The recalibration is the work of locating the other categories of harm, the ones the body had not been the medium of, and learning to recognize them.

Somewhere in those years, in the way that the right book finds a person at the right time, I came across the work of Masaru Emoto.

Emoto was a Japanese researcher who had spent years photographing water at the moment of freezing. He would take samples from different sources, expose them to different conditions, and chill them slowly under a microscope to capture the shape the ice formed at the instant of crystallization. The shapes were different. Water from a clean mountain spring formed delicate, six-pointed crystals, symmetrical and articulate. Water from a polluted river formed nothing in particular, or formed broken half-shapes, or formed a kind of muddy cloud that never resolved. So far this was not surprising. What was surprising was what happened when Emoto exposed water to things other than chemistry. Water that had been spoken to with kindness, or had a label of a loving word taped to its jar, or had been played a piece of music a person loved, formed clean crystals. Water that had been spoken to with cruelty, or labeled with a word of hatred, or played harsh and chaotic sound, formed nothing, or formed broken things.

I knew that mainstream science did not endorse Emoto's experiments. The methodology had been questioned. The photography had been questioned. The results had not been cleanly reproduced in the way real science asks results to be cleanly reproduced. I am not here to defend the experiments. The reader can take Emoto on whatever terms the reader wants. What matters, for the chapter, is what the work did inside me when I encountered it.

It told me that words could hurt a body the way a fist could. I had known, since childhood, that words could hurt. Most people know that words can hurt. What I had not understood, until I read Emoto, was the degree to which they could hurt. The water in a body, which is most of what a body is by weight, was holding the shape of what had been said to it. Not just metaphorically. Structurally. The household I had grown up inside had been a household of words as well as hands, and the words had been writing into the body the same way the hands had. The years of being told what I was, by the people who were doing the things they were doing, had been laying down a record. The record was physical. It was in the water, in the cells, in the patterns the body had built around what it had been told to be.

This was a recalibration. The work I had done in the military had assumed that the body was the primary medium of harm, because the body was what Pararescue was equipped to address. The reading of Emoto, after I came home, told me there was a second medium I had not been equipped to address, and that the second medium was at least as large as the first, and that the people I had been around in childhood had been working in that second medium continuously, without anyone calling it harm. The reading also told me, by extension, that the work of becoming a man who did not extend that harm into the next generation was not only the work of not putting hands on people. It was also the work of being careful about what came out of my mouth. About what was said in the rooms my daughter would grow up inside. About what was being written, daily, into the bodies of the people I loved.

This is what I came to believe in those years and what I still, in my own life, believe now. I am not asking the reader to believe it. I am saying it because it is the working understanding I have been calibrated by since the forest, and without it the rest of how I live does not quite make sense. The reader is welcome to disagree with every word of this. Many of the people who read this book will. What matters is not whether you agree with how I have come to understand the body. What matters is how you show up, day after day, in the body you have, and in the rooms you are in. The reader who agrees with my framework but does not show up has gained nothing. The reader who disagrees with my framework but shows up, faithfully, across the years, has gained everything the book is trying to give.

One of the things I would tell people, on those phone calls, was about the gurgling.

When the gut is full of parasites, the body sends signals upward that the person experiences as hunger. The gurgling that arrives in the stomach an hour or two after a meal, the small insistent rumble that calls the person back to the kitchen, is not — or is not only — the body asking for food. It is the parasites in your gut asking for food. The hunger a person feels in that moment is, in part, theirs. The decisions a person makes under that hunger are, in part, theirs. A man who reaches for the cupboard at three in the afternoon, and who believes he is reaching for himself, is in a real sense reaching for the organisms that have shaped the reaching. The fast clears them. After a clean fast, the gurgling stops. After a clean fast, the man at three in the afternoon notices that he is not actually hungry, and that what he had been calling his hunger had not, for years, been entirely his.

This was a thing I taught for twelve years. I taught it because it had happened in my own body. After the forest, the gurgling stopped. It stayed stopped for almost ten years. The silence in my gut was, across those years, one of the things I would point to when someone asked me what was different now. The hunger I felt was clean. The decisions I made under it were mine. The kitchen, when I walked into it, was a place I was walking into rather than a place that was calling me.

Then the gurgling came back.

It came back in my thirty-seventh year, three years before this writing. It did not come back loudly. It came back the way these things come back — at the edge of a quiet afternoon, a small rumble that I noticed and did not, at first, make anything of. Then it came back the next afternoon. Then the next. By the end of the first week I had stopped being able to pretend that I was not hearing what I was hearing. The thing I had been teaching for twelve years was now happening in me. The framework I had been calibrated by, that the forest had confirmed and that the long quiet years had confirmed again, was confirming itself a third time, in middle age, in my own kitchen.

I was no longer alone in my gut.

The decisions I had been making across the prior year began to look different in light of this. The small reaches for the cupboard. The eating window that had broadened by an hour, then by two. The fermented foods that had quietly stopped appearing on the plate. None of it had been catastrophic. None of it had registered as a fall. It had registered, when it had registered at all, as the ordinary loosening of a busy man in a busy life. Now I could see what had actually been doing the loosening. The population had returned, and the population had been steering, and I had been calling the steering my own.

What I did, when I understood this, was almost nothing. I noticed it. I named it to myself. I knew what the protocol called for. I had walked thousands of people through that protocol. I did not, for the next nearly three years, do it.

I want to be honest about why.

I was busy. The work of teaching others was real work. The work was steady. The people calling me had real bodies and real questions and real fasts that needed real attention. The channel had its own rhythm of comments and questions. The two communities had their own. The teaching that had begun, in the months after the forest, as a few small videos posted to a quiet corner of the internet had grown, across the years, into a thing that was always there waiting for me when I sat down. I was homeschooling my daughter, which is the kind of daily commitment that fills a life in ways that do not leave much room for the thirty to forty days a man would need to clear what was now in his gut. There were the small administrations of an ordinary life — bills, repairs, the calendar that fills up by itself if a person does not actively keep it from filling. There were trips and obligations and the kinds of weeks that arrive in sequence and do not, as a rule, hand a person a clean window for a fast.

All of those reasons were real. None of them were the actual reason.

The actual reason was that the practice I had been teaching for twelve years had become, in my own life, the thing I taught rather than the thing I lived. I had drifted. Not catastrophically — I had not returned to the man I was before the forest. The food in my house was still mostly clean. The fermented foods reappeared, then disappeared, then reappeared again. The eating window was wider than it should have been but not as wide as it had once been. From the outside, very little had changed. From inside the gut, where the actual reading happens, everything had changed.

My daughter was the rest of what moved me. The same daughter whose homeschooling had been one of the reasons the fast kept getting postponed turned out to be, in the end, one of the reasons it could not be postponed any longer. A man who is teaching his daughter to pay attention to her own body cannot, for very long, fail to pay attention to his.

I began the writing of this book in my thirty-ninth year. I worked at it through the first months of my fortieth. The writing of it returned me to what I had stopped doing. Sentence by sentence, page by page, the book asked me whether I was still living what I was setting down. For a long time the answer was that I was, mostly, and that the gaps were small enough to leave for later. There came a morning, somewhere in the writing of the chapter on the long partnership, when the answer stopped being mostly. I closed the laptop. I made the calendar adjustments I had been putting off for three years. I cleared sixty to seventy-five days, the stretch I would need if the fast went its full length and the rebuilding ran clean afterward. I began.

* * *

It is day twenty-three of the second fast, and I am writing this chapter from inside it.

The body, this morning, is quiet. The hunger that arrives in the first week, and that fights for several days before it begins to thin, has been gone for a long time. The mind is clearer than I have known it to be in years. There is a register of attention available to me on day twenty-three that I had stopped having access to in the years between the two fasts, and that I am only now, quietly, recognizing as something I had lost. The seeing has come back.

The first fast, at twenty-eight, did certain kinds of work that this one is not being asked to do. Twelve years ago I went into the forest to clear what the forest cleared. The body and the framework I had carried in confirmed each other. I came back from those twenty-eight days a different man. This fast is different. The work this time is quieter. The behavioral patterns I am now able to see, sitting at my kitchen table with the notebook open, are patterns the first fast did not reach because the man inside them at twenty-eight had not yet lived inside them long enough for them to have become visible. A man at forty has carried his patterns longer. A man at forty has watched them shape twelve years of choices. The seeing of them, when the gut quiets and the mind clears, is a different kind of seeing than the seeing available to a man at twenty-eight in a forest.

I am not, at the time of this writing, certain how long this fast will run. I know more than I knew at twenty-eight about how to exit a fast cleanly, and I know more than I knew then about what the body is asking for from day to day. The exit will be slower. The breaking will be the simplest vegetable broth a person can make, taken in small amounts, with a little MCT oil. Nothing solid for some time after that. The body that has fasted this long does not need food in the way it thinks it does; it needs the gentlest possible reintroduction of nourishment, run through a gut that has not been asked to do anything for weeks. The bread and apples and goat's milk in a moment of joy on a cliff over the Pacific will not be repeated. I have written the chapters of this book that say what to do instead, and I am going to do what they say.

My daughter is the steadier of the daily reasons this fast is being kept. She is the kind of daily reason a man does not articulate, most days, because articulating it would make it smaller than it is. She is one of the people in this house. She is one of the people I am, by being in the practice rather than only teaching it, attempting to be more available to. The articulation will not improve the work. The work itself will. A daughter watching her father pay attention to his own body is a daughter being shown, without being told, that paying attention to one's own body is what an adult does.

The book is the other reason. I have been writing it through the months that led into this fast. I am writing it through the fast itself. What I have been finding is that the writing and the fast are doing the same work in different forms. The chapters that go on after this one set down what the long practice asks for, what the long partnership produces, what it costs to keep paying attention across decades of an ordinary life. I could not have written those chapters from outside the practice. I have tried. The prose that comes out is correct in its facts and false in its register, and a reader can hear the falseness even when they cannot name it. The fast has been, among other things, the thing returning the register to me as I write.

The marriage frame from the chapter on the long partnership has been sitting with me through these twenty-three days in a way it could not have sat with me before I began. The body, after a fast and a rebuilding, is in roughly the situation of a marriage at year three. Everything new has been encountered. The dramatic phase is over. What remains is the long stretch. I am, today, somewhere near the beginning of my own long stretch with this body for the second time. The first time, at twenty-nine and thirty and the years that followed, I held the practice for a stretch of years and then quietly let it thin. This time the conditions are different. The writing of the book is one of them. The daughter watching from across the kitchen is another. The seeing that has come back on day twenty-three is the third. Between them, they are the conditions under which the second long stretch is being entered.

I do not know, at the time of this writing, what the next twelve years will produce. I know what I am doing this morning. I am sitting with a body that is quiet, with a mind that is clear, with a notebook in front of me, in a kitchen that has begun, again, to be the kitchen the body needs it to be. The fermented foods are in the refrigerator, waiting for the gate to open. The water filter is on the counter. The eating window, when it returns, will close before the light leaves the sky. The kitchen the man in the chapter on the long partnership is sitting in is, in a small way, the kitchen I am sitting in now, on the day the writing of this chapter began.

I am going to keep paying attention.

That is the second marriage vow.

* * *

I told you, at the start of all this, about the four passages that set me walking into a forest. I did not show them to you then. Here they are — and here is what I read in each.

The first named, plainly, what lives in the corrupted gut:

> *And his bowels become full with abominable filthiness, with oozing streams of decay; and multitudes of abominable worms have their habitation there.*

I had read that kind of language before and skimmed past it. This time I did not. The text was not reaching for metaphor. It placed the worms in the bowels the same way it placed blood in the veins and breath in the lungs — a fact of the body, part of what had gone wrong, part of what had to be cleared.

Then came the instruction. Not a prayer, not a symbol — a method, described down to the vessel and the water:

> *Seek, therefore, a large trailing gourd, having a stalk the length of a man; take out its inwards and fill it with water from the river which the sun has warmed. Hang it upon the branch of a tree, and kneel upon the ground before the angel of water, and suffer the end of the stalk of the trailing gourd to enter your hinder parts, that the water may flow through all your bowels.*

A hollowed gourd. Warmed river water. A tube the length of a man. The water run through the bowels and let out again, carrying with it what the first passage had named. I read it as directions. So I followed them, into a forest, and stayed until my body answered.

And a third passage named what the others rested on — and it was this one that first sent me to the trees:

> *Earthly Mother come and serve you. For I tell you truly, except you fast, you shall never be freed from the power of Satan and from all diseases that come from Satan. Fast and pray fervently, seeking the power of the living God for your healing. While you fast, eschew the Sons of Men and seek our Earthly Mother's angels, for he that seeks shall find. Seek the fresh air of the forest and of the fields, and there in the midst of them shall you find the angel of air. Put off your shoes and your clothing and suffer the angel of air to embrace all your body. Then breathe long and deeply, that the angel of air may be brought within you. I tell you truly, the angel of air shall cast out of your body all uncleannesses which defiled it without and within.*

Fasting was the ground the rest stood on. The body emptied first, out under open air, before the water and the gourd could reach what they were meant to reach.

And a fourth line, quieter than the others, told me where all of this was happening:

> *Our bowels are born of the bowels of our Earthly Mother, and are hid from our eyes, like the invisible depths of the earth.*

The bowels, it said, are the hidden interior of the Earthly Mother — her depth, invisible from the outside, the same as the depth of the earth.

What I made of it was this. The tree of life those passages named was the gut, and the worms were the parasites that live in it — and what lives there has a hand in temptation itself, not as a metaphor but as a mechanism. When the body cannot move what it needs to where it is needed, the mind goes dim, and a dim mind is an easy one to lead. The old writers may not have had the words for it, but they saw the pattern: that the appetites of the body could steer the choices of a man. I do not think that makes any of us weak. I think it means we should look underneath a bad choice before we judge the one who made it.

Chapter 2

The Architecture of Your Gut

* * *

There is a length of tissue inside you, twenty-five feet of it, that you have never seen and probably never thought to consider. It runs from your lips to the place where your body finally lets go of what it cannot use. Folded and refolded so densely that, were it spread flat, it would carpet a tennis court, it does the work of keeping you alive.

You eat, and you do not think about it. The work happens anyway. A piece of fruit becomes the sugar that fires the cells of your brain. A handful of greens becomes the iron in your blood and the magnesium that lets your heart contract on its steady rhythm. None of this is your decision. It is the decision of a system so old and so practiced that human beings, for most of our history, did not know it existed. It happens whether you understand it or not. It happens whether you are kind to it or not. But it happens better when you understand. And it happens better still when you are kind.

This is a chapter about that system.

A Tube, and What Lives Along Its Walls

The digestive tract is not, as some imagine it, a stomach with a few attachments. It is a tube. A long, intelligent tube, with two great sections that do entirely different work.

The first is the small intestine — twenty feet of folded tissue coiled within your abdomen, pink and pulsing, lined with what biologists call villi. Picture a forest of upright threads, millions of them per square inch, each one a single cell thick, each one reaching up into the slurry of digesting food to pull out what your body needs. Sugars. Fats. The vitamins that dissolve in oil. The amino acids that will, in time, become your skin and your hair and the muscles of your hands. This is where most of the harvest happens.

The second is the colon — five feet, shorter and broader, the chamber where what remains is pressed and slowed and given over to a different kind of intelligence. Here live the bacteria. Trillions of them. They ferment what you could not break down. They make vitamins your own cells cannot make. They produce a fatty acid called butyrate that keeps the cells of the colon wall alive, and another that calms inflammation throughout the body, and another that signals satiety to the brain. The colon is not, as people sometimes imagine, the place where waste is stored before disposal. It is the place where the last and quietest harvesting is done.

Together they leave nothing behind. The small intestine takes the sun, and the colon gleans the field.

The Villi

If you could look at a healthy small intestine through the right kind of lens, you would see something that looks, at first, like a meadow. Soft. Pink. Moving slightly with the work of absorption. Each blade of that meadow is a villus, and each villus is itself covered in still finer projections — microvilli, so small that ten thousand of them can stand in a single millimeter. The whole surface is called the brush border. It is the place where the food you ate this morning crosses out of your gut and becomes you.

The cells of this surface live for three to five days and then are replaced. The body is constantly building this meadow and constantly tearing it down. Every villus you have right now will be gone by the end of next week, and a new villus will be standing where it stood. You are, at this layer of yourself, a continuous act of becoming.

When the meadow is healthy, it is pink and velvet and damp with a thin protective mucus. When it is not, the villi flatten. The microvilli shorten. The mucus thins or thickens unnaturally. The brush border, viewed under magnification, no longer looks like a meadow. It looks like a field after a long drought.

Most people who have spent their lives eating processed food, taking antibiotics, drinking chlorinated water, and living the ordinary life of an industrialized country are walking around with a meadow that has not been a meadow for some time. They do not know this. They feel tired. They feel inflamed. They feel that something is not quite right and cannot say what. The meadow that is no longer a meadow does not announce itself. It simply fails, slowly, to do the work it was built to do.

The Locks Between the Cells

Between each cell of the intestinal lining there is a connection so small that for most of medical history we did not know it existed. We know now. We call them tight junctions. They are not metaphorical. They are physical structures, gates, and they have two states: closed and open.

When the gates are closed — and in a healthy gut they spend most of their time closed — only the molecules your body has decided to admit are allowed across. Sugars. Amino acids. The smallest fats. Each one ferried across by its own dedicated transporter, each one accounted for, each one logged.

When the gates open without permission — and they will, under enough stress, enough damage, enough chronic inflammation — they admit things they should not. Undigested protein fragments. Bacterial debris. Toxins. The eggs of the parasites we will discuss in a later chapter. Things that should have stayed in the tube find themselves in the bloodstream, and the immune system, never having seen these things in this place before, mounts a defense.

The defense was meant for invaders. It is now being mounted against fragments of yesterday's lunch. Over years, this is what we mean when we use the phrase *autoimmune disease*. Over years, this is what we mean when we say a person has become inflamed. Over years, this is the slow grinding cost of gates that no longer close.

Everything in this book — every herb, every enema, every protocol, every quiet hour of fasting — is, at its deepest level, working toward one goal. To restore the locks on the gates.

The Minerals That Make It All Work

Of all the things your gut needs to function, the most overlooked are the smallest. They are called trace minerals, and the word *trace* describes how much of each you require — a thousandth of a gram, sometimes less, sometimes far less. People think because the amounts are small, the importance must be small. The opposite is the truth.

Zinc activates more than three hundred enzymes in your body, many of them digestive. Magnesium activates more than six hundred. Manganese protects the cells of your intestinal lining from the constant oxidative damage of being on the front line between your body and the outside world. Selenium runs the immune defenses of the gut. Without these minerals — and a dozen others, each in their tiny amount — the enzymes your pancreas and intestines produce sit idle. The gates do not close. The villi do not regenerate. The bacteria do not make their butyrate. The whole intricate system slows down, then slows further, then begins, almost imperceptibly, to fail.

We live in soil that has been farmed for too long without rest. The minerals that should be in our food are no longer reliably there. Industrial agriculture has stripped them. Long-distance shipping and refrigeration have completed what stripping could not. A tomato grown in 1950 contained more zinc, more magnesium, more selenium than a tomato grown today. A carrot, the same. An apple, the same. We eat the same volume of food our grandparents ate and absorb a smaller and smaller fraction of what they absorbed.

This is part of what you are correcting when you fast. This is part of why mineral replenishment during the fast is not a courtesy to the body. It is the foundation that allows everything else in this protocol to work. Without the minerals, the herbs cannot be activated. Without the minerals, the enzymes cannot fire. Without the minerals, the bacteria cannot ferment. The entire chemistry of the gut depends on these tiny amounts of metal that most of us have been quietly running short of for most of our lives.

When you put a pinch of Himalayan salt in your morning water and add a few drops of trace mineral solution, you are not performing a wellness ritual. You are returning to your body what the soil and the water and the food no longer reliably provide.

The Second Brain

There is something inside you that medical science has only recently begun to take seriously. The walls of your intestines contain more than five hundred million neurons — more than your spinal cord. They form a network so complex that researchers have begun calling it the enteric nervous system, or, less formally, the second brain.

This network communicates with the brain in your skull through the vagus nerve, the longest cranial nerve in the body, running from the base of the brainstem down through the chest and into the abdomen. The communication is constant and bidirectional. The brain in your head knows what is happening in your gut, moment by moment. The gut knows what is happening in the brain. The two are not separate organs that occasionally exchange messages. They are two ends of a continuous conversation.

The gut produces, by some estimates, ninety percent of the body's serotonin — the neurotransmitter most directly involved in regulating mood. It produces dopamine. It produces other neuroactive compounds whose names mean little to most readers but whose effects are felt every day in the rise and fall of human consciousness.

This is why a sick gut produces a clouded mind. Why the fog that lifts during a prolonged fast is not just metaphorical but neurochemical. Why people who clean their guts often discover they were carrying, without knowing it, a low-grade depression that resolves once the gut is no longer signaling distress. The conversation between the second brain and the first brain has been disrupted for a long time, in most people, and they did not know that what they were calling a personal problem was actually a biological one.

The Inner Ecosystem

You are not, in the strictest sense, only yourself. By cell count, the bacteria living in your gut outnumber your own cells. By gene count, the microbial genes in your intestines outnumber your own DNA by more than a hundred to one. There are roughly thirty-eight trillion microorganisms inside you right now — bacteria, yes, but also fungi, viruses, archaea, protozoa, all of them living in a balance that has taken hundreds of millions of years to develop.

This partnership is older than your species. It is older than mammals. Some of the bacterial lineages in your gut today were already living in the guts of fish three hundred million years before any human walked the earth. They have been with us for the entire human story. They produced our vitamins before we learned to farm. They protected us from pathogens before we discovered medicine. They have been quietly keeping us alive, generation after generation, asking only that we feed them what they need.

What they need is fiber. Not the supplement kind — the kind that arrives in plants, alongside everything else a plant carries. Resistant starches. Pectins. The complex carbohydrates that our own enzymes cannot break down. We deliver these compounds to the colon untouched, and the bacteria break them down through fermentation, and the products of that fermentation feed not only the bacteria themselves but the cells of the colon wall, the immune system, the brain.

When the partnership is healthy, the bacteria reward us with stable mood, regular elimination, calm immunity, and protection from the organisms that would do us harm. When the partnership is starved — by processed food, antibiotics, chronic stress, chlorinated water — the bacterial diversity collapses. The protective species die back. The opportunistic species expand. The ancient bargain breaks down.

Much of what people call modern disease is what happens when we stop holding up our end of an arrangement that has worked for hundreds of millions of years.

What Goes Wrong, and How

The gut you were born with was, in most cases, exquisite. Pink villi. Closed gates. A diverse and abundant microbial population. A clean mucus layer renewing itself daily. This is the architecture you arrived with, and for the first weeks and months of your life, while you nursed and slept and grew, it was fully intact.

Then life happened. Antibiotics for an ear infection at age four killed off bacterial species that may never have returned. Highly processed school cafeteria food in childhood gave the gut things it had not evolved to handle. Sugary drinks fed yeast that should have stayed in low numbers. The first round of stress hormones in adolescence opened the tight junctions just a little. Birth control pills, in the women's case, altered the ecosystem further. Years of restaurant meals and convenience foods and travel and prescription medications, each with its own small contribution, accumulated.

By middle age, the gut of an average person living in an industrialized country bears almost no resemblance to the gut they were born with. The villi have flattened in places. The mucus layer is too thick in some areas, too thin in others. Biofilms have formed where bacterial overgrowth has settled in. Parasites, which we will discuss in detail in the next chapter, have taken up residence and have been there, sometimes, for decades. The microbiome has lost much of its diversity. The trace minerals have been depleted. The tight junctions are not as tight as they once were.

Most of this happened so gradually that the person carrying these changes never noticed. The body adapted. The fatigue felt normal. The bloating felt normal. The food sensitivities that emerged in their thirties felt like just the way things were now.

This is what we mean when we say the gut accumulates a lifetime of damage. Not damage that announces itself in any single moment. Damage that is the cumulative weight of every meal, every medication, every illness, every stress — applied to a system that was never designed to bear it indefinitely.

The good news is that this same system, given the right conditions, has a deep capacity to heal. Within months, the villi can return to something close to their original state. Within weeks, the tight junctions can begin to close again. Within days, the microbial population can begin to shift back toward diversity. The system was built to recover. It just rarely gets the chance.

What the Gut Is

You have a tube inside you that is doing more work than you knew. It is older than you, in the sense that the system itself is the inheritance of a long line of ancestors who depended on it before you were born. It is a partnership, in the sense that you do not own it alone. It is intelligent, in the sense that it contains a nervous system second only to the brain in your skull. It is fragile, in the sense that the modern world is constantly asking it to function under conditions it was never built for.

The chapters that follow will go deeper. They will look at what lives inside this tube that should not. They will look at the layers that build up over a lifetime and the techniques for clearing them. They will look at how to rebuild what has been worn thin.

But all of it begins here. With this length of folded tissue. This meadow of villi. These locks that do or do not close. This conversation between the gut and the brain that has been quietly shaping your moods for as long as you have been alive. This partnership with organisms older than our species.

This is the system you are about to clean. And to clean it well, you need first to understand what you are cleaning.

Chapter 3

Trace Minerals, Bacteria & Enzymes

* * *

It is morning, and a four-year-old boy is sitting at his mother's kitchen table, with his feet swinging slightly above the floor.

The chair is a little too tall for him. The morning light is coming through the window above the sink, soft and not yet warm. He is in no particular hurry to be anywhere. His mother is at the stove. She has been at it since before he came down, simmering the broth she started the night before — bones, a little salt, the vegetables she pulled from the garden the day before yesterday. She moves around the kitchen the way a person moves who has cooked in this kitchen for a long time, which is to say without looking at most of what her hands are doing. She lifts the lid of the pot. She tastes a spoonful. She adjusts something — a pinch of salt, a few grains of something she keeps in a small jar by the stove, dissolved into the morning's water before any of this began. She is not, as she does any of this, thinking about her son's body. She is thinking, if she is thinking about anything, that the soup is almost ready and that the boy looks tired this morning and that the dog needs to be let out before too much longer.

She ladles the soup into a wide shallow bowl and sets it in front of him. Steam rises from it in the slow, undirected way that steam rises from a soup that has had time to cool slightly. The boy reaches for the spoon. She watches him for a moment. Then she turns back to the stove.

Neither of them knows what is about to happen.

The bowl in front of the boy is a bowl of soup. To him, it is breakfast. To her, it is what she made for her son this morning. To both of them, the bowl is one of the small ordinary objects of a small ordinary life, and there is nothing about it that calls for any particular attention. The soup is good. The morning is quiet. He eats slowly because his feet do not reach the floor and he is in no hurry to be anywhere.

And yet, in the seconds it takes for each spoonful to leave the bowl and arrive in his stomach and begin to be drawn down through the small folded length of his intestine, an enormous amount of work is being done. Not by him. Not by her. By the small living world inside him that has been there since before he can remember, and that has been waiting, this morning, for what she made.

That world is older than he is. Some of it was given to him by her — quite literally, in the moments of his birth, gathered from her body as he passed into the world; and again in the first weeks of nursing, drawn from the milk that came from her chest. Some of it arrived later, from the soil his small hands found in the garden when he was three, from the dog that lived in the house, from the foods of the household he is now growing up inside. Across the years of a life, the inhabitation will accumulate. By the time the boy is grown, by the time he is the man at twenty-eight walking into a forest, by the time he is the man at forty sitting at his own kitchen table on a quiet morning, the community he carries will be layered, the way a forest is layered, with different organisms occupying different parts of the long passage and different parts of the day. There will be species that thrive only in the small intestine, where the chyme is still moving fast and the oxygen is still present. There will be species that live only in the colon, where the work is slower and the air is gone. There will be species that come out at certain hours and recede at others. The whole community will shift across the day in ways the man, eating his soup, will have no awareness of.

Their number will be harder to imagine than to state. There will be more of them in his body than there are cells of his own body. He will be, by count of living things he is carrying, more them than him.

They are not passengers. The word does not fit. A passenger is carried by a vehicle for the passenger's own purposes; this community is carried by a body that depends on what the community does. They are not workers either. The word treats them as labor for hire, and they are not for hire. They are something the language of ordinary commerce does not have a clean word for — a small living community a body has carried since childhood, that has done the body's work for as long as the body has been alive, and that asks, in return, only to be fed and kept.

The community is doing a great amount of work, almost continuously, in the dark of the lower gut.

Some of them are taking apart the long fibers of the vegetables in the morning's soup — fibers his own enzymes have no way of breaking. The carrot the cook diced in the broth, the cellulose of the celery stalk, the tougher parts of the kale that softened only partway in the long simmer; all of these are arriving at the colon largely intact, and the members of the community who specialize in fiber are pulling them apart, slowly, releasing the nutrients the man would otherwise have passed without using. Others, in the same neighborhood, are taking the products of that work and converting them into a class of small molecules called short-chain fatty acids, the most important of which is butyrate. Butyrate is the food the cells of the intestinal lining live on. The lining cannot be fed properly from the bloodstream side; it has to be fed from inside the gut, by what the community makes from what the man eats. Without this work, the meadow of the small intestine begins to thin, the way a meadow thins when the small unseen creatures of its soil stop returning what they take.

Other members of the household, working on different molecules, are manufacturing vitamins his own cells cannot make. B12 is being assembled, slowly and carefully, in places of his body he could not reach with any deliberate act. Folate. Biotin. Quantities of these vitamins he had no idea he was depending on are being delivered, daily, by partners whose names he will never learn.

Others are practicing a quieter kind of work. They are training his immune system. The lining of his gut is where the body's largest population of immune cells lives, and those cells learn the difference between friend and threat by being raised, day after day, in the company of the community that has been there since his birth. A child who grows up without exposure to a healthy diversity of bacterial company has an immune system that learns these distinctions poorly, and reacts badly later, to things it should have learned to ignore. Among everything else they do, the community are the teachers of the body's defenses.

And there is one more thing they are doing. They are producing chemicals that travel up to the brain. A substantial fraction of the body's serotonin is made down here. So is some of its dopamine. So is a quiet portion of the substances that shape the man's mood, his sleep, the steadiness of his thinking across an ordinary morning. The community does not only feed his body. They participate in the chemistry of his mind.

This is the kind of relationship a person spends a lifetime either tending or neglecting. The community will be with him until he dies. He will, across the decades that follow this morning, either learn to read its signals and feed it what it asks for, or he will not. The choice will not arrive as a dramatic moment. It will arrive in tens of thousands of small daily decisions about what is on the plate, what is in the water, what kind of week he is going to ask his body to absorb. The man at twenty-eight, walking into a forest to clear what had accumulated, will be making one of those decisions. The man at forty, sitting at his own kitchen table on a quiet morning forty years from this one, will be making another. What he carries forward, in the long passage of his lower gut, will be the steady record of which decisions he made.

All of this is happening, in the dark, in the long passage of the lower gut, while a four-year-old boy sits at his mother's kitchen table eating his soup. None of it requires his attention. It will continue whether he attends to it or not. What it does require — what every part of this work depends on — is the small thing the soup contains that neither he nor his mother knew was there.

The pinch in the small jar by the stove was a pinch of trace minerals.

They are called trace minerals because the amounts the body needs are so small that for most of human history they could not be measured. Zinc. Magnesium. Manganese. Selenium. Copper. Chromium. Molybdenum. Each of them a metallic element drawn out of the earth and found, in tiny quantities, in the rivers and the soil and the bodies of animals and the green leaves of plants. The amounts are easy to underestimate. A thousandth of a gram in a day. Sometimes less than that. Sometimes far less.

People hear the word trace and assume the importance must be small. The opposite is the truth. The smallness is the entire reason the system can be regulated with precision. Too much of any of these is as harmful as too little, and the body has spent the long ages of its evolution learning to maintain these tiny quantities at exactly the level the work requires. What it has not learned is how to make them. The body does not synthesize trace minerals. It receives them, or it does not.

In the kitchen, the boy does not know any of this. Neither does his mother. The pinch she added to the morning water came from a small habit she picked up years ago, recommended once by someone she trusted, and it has become part of how she cooks without her ever quite thinking about why. The minerals dissolve into the water. The water becomes the broth. The broth carries the minerals into the boy's stomach. They travel down to the long folded length of the small intestine, where the lining receives them, draws them across the boundary between the gut and the body, and distributes them into the bloodstream that feeds every cell.

What they do, once they arrive, is the quiet part of the work that makes everything else possible.

The body is full of small machines that need to be turned on. They are called enzymes, and most of them cannot start their work without a specific trace mineral binding to them first. Zinc activates hundreds of these. So does magnesium, in even greater number; magnesium turns on more of the body's enzymatic machinery than any other element. Manganese protects the cells of the gut lining from the slow oxidative damage of being on the front line between the body and the outside world. Selenium activates the immune defenses of the gut and supports the chemistry by which the body neutralizes the toxic byproducts of its own clearing work. Copper is essential for the small fires inside every cell — the work the mitochondria do to make energy. Chromium quietly steadies the body's relationship with sugar, holding insulin's responsiveness even, across a meal and across a day. Molybdenum activates the liver's deeper detoxification systems, the ones that handle what the lighter ones cannot.

Each one has a specific job. Each one is small. Each one is essential.

And in the soil and the water and the food of the modern world, each one is increasingly absent.

The minerals are not made on farms. They are pulled from the ground by plants whose roots reach into earth that, in earlier centuries, was rich and continuously replenished. The earth a vegetable now grows in is, in many places, soil that has been farmed continuously for decades and replenished only with the three or four minerals the industrial fertilizer industry has decided are worth replacing. The vegetable that arrives at the kitchen looks like a vegetable. It tastes, more or less, like a vegetable. It is missing the small invisible content that made the vegetable, in earlier times, a complete delivery of what the body required. The water that arrives at the tap has been treated, filtered, cleaned of many things, including some of the trace minerals it once carried. The salt on the table is, in most households, an industrial product that has been stripped of the small natural complement of other minerals it once contained, leaving only sodium and a few additives.

The result is a population of bodies that are not, by ordinary measure, malnourished. They are eating. They have weight. They produce, on a blood test, levels of the major nutrients that look acceptable. What they are missing is the smaller substrate beneath all of that — the trace cofactors without which the enzymes the body builds cannot do their work. The lining cannot be properly maintained. The bacteria cannot do their full share. The fires inside the cells burn dimly. None of this announces itself. It manifests as a slow tiredness, a slow inflammation, a slow drift away from the body the person was meant to inhabit, that no single test will ever quite locate.

The pinch the boy's mother added to the morning water was, without her knowing it, a small act of resistance against this drift. The minerals dissolved in the broth will reach his lining. His enzymes will be activated. The community in his gut will receive what it needs to do its work. None of this is visible. None of it is dramatic. It is the small daily act by which a body is kept whole.

Whether the boy will, as a man, continue to receive this small daily act is another question. The decades that follow this morning will tell. For now, the soup is on the table, and the work is being done.

The work itself is done by the enzymes.

If the trace minerals are the small invisible conditions, and the bacterial neighbors are the living community of the lower gut, then the enzymes are the work each of them performs across an ordinary day. The body has thousands of enzymes. The reader does not need to know their names. What the reader needs to know is what kind of thing an enzyme is, and what an enzyme is doing inside the boy's body in the seconds it takes for him to swallow another spoonful.

An enzyme is a small folded protein. It is shaped, with exact precision, to fit one specific molecule and do one specific thing to it. There is an enzyme that recognizes the link between two amino acids in a protein and severs it, and severs nothing else. There is another that recognizes the link between two sugars in a carbohydrate and breaks only that. There are enzymes that fit fats and split them. There are enzymes that fit larger molecules and assemble them. Each one is a tiny tool, made for a single job, manufactured by the body in enormous quantity, sent out across the gut and the bloodstream and the cells of every organ to do its single work without rest.

The work happens fast. A digestive enzyme can act on tens of thousands of molecules in a single second. The chemistry that, without enzymes, would take hours or days, takes the body a fraction of a moment. This speed is not optional. The body cannot wait for slow chemistry. A meal arriving in the stomach has to be reduced to its small parts, those parts have to be drawn across the lining of the gut, and the parts have to reach the cells that need them, in time for the cells to do whatever they were going to do next. The whole intricate timing of being a living animal depends on chemistry happening at the speed enzymes make possible.

And here is the small fact that the rest of this work depends on. An enzyme, on its own, sitting in the lining of the gut without anything else, does not work. It is folded correctly, manufactured correctly, sent to the right place — and it sits inert. It cannot start. The bond it was made to break sits in front of it, and the enzyme does nothing.

What the enzyme is waiting for is a single atom of a trace mineral.

The mineral fits into the enzyme — a particular atom of zinc, or of magnesium, or of one of the other five — and the fitting is the activation. The folded protein, in the moment the mineral arrives in its socket, becomes a working tool. The enzyme begins. The bond is broken. The chemistry happens. Without the mineral, the chemistry does not happen. With the mineral, it happens at the speed of life.

This is why the trace minerals matter so much, in such tiny amounts. They are not consumed in the work. A single atom of zinc can sit in an enzyme and activate that enzyme through tens of thousands of cycles of work before it is, eventually, exchanged out for a fresh atom from the bloodstream. The body's stored minerals are a working inventory, drawn on continuously, replenished only by what comes in through the food and the water. A body with a thinning supply of trace minerals is a body whose enzymes are sitting inert in greater numbers than the system was built to tolerate. The work that should be happening — the digestion, the absorption, the cellular maintenance, the immune response — slows. None of this is visible. The bowl is still being eaten. The body is still functioning. But the chemistry that the body depends on is happening at a fraction of the speed it was meant to happen at.

And here, also, the bacterial neighbors enter the work.

Many of the enzymes that operate in the lower gut are not made by the body at all. They are made by the bacterial community, manufactured by the partners that live there, sent out into the chyme to do work the body's own enzymes cannot do. The fiber-breaking enzymes of the colon are bacterial enzymes. The vitamin-assembling enzymes are bacterial enzymes. Some of the enzymes that prepare nutrients for absorption across the lining are bacterial enzymes. And those enzymes, like the body's own, are inert without their mineral cofactors. The bacteria, to do their work, need the trace minerals as much as the body does. The minerals dissolved in the morning's broth feed two populations of enzymes at once — the body's, and the partners'.

This is the cycle that has been assembling, quietly, beneath the boy's bowl of soup. The minerals activate the enzymes. The enzymes break down the food. The food feeds the bacterial neighbors. The bacteria produce more enzymes that need more minerals. The lining is fed, the bacteria are fed, the body is fed. One integrated arrangement, three interlocking partners, none of which works on its own.

And here is the harder thing.

Across most of the developed world, in the years that contain this kitchen, this cycle has been quietly coming apart.

The soil began it. The earth a vegetable now grows in is, in many places, soil that has been farmed continuously for sixty or seventy years and replenished only with the three or four minerals the industrial fertilizer industry decided were worth replacing. The vegetable that arrives at the kitchen looks like a vegetable. It tastes, more or less, like a vegetable. It is missing the small invisible content that made the vegetable, in earlier times, a complete delivery of what the body required. A carrot pulled from the ground a hundred years ago carried, by careful measurement, several times the trace mineral content of a carrot pulled from a modern field. This is not a contested figure. The agricultural records show it. The reader's grandmother knew, without needing the records, that the food in her kitchen was not the food in her grandmother's kitchen.

The water began it too. The rain that once carried trace minerals from the high places to the low has been falling on land whose surface chemistry has changed; the rivers that once delivered the small dissolved complement to the towns along their banks have been cleaned of many things, including the things that were good for a body. The salt on most kitchen tables is, in most households, an industrial product that has been stripped of the small natural complement of other minerals it once contained, leaving only sodium and a few additives. None of this is malice. Each step of it was, in its own time, a reasonable response to a real problem. The cumulative effect was a slow thinning of what was reaching the body at every meal.

The bacterial community has been thinning in parallel.

The friends a person carries in their gut are sustained, day after day, by the food they receive. When the food is varied, when it contains the fibers and the polyphenols and the small living foods the community evolved on, the community thrives. When the food becomes narrow — when the diet shrinks to a few processed staples, when the antibiotic course in childhood was followed by no period of careful re-establishment, when the fermented foods that sustained generations of human guts disappeared from the household — the community shrinks. Whole species, present in the gut of a child a century ago, are now missing from the gut of the average child in a developed country. They are not endangered in the gut alone. They are gone. A modern body is carrying a smaller, less diverse population than any human body has carried for as long as humans have been keeping records of what is inside them.

And the enzymes, in the middle of all this, sit in greater numbers inert.

A body whose trace mineral supply is thin has fewer activated enzymes. A body whose bacterial company has grown small has fewer of the enzymes the bacteria would have made on its behalf. The chemistry slows. Not all at once. Not in any way that a single doctor's appointment would catch. The work that should be happening continuously across the lining of the small intestine, in the cells of the colon, in the cells of every organ — happens at a fraction of the speed it was meant to happen at. The body, like a garden whose soil is failing, looks from a distance like the same garden it always was. The plants are still there. The flowers still come. But the deeper layer beneath the surface is no longer doing what it once did, and the slow signs of the failure show up only across the years.

The result is a population of bodies that are not, by ordinary measure, malnourished. They are eating. They have weight. Their blood tests show levels of the major nutrients that look acceptable. What they are missing is the smaller substrate beneath all of that — the trace cofactors, the diverse community, the activated enzymes, the steady delivery of what the cycle was built to deliver. None of this announces itself. It manifests as a slow tiredness, a slow inflammation, a slow drift away from the body the person was meant to inhabit, that no single test will ever quite locate.

This is the condition of the modern body in the modern world. It is not the condition the body was made for. It is the condition the body has come to live in, across two or three generations of changing soil and changing water and changing food, in ways no one quite chose and no one quite knows how to undo at scale.

And it is the condition the boy at his mother's kitchen table will, in some measure, grow up inside.

The pinch of trace minerals in his morning broth is one small refusal of this condition. The bone broth his mother started the night before is another. The vegetables from the garden the day before yesterday are a third. None of these are dramatic. None of them, on their own, are a complete answer. Together, repeated across the years of a childhood, they are something. They are a household where one form of the long thinning is being held back, slightly, by a woman who does not call what she is doing a practice and would not know what to say if asked why she does it the way she does. She does it because her mother did it that way, or because something in her body knew what to ask for, or because someone she trusted recommended the small jar by the stove and the careful broth and the garden out back, and she found, over the years, that her family was steadier when she kept up these small things.

Whether the boy will, as a man, keep them up himself is the question the rest of his life will answer.

What the fast does, at the larger scale of years, is the deliberate version of what his mother was doing in the small scale of a morning.

The body that has been living for decades inside the modern conditions — the thinning soil, the stripped water, the narrowing community in the gut, the enzymes sitting in greater numbers inert — does not, on its own, recover. It does not have the room to do so. The continuous arrival of food, even of clean food, keeps the digestive system in continuous operation; the system never gets the long quiet stretch it would need to do its deeper repair work. The bacterial company, once thinned, does not re-diversify on its own while the same daily food is arriving. The lining, once weakened, cannot rebuild itself while it is continuously being asked to absorb. The trace mineral inventory, once depleted, does not rise on its own while the mineral content of the food coming in is too small to keep up with what the work is using.

The fast opens the room.

During a prolonged fast, the digestive system slows nearly to a stop. The lining, no longer occupied with the absorption of new food, turns to its own repair. The bacterial community, freed from the constant arrival of whatever the modern diet was bringing, has the chance to recompose itself. The enzymes, no longer being asked to handle a continuous load, settle into a different rhythm. And into this opened room, taken with the morning's water, a small daily pinch of trace minerals — the same kind of pinch the boy's mother dropped into her broth — keeps the body's cofactor inventory steady through the deeper work. The minerals are not absorbed in the way food is absorbed. They cross the lining quietly, by a mechanism that does not require the lining to be at full strength. They reach the enzymes that are still doing the maintenance work the body never quite stops doing. They reach the bacterial company that is re-establishing itself in the slowed dark of the lower gut. They keep the cycle alive while everything else around the cycle is given permission to reset.

This is why a single small jar of dissolved trace minerals can sit on the counter beside a fasting body for many days, and quietly do work that no other intervention would do as well. The body is not being fed. The body is being kept.

The boy at his mother's kitchen table is finishing his soup.

The morning is quiet. He swings his feet a little. The bowl in front of him is almost empty, and the steam has thinned to nothing, and the sounds of his mother moving around the kitchen behind him are the small unremarkable sounds of an ordinary day. He does not know any of what has been happening across the long passage of his lower gut while he ate. He does not know that the pinch his mother dropped into the morning's water has reached the deepest cells of his body. He does not know that the community he will carry for the rest of his life has just been fed, and will continue to be fed, day after day, across the decades that follow this one.

And yet across those decades, in a body that nobody is watching from inside, he will be quietly building what no one will quite have a name for. A community. A neighborhood. A circle of partners who will know his rhythms before he knows them himself. A household of friends whose work he will live on for as long as his body draws breath. None of this will be planned. None of this will be intended. He will become, by the small accumulated weight of bowl after bowl, the kind of body inside which a long living world has been carefully kept.

That is what a fed body becomes, in the end. A small kept world.

The seven below are the trace minerals most often named in the prose above. They are not the whole story. The human body draws on as many as a hundred ionic sulfated trace minerals across its work, and an enzyme made by any one of them needs the right one of them to begin. The food sources listed for each are honest sources, but in a modern food system the amounts are uneven and often thin. Liquid ionic sulfated trace mineral products, taken according to the directions on the bottle, deliver many of the hundred at once, in small daily doses that the body excretes what it does not need from. The chart below is a reference, not a complete catalog.

Trace mineral	Role and food sources
Zinc	Activates hundreds of digestive and immune enzymes. Found in oysters, grass-fed beef, pumpkin seeds, lentils, eggs.
Magnesium	Activates more enzymatic work than any other element; supports muscle relaxation and the energy work of the mitochondria. Found in dark leafy greens, pumpkin seeds, almonds, dark chocolate, avocado, fish.
Manganese	Protects the cells of the gut lining from oxidative damage. Found in pineapple, pecans, brown rice, leafy greens, whole grains.
Selenium	Activates immune defenses of the gut and supports the chemistry of detoxification, particularly during parasite die-off. Found in Brazil nuts (one or two a day is sufficient), seafood, eggs, organ meats.
Copper	Essential for the small fires of the mitochondria; supports connective tissue and iron metabolism. Found in shellfish, organ meats, dark chocolate, sesame seeds, cashews.
Chromium	Steadies the body's relationship with sugar; holds insulin's responsiveness across the day. Found in broccoli, grass-fed meats, whole grains, brewer's yeast.
Molybdenum	Activates the liver's deeper detoxification systems. Found in legumes, leafy greens, organ meats, whole grains.

A note on iodine. The liquid ionic sulfated trace mineral products described above deliver many minerals but typically do not include iodine. This is by design. Iodine sits in a category of its own, with its own narrow window between the amount the thyroid needs and the amount that begins to interfere with the thyroid's work. Most people do best with iodine handled separately from the daily mineral mix — through the food they eat, primarily, and through occasional considered intake when the diet runs thin in iodine-rich sources. Seafood and seaweed are the richest natural sources. Eggs and dairy carry meaningful amounts. Iodized salt, where it is still used, was the public-health intervention that solved the iodine deficiencies of the early twentieth century and continues to do quiet work in the kitchens that still keep it on the table.

The fast itself is not the time for added iodine. During a prolonged fast the thyroid downshifts as part of the body's deeper rest, and pushing iodine into a downshifted thyroid can produce the opposite of what the supplementation was meant to give. The note here is for the long stewardship that follows the fast — the years of careful eating, the seasonal returns, the household where these small things are kept. If a reader's ordinary diet runs thin in seafood, seaweed, dairy, eggs, and iodized salt, considered iodine intake paired with selenium is worth a conversation with someone who knows the reader's particular body. The chart above does not address it. The chart above stays with what the trace mineral mix actually delivers.

Chapter 4

What Lives Inside You

* * *

You have never eaten alone. Every meal you have ever consumed, every nutrient your body worked to absorb, has been shared. Not by your choice. Not with your knowledge. But shared nonetheless.

Inside your gut right now lives a community of organisms. Some of them are partners — the trillions of bacteria that ferment your fiber and produce your vitamins, the ones we discussed in the previous chapter. They are old, they are useful, and they are welcome. But the gut is also home to others. Organisms that have been quietly taking from you for years. Organisms whose presence you cannot feel and whose work you cannot see, but whose effects accumulate, generation after generation, in the slow erosion of vitality that most people in the modern world have come to think of as ordinary aging.

The pages that follow are about the ones that take.

Before we go further, release any judgment about this. Parasitic infection is not a reflection of cleanliness, intelligence, or moral worth. It is a fact of living on Earth. Conservative estimates suggest that more than three and a half billion people worldwide carry some form of gut parasite — a third of every human alive — and most of them have no idea. The organisms are in the soil where vegetables grow. They are in water that has not been adequately filtered. They are on the surfaces of fruit. They have been part of the human experience since the beginning of the human experience. Knowing they are there is not cause for alarm. It is cause for action.

What follows is a description of the organisms most commonly found in human guts. There are four families, each with distinct characteristics, distinct preferred locations within the body, and distinct methods of doing the work they do.

The Roundworms

The roundworms — what biologists call nematodes — are the most common parasites on earth. They are also among the most ancient. Versions of these organisms have been living in the guts of vertebrates since long before mammals existed, and the species that infect humans today have been adapting to us, specifically, for the entire span of our evolutionary history. They know us very well.

The largest of them is *Ascaris lumbricoides*, the giant roundworm, which can grow to thirteen inches in length inside the human small intestine. This is not an exaggeration. A mature Ascaris is the size and approximate weight of a thick pencil, pink and translucent, and a single female lays up to two hundred thousand eggs each day, every day, for the entire span of her one-year life. Most people who carry Ascaris carry a small number — three or four worms, perhaps — and never know. In regions of the world where contamination is heavy, people sometimes carry hundreds, and the worms tangle into masses inside the intestine that block its function. The first time Ascaris was discovered in the modern era, it was found in numbers that astonished the surgeons who removed it. They had not believed, before they saw it, that something so large could live inside a human being without producing obvious symptoms. It can. It does.

The whipworm, *Trichuris trichiura*, is smaller — about an inch and a half long — and lives in a different part of the gut. It threads its long thin front end into the wall of the large intestine, where it embeds and feeds on tissue secretions and blood. Imagine a length of sewing thread driven into a soft surface and you have something close to the picture. The eggs, when seen under a microscope, are perhaps the most distinctive in all of parasitology — barrel-shaped, with a small plug at each end, like miniature lemons. Once you have seen one you cannot mistake it for anything else.

Hookworms — *Ancylostoma* and *Necator* are the genera most often found in humans — enter through the skin. They live as larvae in soil and, when bare skin makes contact with that soil, they bore directly through. From the skin they enter the bloodstream and ride to the lungs, where they crawl up the airways, are coughed up, are swallowed, and arrive finally in the small intestine. There they bite into the wall with mouth parts that look, under sufficient magnification, like the cutting plates of a small machine. They are blood-feeders, and a heavy hookworm load is the leading cause of iron-deficiency anemia worldwide. Their entire migration through the human body — from the soil-walking foot to the intestinal wall — takes about six weeks.

Strongyloides stercoralis is the threadworm, and it deserves a moment of particular attention. Most parasites need to leave the body and pass through some external environment before they can infect again. Strongyloides does not. It can complete its entire lifecycle inside one human host, generation after generation, without the parasite ever leaving the body. This means that an infection acquired in childhood — perhaps from a single barefoot afternoon in contaminated soil — can persist for the entire lifetime of the host. People in their seventies and eighties have been found carrying Strongyloides infections that they acquired during military service half a century earlier. The organism is one of the most under-diagnosed parasites in developed countries, and its capacity for indefinite persistence makes it among the most consequential.

The pinworm, *Enterobius vermicularis*, is the parasite most likely to be in your home right now. Estimates suggest that one in five children in industrialized countries carry it at any given time, and it is so common in adults that most adult cases are simply never diagnosed. It is small, white, threadlike — perhaps half an inch in length for the females, smaller for the males — and it lives in the large intestine and rectum. Its lifecycle has a peculiar feature whose details belong to the larger account of pinworms specifically: at night, the gravid females migrate out of the anus and lay their eggs on the perianal skin, where they become infective within hours. The cycle of pinworm transmission is fundamentally different from every other parasite covered here, and it is the reason pinworms receive separate, fuller treatment of their own.

Anisakis is the worm of raw fish. It is acquired most commonly through sushi made with insufficiently frozen fish, and increasingly through ceviche and other preparations of marine origin. The larvae, which can be visible to the naked eye if you know where to look in the flesh of an infected fish, attempt to embed themselves in the human stomach or intestinal wall once swallowed. The body's response is severe — sharp pain, sometimes vomiting, often an allergic reaction — and the diagnosis is sometimes made through endoscopy, when the small white worm is seen, alive, in the act of attempting to bore into the gastric lining. As global consumption of raw fish has grown, anisakiasis has grown with it. The cuisine that defined Tokyo for centuries has now followed the city's emigrants and travelers around the world, and the parasite has come along.

The Tapeworms

The tapeworms are different from the roundworms in nearly every way. They are flat — ribbon-like, as the common name suggests — and they have no digestive system of their own. They do not need one. They live, throughout their entire adult life, inside the human small intestine, bathed in the partially digested products of human meals, and they absorb their nourishment directly through their outer surface. They are, in this sense, the most fully adapted parasites we know. Everything about them has been simplified to the single purpose of absorbing nutrients and producing eggs.

Tapeworms anchor themselves to the intestinal wall by a head called a scolex — a structure equipped, depending on the species, with hooks, suckers, or specialized grooves. From the scolex grows a chain of segments called proglottids. New segments form continuously near the head; old segments break off at the far end and are passed in the stool. A mature tapeworm is, in this sense, a continuously renewing organism. The worm you carry today contains some segments that are only days old and some that have been growing for months. Over the lifetime of the parasite, the tapeworm produces an astonishing total: a single beef tapeworm can release several hundred million eggs over its twenty-five-year life inside a human host.

Taenia saginata, the beef tapeworm, is acquired through undercooked beef from cattle that have grazed on contaminated land. It can grow to twenty-five feet in length inside the human small intestine — long enough to span the length of a small house — and many of its hosts experience no symptoms beyond an occasional sense that something is not quite right. Some people discover their infection only when a segment of the worm passes in stool and is recognized for what it is. The discovery is, by all reports, unforgettable.

Taenia solium, the pork tapeworm, is the more dangerous cousin. The adult worm in the gut is similar to the beef tapeworm in size and behavior. The danger lies in what happens when the eggs of *T. solium* are swallowed by a human, rather than the meat containing its larvae. The eggs hatch in the small intestine, and the larvae do something that *T. saginata* never does: they migrate out of the gut, through the bloodstream, into the body's tissues — including, often, the brain. There they form cysts. The condition is called neurocysticercosis, and it is the leading cause of acquired epilepsy in many parts of the world. It is a condition that deserves careful attention, and any account of tapeworms that omits it is incomplete.

Diphyllobothrium latum, the fish tapeworm, is the longest of the human tapeworms — capable of reaching thirty feet inside its host. It is acquired through raw freshwater fish and is particularly common in regions where such consumption is traditional. It has a peculiar nutritional habit that distinguishes it from the other tapeworms: it directly consumes vitamin B12 from the host's small intestine, in such quantity that long-term infection produces severe and characteristic B12 deficiency. The diagnosis is sometimes made backward, from a megaloblastic anemia of unclear origin in a person who has eaten raw fish regularly.

The dwarf tapeworm, *Hymenolepis nana*, is the smallest of the human tapeworms — only an inch or two in length — but it has a feature that makes it unusually transmissible. It can complete its entire lifecycle inside a single human host, without an intermediate host, which means it can spread directly from person to person and can even auto-infect within a single individual. It is particularly common in children and in households where any single member is infected.

The Flukes

The flukes are the third family, and they are different in nearly every way from the worms we have discussed so far. They are flat and leaf-shaped, often quite small, and they live not always in the gut but sometimes in the bile ducts, the liver, the lungs, even the bloodstream. They have, perhaps, the most complex lifecycles of any parasite that infects human beings — most of them require multiple intermediate hosts, including specific species of freshwater snails, before they can complete their development and reach the human gut. They are also, by reputation and by clinical experience, the most stubborn parasites to clear. The work of removing them requires its own careful protocol, addressed at length in the practical chapters of this work.

But here is what you need to know about who they are.

Fasciolopsis buski, the giant intestinal fluke, lives in the small intestine and reaches up to three inches in length — visible to the naked eye, leaf-shaped, with a body broad enough that it can be seen distinctly in surgical specimens. It is the largest intestinal fluke that infects humans. It attaches to the intestinal wall and feeds, and a mature population of these flukes inside one host can produce significant inflammation and intermittent obstruction.

Fasciola hepatica, the liver fluke, lives somewhere far less accessible. After being swallowed in the form of a microscopic cyst on contaminated produce, the larvae penetrate the wall of the small intestine, migrate through the abdominal cavity, bore through the capsule of the liver, and travel through the liver tissue itself until they reach the bile ducts. There they take up permanent residence. They can live for nine to thirteen years in the bile ducts, laying eggs that travel down the bile and out through the stool, perpetuating the cycle. They are essentially beyond the reach of any cleansing protocol that does not specifically address the bile ducts — which is why coffee enemas occupy the central place they do in the practical work of clearing.

Clonorchis sinensis, the Chinese liver fluke, is similar in habitat to *Fasciola hepatica* but smaller, more slender, and considerably longer-lived. Records exist of *Clonorchis* infections persisting for thirty years inside a single host. Thirty years. The fluke that you might acquire at twenty-five would still be alive and laying eggs at fifty-five. Chronic *Clonorchis* infection is associated with bile duct cancer in regions where it is endemic, and the World Health Organization has classified it as a carcinogen.

There are smaller flukes, too. *Heterophyes heterophyes* is one of them — less than two millimeters in length, almost too small to see without magnification — but capable of penetrating the intestinal wall and entering the bloodstream, where its eggs can lodge in the heart and brain in cases of heavy infection. The smallness of a parasite does not predict the size of the trouble it can cause.

What unites the flukes, across their many species and habitats, is endurance. They live for years, sometimes for decades. They occupy locations that are difficult to reach. They reproduce continuously, and their eggs are protected by shells more resistant than those of any other parasite group. The work of clearing flukes, when it is undertaken seriously, is the work of weeks of consistent protocol, not days.

The Protozoa

The fourth family is invisible to the naked eye. The protozoa are single-celled organisms — much closer in size to the bacteria of the gut microbiome than to the worms we have been discussing — but they are very much animals, with cellular machinery similar to ours, and they cause some of the most consequential gut infections in modern medicine.

Giardia lamblia is perhaps the most well-known of them. It is a tear-drop-shaped organism with two nuclei that, under the microscope, look strikingly like a pair of eyes staring back. It has a flat ventral surface called a sucking disc that allows it to attach to the lining of the small intestine, where it covers stretches of villi like a carpet of clinging cells. Where Giardia attaches, nutrient absorption fails. The infection is one of the most common waterborne illnesses in the world, and it is increasingly common in developed countries through contamination of municipal water supplies and recreational lakes and streams. The symptoms — chronic diarrhea, bloating, fatigue, weight loss — often persist for months in the people who develop them, and the diagnosis is missed in a substantial fraction of cases.

Entamoeba histolytica is the protozoan that does what its species name suggests: it lyses, or dissolves, tissue. It lives in the large intestine, and in its invasive form it actually consumes the intestinal lining cells one by one, leaving the characteristic flask-shaped ulcers that pathologists recognize as the signature of amebic infection. In severe cases, the organism enters the bloodstream and travels to the liver, where it forms abscesses — pockets of liquefied tissue that, on ultrasound, appear as dark voids in the body of the organ. Untreated, advanced amebic infection can be fatal, though the more common picture is chronic, low-grade dysentery that the patient lives with for years.

Cryptosporidium parvum lives inside the cells of the small intestine — a true intracellular parasite — and is famous for its resistance to chlorine. The municipal water-treatment systems that protect against most pathogens do not protect against Crypto. It survives chlorination at standard levels and has caused mass outbreaks in major cities, the most famous of which was the 1993 outbreak in Milwaukee that infected an estimated four hundred thousand people through the city's drinking water. In immunocompromised individuals it can be devastating; in healthy adults it produces a watery diarrhea that, while severe, usually resolves over weeks. The cysts of Crypto, like those of Giardia, persist in the environment for months.

Blastocystis hominis is one of the most common gut parasites in developed countries — it has been found in the stool of an estimated twenty percent of healthy adults — and yet its clinical significance is still debated. Some carriers have no symptoms whatsoever. Others have chronic digestive distress, skin conditions, and fatigue that resolve when the organism is cleared. The current clinical view is that Blastocystis matters in some people and not in others, and the difference may have to do with the strain, the host's immune state, or other factors not yet understood.

Dientamoeba fragilis is another organism that has been quietly common and quietly missed. It does not form cysts of the type that standard stool tests detect, which means most laboratory testing fails to find it. It causes chronic gut symptoms that are often misdiagnosed as irritable bowel syndrome. It is a parasite that has been hiding in plain sight for decades, recognized as common only as testing methods have improved.

Where They Live

Each parasite has its preferred location. The roundworms occupy primarily the small and large intestines. The tapeworms attach in the upper small intestine. The intestinal flukes live in the small intestine, while the liver flukes inhabit the bile ducts and liver tissue itself. Giardia takes the upper small intestine; Entamoeba and Blastocystis live in the large intestine; Cryptosporidium burrows into the small intestine lining; the smaller flukes can travel to the heart and brain.

What this means, practically, is that a thorough cleansing protocol must reach all of these locations. An enema reaches the large intestine but not the small. An oral herbal tincture reaches the small intestine through digestion but does not penetrate to the bile ducts effectively. A coffee enema, through its stimulation of bile flow, reaches the bile ducts in a way nothing else easily can. Each tool in this protocol exists because some specific organisms could not otherwise be reached.

What They Have in Common

Different families. Different locations. Different methods of attachment, of feeding, of reproduction, of evading the immune system. But every single one of these organisms, across all four families, shares one fundamental characteristic. They take.

They take your nutrients before you can absorb them. They take your energy by forcing your body to maintain a constant low-grade immune defense. They damage the lining of your intestine through their feeding activities. They alter the composition of your microbiome by competing for resources with the beneficial bacteria. They release waste products into the gut that your liver then has to process. They consume your vitamins and minerals, and in some cases they consume them in such quantity that they create deficiencies the diet alone cannot correct.

And most of them do this quietly. For years. Sometimes for decades. Without any obvious symptom that would lead the host to suspect what is happening.

The symptoms, when they appear, are often the kind that get attributed to other causes. Chronic fatigue is dismissed as stress. Bloating and irregular elimination are labeled irritable bowel syndrome and treated with prescriptions that mask the symptoms without addressing the cause. Skin conditions are pursued through dermatology rather than through the gut from which they often originate. Brain fog and mood disturbance are treated as primary mental health conditions rather than as downstream consequences of an inflamed and disrupted gut. Sleep disruption — particularly the nighttime restlessness and itching produced by pinworm activity — is rarely connected to its actual cause.

The absence of obvious symptoms does not mean the absence of parasites. It means the parasites have found a comfortable home and are doing their work without disturbing the host enough to be noticed.

What Living With Them Looks Like

You are not alone in your gut. You have never been alone in it. These organisms, in some combination and in some quantity, are very probably present in you right now, as they are present in roughly a third of all human beings on earth. Knowing they are there does not require alarm. It requires only the willingness to look honestly at what is, and to do the work of clearing what should not be.

Each of these parasites will be traced, in its turn, back to its source — how it enters the body, how it establishes itself, what it does once it has settled in. The lifecycles, the transmission routes, the damage done over years of unrecognized residence: each can be followed, named, and understood. And then there is the work of clearing them out.

A reader who came to fasting wanting to understand what it could do for the body finds, here, that the answer involves these organisms more than they knew. They are the unwelcome inheritance of human life on earth, and the protocol that follows is the inheritance of all the cultures that figured out, over thousands of years, how to set them down.

Figure References — by Parasite Family

(See the online Figure Guide for all figures referenced above.)

Family 1 — Roundworms (Nematodes)

Figures 4.1–4.19 *online Figure Guide

Family 2 — Tapeworms (Cestodes)

Figures 4.20–4.31 *online Figure Guide

Family 3 — Flukes (Trematodes)

Figures 4.32–4.40 *online Figure Guide

Family 4 — Protozoa (Single-Celled Parasites)

Figures 4.41–4.57 *online Figure Guide

Chapter 5

How Each Parasite Gets In

* * *

Every uninvited guest found a door. The doors are not exotic. They are the ordinary openings of human life — the food we eat, the water we drink, the soil we walk across, the surfaces we touch, the people we live alongside. Each parasite has its preferred route, and most of them are routes you cross without noticing.

This chapter traces every route, for every parasite, so you understand exactly how transmission happens and what genuine protection looks like. You will see your own life inside these pages — the meal that was a little undercooked, the salad washed in tap water, the swim in the lake, the barefoot walk through warm grass. None of these things are sins. They are simply human. But once you understand them as transmission events, you can decide which doors to keep open and which to close.

* * *

The Five Routes

Before we look at each parasite individually, every transmission route falls into one of five categories. The categories are worth knowing because the same protective habits address multiple parasites at once.

1. Fecal-oral. Contaminated feces reaches the mouth through food, water, or unwashed hands.

2. Skin penetration. Larvae in soil or water penetrate directly through bare skin.

3. Consumption of infected food. Undercooked meat, fish, or raw produce carrying larvae or eggs.

4. Contaminated water. Drinking, swimming, or incidental contact with infected water sources.

5. Person to person. Direct contact or shared surfaces carrying infectious stages.

Most people are exposed through multiple routes over a lifetime — often without ever knowing it. The atlas tables that follow show every parasite in this book with its route, its specific transmission vehicles, and the one fact about it most worth carrying in your head.

* * *

Roundworms

The roundworms are the most common parasitic infections on earth. They are also the most varied in how they reach you — some through the soil, some through the skin, some through ordinary household contact. The table below covers the six most clinically significant roundworms in the human gut.

Parasite	Common name	Primary route	Vehicles & specifics
Ascaris lumbricoides	Giant roundworm	Fecal-oral via soil	Eggs in human feces contaminate soil and produce. Eggs survive in soil up to 6 years. Unwashed produce, dirty hands, contaminated water are the primary vehicles. Children playing in soil are particularly vulnerable.
Trichuris trichiura	Whipworm	Fecal-oral via soil	Identical route to Ascaris. Eggs deposited in feces, survive in warm moist soil, transmitted through contaminated produce and water. Often contracted alongside Ascaris in the same environment.
Ancylostoma & Necator	Hookworms	Skin penetration	Eggs hatch in warm moist soil within 1–2 days. Larvae actively seek body heat and penetrate the skin of bare feet. Travel via bloodstream to lungs, are coughed up, and swallowed. Also possible through hand contact with infected soil.
Strongyloides stercoralis	Threadworm	Skin penetration + autoinfection	Larvae in contaminated soil penetrate bare skin, like hookworm. Uniquely, can also reinfect from within the body — larvae in the gut penetrate the intestinal wall and restart the cycle internally without external reexposure.
Enterobius vermicularis	Pinworm	Person-to-person, surfaces	Female worms migrate to anal area at night to lay eggs. Itching deposits

Parasite	Common name	Primary route	Vehicles & specifics
			eggs on hands and under fingernails. Hand-to-mouth transfer reinfects same person or others. Eggs survive on bedding, towels, toilet seats, door handles for up to 3 weeks. Airborne transmission possible.
Anisakis	Fish worm	Raw or undercooked fish	Larvae live in flesh of cod, salmon, herring, mackerel, halibut, and squid. Visible as small coiled worms but easily missed. Killed by thorough cooking or by freezing at −20°C for 7 days. Sushi, sashimi, ceviche, pickled and cold-smoked fish are primary risks.

Two things about this family deserve a closer look.

Hookworm is one of the most striking transmission routes in human parasitology. You do not eat them. They come to you. The larvae detect body heat, move toward it, and penetrate skin on contact. A walk through warm grass with bare feet is enough.

Strongyloides is the parasite that breaks the rules. Once it is in, it can stay in — sometimes for decades — without ever being re-exposed. The biological reason is covered in the next chapter, with the rest of its lifecycle.

And pinworm. Of all the parasites in this chapter, pinworm is the one most likely to be in your immediate environment right now regardless of your lifestyle. It does not care about hygiene the way the soil-transmitted parasites do. It travels through families, through schools, through any environment where people share surfaces — and entire households are typically infected once one person is.

* * *

Tapeworms

The tapeworms are different. They do not enter through soil or skin or contaminated water. They enter through meat. Each species of human tapeworm has a specific intermediate host — the animal that carries the larval stage — and the meat of that animal, eaten undercooked, is the route in. There is one critical exception, covered after the table.

Parasite	Common name	Primary route	Vehicles & specifics
Taenia saginata	Beef tapeworm	Undercooked beef	Cattle graze on pasture contaminated with human feces containing tapeworm eggs. Larvae encyst in beef muscle as cysticerci. Humans consume undercooked beef containing living cysts. No person-to-person transmission — cattle intermediate host required.
Taenia solium (route 1)	Pork tapeworm — adult worm	Undercooked pork	Pigs consume food or water contaminated with human feces containing eggs. Larvae encyst in pork muscle tissue. Humans infected by eating undercooked pork — an intestinal tapeworm develops in the gut.
Taenia solium (route 2)	Pork tapeworm — eggs directly	Contaminated food/water with eggs	Humans become intermediate hosts (instead of definitive hosts) by consuming food or water contaminated with the eggs themselves rather than larval cysts. Eggs hatch and larvae migrate to tissues including the brain, eyes, and spine. This is the dangerous route. See standalone warning below.
Diphyllobothrium latum	Fish tapeworm	Raw/ undercooked freshwater fish	Complex lifecycle involving microscopic crustaceans and freshwater fish. Larvae encyst in flesh of pike, perch, salmon, trout. Common in Scandinavian, Eastern European, Asian, Latin American traditional dishes. Sushi prepared with freshwater fish is a primary contemporary route.
Hymenolepis nana	Dwarf	Fecal-oral,	Eggs passed in feces of infected

Parasite	Common name	Primary route	Vehicles & specifics
	tapeworm	person-to-person	person. Direct person-to-person transmission — no intermediate host required. Beetles and fleas can serve as intermediate hosts. Most common in institutionalized settings and areas with poor sanitation.

The pork tapeworm route 2 — eggs ingested directly rather than larval cysts in meat — is the chapter's most important warning. Larvae from these eggs do not stay in the gut. They migrate to tissues throughout the body, including the brain. This is neurocysticercosis, the most dangerous parasitic brain infection in the world, and it is the reason T. solium gets a chapter of its own in this book — Chapter 8 — before any of the protocol instructions begin. If you have any reason to suspect brain involvement, that chapter must be read before anything else in this book is acted on.

* * *

Flukes

The flukes have the most complex transmission routes of all gut parasites. They always involve at least one — and often two — intermediate hosts before reaching humans. Almost every fluke route involves freshwater snails as the first intermediate host, with the parasite emerging from the snail and either encysting on aquatic plants or penetrating fish before reaching the human consumer.

Parasite	Common name	Primary route	Vehicles & specifics
Fasciolopsis buski	Giant intestinal fluke	Raw aquatic plants	Eggs pass into water, hatch into miracidia, penetrate freshwater snails. Cercariae emerge and encyst on water chestnuts, water caltrop, lotus root, water bamboo. Humans infected by eating these plants raw or peeling them with their teeth. Common in Southeast and East Asia.
Fasciola hepatica	Liver fluke	Raw aquatic vegetation,	Eggs from infected cattle, sheep, or humans pass into water, hatch,

Parasite	Common name	Primary route	Vehicles & specifics
		especially watercress	penetrate snails, and cercariae encyst on aquatic plants. Wild watercress gathered from streams is highest-risk; commercially grown is occasionally implicated. Contaminated water used to wash salad vegetables also transmits.
Clonorchis sinensis	Chinese liver fluke	Raw/ undercooked freshwater fish	Eggs enter water, hatch, enter snails, cercariae penetrate freshwater fish (carp, bream, roach), encyst in fish muscle. Humans infected by eating raw or undercooked freshwater fish. Traditional dishes in China, Korea, Vietnam are primary risks. Migrates through bile duct to liver.
Heterophyes heterophyes	Heterophyes	Raw/ undercooked saltwater fish	Lifecycle involves snails and saltwater or brackish-water fish — mullet, tilapia, others. Transmission through raw, pickled, or inadequately cooked fish. Common in Egypt, the Middle East, the Far East, and Mediterranean regions.

Of these, Fasciola hepatica deserves a special note. It does not stay in the bile ducts the way other flukes do — it migrates through liver tissue itself on the way there. The full destructive path is covered in the next chapter. The relevant point here is that the flukes are the parasites that demanded the additional protocol layers described later in this book. They are the reason the basic herbal triad alone is sometimes not enough.

* * *

Protozoa

The protozoa are different from everything else in this chapter. They are single-celled. They are far smaller than the smallest worm — invisible without a microscope. They divide rapidly inside the host, sometimes every eight to twelve hours, which means a single organism can become a population in a matter of days. And they have evolved cyst forms that survive outside the body for weeks or months, resistant to drying, to chlorination, to most of the conditions that kill worms and their eggs.

The result is that protozoa transmit through routes that look ordinary. Treated municipal water. A swimming pool. A salad. A handshake. They do not require warm soil or undercooked meat or raw fish. They require the conditions of everyday life in the developed world, and they find them.

Parasite	Common name	Primary route	Vehicles & specifics
Giardia lamblia	Giardia	Contaminated water, fecal-oral	Cysts in feces of infected humans and animals. Survive in cold water for months — resistant to standard chlorination. Streams, lakes, poorly treated municipal water are primary sources. Hiking and camping are common transmission events. Survives chlorine in swimming pools and water parks. Daycare centers are well-documented transmission environments.
Entamoeba histolytica	Amoeba	Contaminated food and water	Cysts passed in feces; survive weeks in environment. Contaminated drinking water is the primary route in developing regions. Raw produce washed or grown with contaminated water. Travel to regions with inadequate sanitation is the most common exposure for people in developed countries.
Cryptosporidium parvum	Crypto	Contaminated water, animal contact	Oocysts passed in feces of humans and animals (cattle particularly). Resistant to chlorine at standard treatment levels. Drinking water in developed countries. Swimming pools and water parks. Contact with infected farm animals. Person-to-person in healthcare and childcare.
Blastocystis hominis	Blasto	Contaminated	Cysts passed in feces. Contaminated

Parasite	Common name	Primary route	Vehicles & specifics
		water and food	water and food are the primary routes. Person-to-person through poor hand hygiene. May spread through flies and cockroaches as mechanical vectors. One of the most prevalent gut parasites in developed countries despite good sanitation.
Dientamoeba fragilis	Dientamoeba	Fecal-oral, possibly via pinworm eggs	Exact route still being studied. Fecal-oral through contaminated food and water. May travel inside pinworm eggs as a protected passenger — which would explain why Dientamoeba and pinworm infections so frequently occur together. Person-to-person in close-contact settings.

Giardia is one of the most successful parasites on earth precisely because of its environmental resilience. The cyst form is what makes the difference — it is what allows Giardia to survive in cold mountain streams for months at a time, what allows it to pass through swimming pool chlorine and municipal water treatment, and what makes it the most common cause of waterborne diarrheal illness in the United States.

Cryptosporidium has caused some of the largest waterborne disease outbreaks in history — including the 1993 Milwaukee outbreak that affected an estimated 400,000 people and killed more than a hundred immunocompromised patients. The municipal water treatment was working as designed. Cryptosporidium passed through it anyway.

* * *

Quick Reference — By Route of Entry

The atlas tables above are organized by parasite. The table below is organized the other way around — by transmission route — for the reader who wants to know what comes from a specific source.

Route	Parasites
Contaminated water (drinking, recreational)	Giardia, Cryptosporidium, Entamoeba, Blastocystis, Ascaris, Whipworm, Flukes

Route	Parasites
Raw or undercooked saltwater fish	Anisakis, Heterophyes
Raw or undercooked freshwater fish	Fish tapeworm, Chinese liver fluke
Raw or undercooked beef	Beef tapeworm
Raw or undercooked pork	Pork tapeworm (adult worm)
Raw aquatic plants (watercress, water chestnut, lotus root)	Intestinal fluke, Liver fluke (Fasciola)
Contaminated produce (soil-grown, washed in unsafe water)	Ascaris, Whipworm, Entamoeba, Cyclospora
Skin penetration in warm moist soil	Hookworm, Strongyloides
Person to person, shared surfaces	Pinworm, Dwarf tapeworm, Giardia, Dientamoeba, Pork tapeworm (eggs)
Animal contact (especially livestock)	Cryptosporidium, Echinococcus

* * *

Protecting Yourself Going Forward

After your cleanse, this knowledge becomes your shield. The parasites that came in once can come in again, through the same doors that were open to them before. Closing the doors does not require an obsessive lifestyle. It requires attention to a few specific habits.

The simplest and most effective protective habits:

• Filter all drinking water. Standard carbon filters remove most parasites; reverse osmosis removes all of them.

• Wash all produce thoroughly. Soak in filtered water with apple cider vinegar for 10 minutes before consumption.

• Cook meat and fish thoroughly. Internal temperature matters. Use a thermometer until you know what done looks like.

• Wash hands consistently — particularly before eating and after outdoor contact.

• Wear shoes outdoors, especially in warm moist climates.

• Be cautious with raw fish. Know the source and the freezing protocol. Restaurants required to use commercially flash-frozen fish are safer than informal sources.

• Travel awareness. Water and produce vigilance increases significantly when abroad. The local immune systems of residents are not your immune system.

• Quarterly herbal maintenance, as covered in Chapter 32, catches any new exposure before it can establish.Chapter 33Chapter 33

Knowledge closes the doors that ignorance leaves open. You now know every road they travel. You know how to close every one of them. The chapter that follows traces what happens once the doors have been crossed — the lifecycles of these organisms once they have arrived, and the long invisible work they do inside their hosts before anyone knows they are there.

*Figures referenced in this chapter: 5.1–5.36 **(online Figure Guide)*

Chapter 6

The Parasite Lifecycle

* * *

Every parasite you carry began as something almost invisible. An egg. A cyst. A microscopic larva. A speck so small that the soil or water carrying it gave no indication anything was there. From that beginning, every parasite runs a lifecycle — a sequence of stages, each with its own location in the body, its own duration, its own vulnerabilities.

Understanding that journey — from invisible beginning to fully established adult — is not just fascinating biology. It is the key to eliminating these organisms. Every herb in this protocol, every enema, every day of the fast, targets a specific stage of these lifecycles. Without understanding which stage you are reaching, the work would be guesswork.

When people attempt cleanses that fail, the reason is almost always the same. They killed the adults. They ignored the eggs. Weeks later, new adults emerge from eggs that the protocol never reached, and the infection appears to have returned. It did not return. It was never fully removed.

This chapter focuses entirely on what happens once a parasite is inside you. For how each parasite gets in — the routes, vehicles, and protective habits — see Chapter 5.

* * *

The Universal Stages

Almost every gut parasite passes through the same fundamental stages, regardless of family. Understanding these three stages is the foundation of understanding the entire protocol.

1. The egg or cyst. The most resilient stage — protected by a tough outer shell designed to survive harsh environments for extended periods. The egg is what makes parasitic infections so difficult to eliminate, because eggs are immune to most herbs and harsh conditions.

2. The larva. The developmental stage — actively growing, migrating, and maturing. Often the most vulnerable stage to herbal intervention because the larvae are metabolically active, taking in compounds from their environment as they develop.

3. The adult. The reproductive stage — the organism reaches sexual maturity and begins producing eggs, restarting the cycle.

Your protocol must address all three stages simultaneously. This is precisely why the triad of black walnut, wormwood, and clove works so effectively. Each one targets a different stage, and together they break the cycle at every point. Without all three, the cycle continues.

What follows is a parasite-by-parasite map of the lifecycle each organism runs, organized by family. The lifecycle tables are presented in landscape orientation so all six biological columns can be read side by side.

* * *

Roundworm Lifecycles

The roundworms have the most varied lifecycles of any family in this chapter. Some run their entire cycle inside one host. Some require a journey through the lungs as part of normal development. One — Strongyloides — can reproduce inside the body indefinitely without ever needing to leave.

Parasite	Egg stage	Larval path	Adult location	Adult lifespan	Eggs per day
Ascaris lumbricoides	Develops to infective inside shell in soil; survives 6 years	Hatches in small intestine, penetrates wall, travels via portal vein to liver, then bloodstream to lungs (10–14 days), coughed up, swallowed	Small intestine	1–2 years; females grow up to 13 inches	200,000
Trichuris trichiura (Whipworm)	Develops in soil over 3–6 weeks; barrel-shaped with plugs	Hatches in small intestine, migrates immediately to large intestine; no tissue migration	Cecum, embedded in intestinal lining	1–3 years	3,000–20,000
Hookworms (Ancylostoma & Necator)	Hatches in warm moist soil within 1–2 days; not infective until hatched	First-stage larvae feed on soil bacteria, develop into infective third-stage larvae in 5–10 days, penetrate skin, travel to lungs, are coughed up and swallowed	Small intestine, attached to wall via cutting plates	1–5 years; feeds on blood	10,000–30,000
Strongyloides	Eggs hatch	Two paths:	Small	Decades via	Continuous

Parasite	Egg stage	Larval path	Adult location	Adult lifespan	Eggs per day
stercoralis	inside intestine — released as larvae directly, not eggs	external (passes in feces, develops in soil, penetrates new host) OR internal autoinfection (penetrates intestinal wall directly, restarts cycle inside host)	intestine, embedded in lining; reproduces by parthenogenesis	autoinfection	
Enterobius vermicularis (Pinworm)	Laid on perianal skin; infective in 4–6 hours — the fastest of any parasite egg; survives on surfaces 3 weeks	Hatches in small intestine, migrates to colon and matures there	Colon and rectum; females migrate to perianal skin at night to lay eggs and then die	Adults only 5–13 weeks; environmental autoinfection sustains generations	Thousands per laying

Three lifecycle features in this family are worth dwelling on.

Ascaris briefly leaves the gut and then returns. The lung migration phase — ten to fourteen days during which the larvae develop in the respiratory tissue — is part of the parasite's normal development, and it is also the phase where systemic herbal absorption through the bloodstream reaches them most effectively. Cough, fever, and respiratory symptoms during a fast are sometimes the body responding to dying larvae in the lungs, not a separate illness.

Strongyloides is the parasite that breaks the rules. Most parasitic infections require external reexposure to persist — clear the current infection and the cycle is broken. Strongyloides does not need that. Its larvae develop into the infective stage inside the intestine itself, penetrate the intestinal wall or perianal skin directly, re-enter the bloodstream, travel to the lungs, get swallowed, and return to the intestine. The full cycle runs without ever leaving the body. A single exposure decades ago can still be present today, quietly reproducing, with the host never having encountered the parasite again. Immunocompromised individuals are at particular risk of overwhelming internal reinfection. This is why Strongyloides requires the most sustained herbal protocol of all the roundworms — the protocol you are running is one of the few approaches that addresses both the external and internal cycles together.

Pinworm is biologically simple but environmentally relentless. The adult lives only five to thirteen weeks — short enough that without reinfection, the population would collapse on its own. But the eggs are so contagious, and so persistent on shared surfaces, that environmental reinfection happens constantly within a household. This is why Chapter 23 is dedicated entirely to working with pinworm's peculiar lifecycle — the protocol must address the home environment, not just the host.

* * *

Tapeworm Lifecycles

The tapeworms differ from the roundworms in nearly every way. Their lifecycles always involve at least one intermediate host — an animal in which the larval stage develops before the adult can establish in a human. The adult tapeworm itself is unusual in scale: a single specimen can grow for decades, reach lengths measured in feet, and produce eggs in numbers that defy ordinary biological intuition.

Parasite	Egg stage	Intermediate host	Larval form / location	Adult location & size	Adult lifespan
Taenia saginata (Beef tapeworm)	Released in proglottid segments; survives on pasture for months	Cattle ingest eggs from contaminated grazing	Cysticerci encysted in beef muscle, dormant for years	Human small intestine; up to 25 feet, attaches via scolex	Up to 25 years
Taenia solium (Pork tapeworm)	Released in feces; resistant to most environmental conditions	Pigs ingest eggs from contaminated feed/water	Cysticerci encysted in pork muscle. (Eggs ingested directly by humans cause neurocysticercosis — see Ch 8)	Human small intestine; up to 12 feet, attaches via scolex	Up to 25 years
Diphyllobothrium latum (Fish tapeworm)	Must reach water to develop; hatches into free-swimming larvae	Two hosts: copepods (microscopic crustaceans) then freshwater fish	Plerocercoids encysted in fish muscle	Human small intestine; up to 30 feet long	Up to 20 years
Hymenolepis nana (Dwarf tapeworm)	Immediately infective; no intermediate host required	None required (direct fecal-oral transmission); beetles/fleas can serve as accessory hosts	Cysticercoid develops directly in the human intestinal wall	Human small intestine; only about 1–2 inches	Several weeks; rapid turnover

Two facts about the tapeworm lifecycle are worth carrying.

A single beef or pork tapeworm that has lived inside one human for twenty-five years has produced an almost incomprehensible number of eggs over that time — millions, year after year. This is why the clove protocol matters so deeply. The adult worm is the visible problem, but the legacy of an old tapeworm infection is eggs and cysts seeded throughout the host's tissues, and only an egg-killing herb can address them. Killing the adult does not finish the work.

The fish tapeworm has one additional and unusual capability: it actively competes for vitamin B12. The adult worm absorbs B12 from the host's intestine before the host can absorb it, which over years of infection can produce a measurable B12 deficiency — sometimes severe enough to cause neurological symptoms. A long-term B12 deficiency without obvious dietary cause is one of the older clinical signals of fish tapeworm infection.

* * *

Fluke Lifecycles

Fluke lifecycles are the most complex in human parasitology, always involving snails and often a second intermediate host. The freshwater snail is the obligatory first host for nearly every human fluke — the parasite cannot complete its development without it. Once the cercariae emerge from the snail, they either encyst on aquatic plants or penetrate fish, depending on species, before reaching the human consumer. Inside the human, fluke adults take up residence not in the gut itself but in the bile ducts of the liver, where they are particularly difficult for herbs alone to reach.

Parasite	Egg & first developmen t	First intermediate host	Second intermediat e host / vehicle	Migration into human	Adult location & lifespan
Fasciolopsis buski (Giant intestinal fluke)	Eggs into water, hatch into miracidia in 3–7 weeks	Freshwater snails (development inside takes weeks)	Encyst on aquatic plants — water chestnut, lotus root, water bamboo	Excysts in small intestine; remains in intestinal lumen (no liver migration)	Small intestine; lives 2–3 years
Fasciola hepatica (Liver fluke)	Eggs into water, hatch into miracidia in 2–4 weeks (must find snail within hours)	Freshwater snails (6–8 weeks of development inside)	Encyst on aquatic vegetation — watercress is the primary vehicle	Larvae penetrate intestinal wall, migrate through abdominal cavity, burrow through liver tissue itself, then enter bile ducts	Bile ducts; lives 9–13 years
Clonorchis sinensis (Chinese liver fluke)	Eggs into water, hatch into miracidia in 1–2 weeks	Freshwater snails (several weeks of development)	Encyst as metacercariae in freshwater fish — carp, bream, roach	Migrates through common bile duct into liver biliary system (no tissue burrowing)	Bile ducts; up to 30 years
Heterophyes heterophyes	Eggs into water, hatch	Snails in saltwater or	Encyst in saltwater/bra	Excysts in small	Small intestine; lives about 1

Parasite	Egg & first developmen t	First intermediate host	Second intermediat e host / vehicle	Migration into human	Adult location & lifespan
	in 1–2 weeks	brackish-water environments	ckish-water fish — mullet, tilapia	intestine; remains in intestinal lumen	year

Two lifecycle features in this family deserve particular attention.

Fasciola hepatica's migration through liver tissue is what makes it uniquely damaging. By the time the adult is established in the bile duct, it has already left a trail of damage through the liver itself — inflammation, scarring, sometimes hemorrhage. The damage of this fluke is not only the chronic presence of an adult organism in the bile system but the migration that put it there. This is why Fasciola, more than any other fluke, demands the support of the coffee enema as part of the protocol — the herbs alone cannot reach the parasite efficiently while it is migrating, and the bile-flushing action of the enema is what makes the difference.

Clonorchis sinensis, the Chinese liver fluke, takes a different path — it migrates through the common bile duct rather than through liver tissue, so the acute damage is less. But its unusual lifespan of up to thirty years means cumulative damage over decades. Chronic Clonorchis infection is associated with cholangiocarcinoma — cancer of the bile duct — in regions where it is endemic. The slow burn over many years is what does the harm.

* * *

Protozoa Lifecycles

Protozoa lifecycles differ fundamentally from worms. They reproduce by cellular division rather than by laying eggs. A single protozoan that establishes itself in a host can become a population of millions within days. There is no larva, no adult, no maturation in the way the worms have it — there is only the resilient cyst stage that survives outside the host, and the active dividing form that lives inside.

Parasite	Cyst / oocyst stage	Active form	Reproduction inside host	Division speed	Distinguishing feature
Giardia lamblia	Infective and environmentally resistant; survives cold water for months	Trophozoite — attaches to intestinal villi using a ventral disc, like a suction cup	Binary fission (one cell splits into two); some trophozoites transform back into cysts and pass in feces	Every 8–12 hours	As few as 10 cysts can establish infection
Entamoeba histolytica	Four-nucleus cyst; survives in environment for weeks	Trophozoite — may live non-invasively in the lumen, OR penetrate the intestinal wall and enter bloodstream	Binary fission within the host; two distinct behavioral states	Rapid (hours)	Invasive form can travel to liver, lungs, brain
Cryptosporidium parvum	Oocyst; immediately infective; resistant to chlorine at standard treatment levels	Sporozoites — invade intestinal lining cells and reproduce inside them	Asexual reproduction inside host cells; produces both thin-walled (internal reinfection) and thick-walled (passes in feces) oocysts	Extremely rapid intracellular	As few as 10 oocysts establish infection; internal reinfection cycle
Blastocystis hominis	Multiple morphological forms including cyst-like;	Vacuolar form — lives in the colon, often without obvious	Binary fission; multiple morphological forms make	Every 12 hours	One of the most prevalent gut parasites in developed

Parasite	Cyst / oocyst stage	Active form	Reproduction inside host	Division speed	Distinguishing feature
	survives outside host	symptoms	study difficult		countries
Dientamoeba fragilis	Recently confirmed cyst form; previously thought to lack one	Trophozoite — lives in the colon	Binary fission; transmission still partly being studied	Moderate	May travel inside pinworm eggs as a protected passenger

Three protozoa-specific points are worth noting.

Giardia's infectious dose is shockingly small. As few as ten cysts can establish a clinical infection. This is part of why Giardia is so common despite its simple-looking lifecycle — a tiny amount of contaminated water, drunk once, is enough.

Entamoeba histolytica's two behavioral states are one of the more puzzling features of human parasitology. The same organism, with the same genetics, can live as a non-invasive lumen-dweller causing minimal symptoms in one host — and as a tissue-invading destroyer in another. The factors that determine which state it takes are not fully understood. The same organism can shift between both states depending on host immune status and other unknown factors.

Cryptosporidium has its own version of the autoinfection cycle that makes Strongyloides so persistent. Some of the oocysts produced inside the host are thin-walled rather than thick-walled — these excyst immediately and reinfect the same host without ever leaving the body. This internal reinfection cycle is why Cryptosporidium can be particularly difficult to clear, even when the source of original exposure has long since been removed.

* * *

The Complete Lifecycle Comparison

For quick reference, the parasites organized by their reproductive parameters and most vulnerable stage. This is the table to consult when running the protocol — the "most vulnerable stage" column tells you which protocol element is doing the work for that parasite.

Parasite	Family	Egg/cyst to infective	Adult lifespan	Reproductive output	Most vulnerable stage
Ascaris lumbricoides	Roundworm	2–3 weeks in soil	1–2 years	200,000 eggs/day	Larvae during lung migration
Trichuris trichiura (Whipworm)	Roundworm	3–6 weeks in soil	1–3 years	3,000–20,000 eggs/day	Larvae in intestine
Hookworms	Roundworm	5–10 days in soil	1–5 years	10,000–30,000 eggs/day	Larvae penetrating skin
Strongyloides stercoralis	Roundworm	Hours	Decades via autoinfection	Continuous	Larvae in intestine
Pinworm (Enterobius)	Roundworm	4–6 hours — fastest of any	5–13 weeks	Thousands per laying	Eggs on surfaces
Anisakis (fish worm)	Roundworm	Cannot mature in humans	3–4 weeks (does not establish)	None in humans	Larvae in fish flesh
Beef tapeworm (T. saginata)	Tapeworm	Immediately infective in muscle	Up to 25 years	Millions over lifetime	Cysticerci in meat
Pork tapeworm (T. solium)	Tapeworm	Immediately infective in muscle (or as eggs directly)	Up to 25 years	Millions over lifetime	Cysticerci in meat / eggs
Fish tapeworm (Diphyllobothrium)	Tapeworm	Weeks in water, then in fish	Up to 20 years	Millions over lifetime	Plerocercoid in fish
Dwarf tapeworm (Hymenolepis nana)	Tapeworm	Immediately infective	Several weeks	Continuous fecal-oral cycle	Eggs in environment
Intestinal fluke (Fasciolopsis)	Fluke	3–7 weeks (egg + snail)	2–3 years	Thousands of eggs	Metacercaria on plants
Liver fluke (Fasciola hepatica)	Fluke	8–12 weeks (egg + snail)	9–13 years	Thousands of eggs	Metacercaria on plants
Chinese liver fluke (Clonorchis)	Fluke	Several weeks (egg + snail)	Up to 30 years	Thousands of eggs	Metacercaria in fish

Parasite	Family	Egg/cyst to infective	Adult lifespan	Reproductive output	Most vulnerable stage
Heterophyes	Fluke	5–7 weeks (egg + snail)	About 1 year	Thousands of eggs	Metacercaria in fish
Giardia lamblia	Protozoan	Immediate	Continuous division	Millions of cysts	Trophozoite in intestine
Entamoeba histolytica	Protozoan	Immediate	Continuous division	Millions of cysts	Trophozoite in intestine
Cryptosporidium parvum	Protozoan	Immediate	Continuous division	Millions of oocysts	Sporozoite in cell

* * *

Why Your Protocol Is Designed the Way It Is

Every element of what you are doing maps directly onto this lifecycle knowledge. Once the cycles above become familiar, the design of the protocol stops looking arbitrary and starts looking inevitable.

• Fasting — removes the food source that sustains adult organisms and the conditions that protect biofilm communities.

• Wormwood — targets larvae and juvenile organisms.

• Black walnut — targets adult organisms.

• Clove — targets eggs and cysts, the stage everything else misses.

• Enemas — physically expel dead and dying organisms at every stage.

• Coffee enemas — flush bile ducts where fluke adults and eggs accumulate.

• Daily consistency — maintains lethal conditions through multiple complete lifecycle rotations.

You are not randomly attacking parasites. You are systematically dismantling their lifecycle — stage by stage, week after week — until there is nothing left to restart the cycle.

What you have learned in this chapter is not just biology. It is the architectural blueprint of the work you are doing. Every herb, every enema, every consistent day of the protocol has its place in the design. The chapters that follow describe what these organisms do to you over time — the symptoms, the damage, the long invisible cost of carrying them — and then turn to the protocol itself.

*Figures referenced in this chapter: 6.1–6.32 **(online Figure Guide)*

Chapter 7

What They Do To You

* * *

You have met them. You know where they came from. You know how they got in. Now it is time to understand what they have actually been doing while they were there.

What follows is not meant to alarm. It is meant to make plain why the transformation that follows a deep cleanse can feel as marked as people describe it. When you understand what was being taken from you over the years, you begin to understand why getting it back can feel like recovering a self you had not known you had lost.

The damage these organisms do is rarely dramatic. It is rarely the kind of thing that produces a moment of clear diagnosis, a single symptom that points to a single cause. It is, instead, accumulated. Erosion rather than catastrophe. Year after year, a small daily theft of nutrients, a small daily inflammation, a small daily disruption of the conversation between gut and brain. The damage is the new normal in the bodies of the people who carry these organisms, which is to say, the new normal in most of the human population.

The absence of dramatic symptoms does not mean the absence of damage. It means the damage has become invisible to the person living inside it.

What the Roundworms Take

Ascaris does not attack the tissue of your intestine. It does not feed on blood. It simply lives where you absorb your food, and it intercepts that food before your body can claim it. A heavy *Ascaris* infection — a hundred worms or more, which is common in regions where contamination is heavy — can cause meaningful caloric malnutrition in a person eating a perfectly adequate diet. The food enters. The food is partly digested. And then a third of the nutrients, perhaps more, are absorbed by the worms instead of by the host.

The most consequential nutritional theft is of vitamin A, which the worms consume in disproportionate quantity. Vitamin A is required for vision, for immune function, for the integrity of every epithelial surface in the body. Children with heavy *Ascaris* loads in regions of the world where reinfection is constant develop characteristic vitamin A deficiency that affects their growth, their resistance to infection, sometimes their eyesight. The protein deficit follows close behind: the worms take their share of dietary protein, and the host, especially if a child, develops the muscle wasting and immune compromise that chronic protein insufficiency produces. None of this is dramatic. All of it is real.

In addition to the daily theft, *Ascaris* can produce mechanical trouble. A heavy infection can tangle into a mass that physically obstructs the small intestine, and in children with severe loads this is sometimes life-threatening. The worms can migrate into the bile duct or the pancreatic duct and lodge there, producing pain that surgeons sometimes mistake for gallstones until they look inside and find what is actually there. The lung migration phase can produce respiratory symptoms — cough, fever, wheezing — that are routinely misdiagnosed as asthma or bronchitis. A child whose persistent cough resists every treatment may be carrying a population of larvae moving through the alveoli, and the child's pediatrician may never know.

The whipworm, *Trichuris trichiura*, does its work differently. It lives in the wall of the large intestine, with its long thin front end embedded in the tissue, and it feeds on tissue secretions and blood at the point of attachment. Each whipworm is a tiny chronic wound. The wounds inflame the surrounding tissue. The inflammation produces local damage to the intestinal lining's ability to absorb water and nutrients properly, which is why heavy whipworm infections can produce diarrhea that resists every dietary intervention. In severe cases the rectum prolapses — protrudes outside the body — from the chronic inflammation and straining. This last presentation is uncommon in adults but is sadly common in children in regions of heavy infection. The children, often, look perfectly healthy at a casual glance. The damage is internal and the consequences are slow.

Hookworms drink blood directly. Each adult worm consumes a small but consistent amount of blood every day, and a heavy hookworm load — a hundred worms, two hundred — produces measurable anemia from cumulative blood loss alone. The anemia is iron-deficient. It produces fatigue and weakness that build over months and years until the person carrying the infection cannot remember when they last felt fully energetic. In children, the anemia is more devastating still: it impairs cognitive development in ways that may not fully recover even after the parasites are eliminated. The global burden of hookworm on human development is, by some measures, one of the most significant of any parasitic disease — a quiet drag on the intellectual potential of entire populations.

There is, additionally, the skin damage where the larvae enter. The intense itching at the site of penetration is called, in the older medical literature, ground itch, and it is the body announcing that something has just bored through it. The track of the migrating larva sometimes shows visibly under the skin — a winding red line that moves over the course of days, called cutaneous larva migrans. The track is the parasite's path through the dermis, not yet finished with its journey to the gut.

Strongyloides does its work over decades. The autoinfection cycle of this parasite — its capacity to complete its lifecycle inside one host without ever leaving the body — means that an infection acquired in childhood can persist into old age. The damage in the immunocompetent host is often subtle: chronic villous atrophy where the worms embed, intermittent skin rash from larval migration, mild digestive irregularity, occasional respiratory symptoms when larvae move through the lungs. The carrier feels, generally, fine. Or rather — the carrier has felt this way for so long that they take it as their baseline.

The danger of *Strongyloides* arrives if the immune system is later suppressed. A course of corticosteroids for an unrelated condition, an organ transplant requiring immunosuppression, a chemotherapy regimen for a cancer — any of these can collapse the equilibrium that has held the parasite in check, and the autoinfection accelerates dramatically. In the worst cases, the parasite disseminates throughout the body, carrying gut bacteria into the bloodstream, producing sepsis that can be fatal. The original infection, decades old, suddenly becomes the dominant medical event of the patient's life. Cases like this are rare but documented, and they are the reason any patient about to begin immunosuppressive therapy in regions where *Strongyloides* exists should be screened first.

Pinworms, the most common parasite in the developed world, rarely cause serious physical damage. What they take is sleep. The female pinworms migrate to the perianal skin at night to lay eggs, and the host, often a child, wakes scratching, rolls over, scratches again, dozes, scratches more. The chronic sleep disruption in heavily infected children produces behavioral effects — irritability, poor concentration, learning difficulties — that are routinely misattributed to other causes. In adults the same disruption produces the kind of low-grade chronic fatigue that becomes simply how a person feels. They do not connect it to the cause. They never knew there was a cause.

In rare cases — uncommon enough that pediatricians may go a career without seeing it — pinworms migrate into the female reproductive tract, producing pelvic pain and discharge that is often misdiagnosed before someone identifies the actual organism. The psychological impact of pinworm infection, particularly in adults who discover it, is often greater than the physical impact. Shame is a common response, and shame delays treatment. All of this is treated more fully in the longer account of pinworms.

What the Tapeworms Take

A twenty-five-foot tapeworm living inside your small intestine for twenty-five years, producing hundreds of millions of eggs across its lifetime, consuming your nutrients every day — and often producing no symptoms whatsoever. This is perhaps the most striking biological reality in any of the parasites described here. The body adapts. The parasite is so well co-evolved with its host that it takes only what the host can spare without obvious distress. The host carries the worm and does not know.

What is taken nonetheless is real. Continuous nutrient competition. Daily theft of proteins and fats and carbohydrates that the host's body would otherwise have absorbed. The fish tapeworm, *Diphyllobothrium latum*, deserves a particular mention here for its specific dietary habit: it consumes vitamin B12 directly from the host's small intestine, in such quantity that long-term infection produces severe and characteristic B12 deficiency. The deficiency manifests as fatigue and memory problems and the numbness and tingling in the extremities that characterize subacute combined degeneration of the spinal cord. The diagnosis is sometimes made backward, from a megaloblastic anemia of unclear origin in a person who has eaten raw fish regularly for years, and the treating physician thinks at last to ask the right question.

Beyond the daily nutritional theft, tapeworms can produce mechanical trouble in heavy infections. Intestinal obstruction. Abdominal discomfort. Nausea. Weight loss despite adequate food intake. Some people first discover their infection by seeing a segment of the worm in their stool — a flat, rice-like piece, sometimes still moving — and the discovery is, by every account, unforgettable. The psychological response can persist for years afterward. People who have seen a tapeworm segment in themselves speak of it the way people speak of car accidents. The image stays.

The pork tapeworm, *Taenia solium*, requires its own consideration. The adult worm in the gut is not the most consequential aspect of *T. solium* infection. The danger lies in cysticercosis — the migration of the larvae, when eggs of the worm are swallowed, into the body's tissues, and especially into the brain. Once a cyst forms in brain tissue, it can sit there for years, sometimes for decades, sometimes producing no symptom until it doesn't. The first sign is often a seizure. *T. solium* is, by some estimates, the leading infectious cause of acquired epilepsy worldwide. The brain implications of certain parasites — and the limits of any cleansing protocol that does not involve a hospital — deserve their own treatment, given separately. For now, you need only know that the pork tapeworm can do something the other tapeworms cannot, and it is the reason undercooked pork has been forbidden in so many cultures across so many centuries.

What the Flukes Take

The intestinal flukes attach to the wall of the small intestine and live there for years. Each attachment site is a small chronic wound. Each wound inflames. Each inflammation reduces, in its small way, the absorptive function of the segment of intestine that should have been doing its quiet work of taking in nutrients. Heavy infections produce mechanical irritation, intestinal obstruction in some cases, the chronic diarrhea and abdominal pain that accompany any condition in which the intestinal lining cannot recover faster than it is being injured. In the heaviest *Fasciolopsis* infections, the toxic metabolic products of the flukes are absorbed into the bloodstream in sufficient quantity to produce facial edema and other systemic effects — the body responding to the burden of carrying so much foreign tissue inside it.

The liver flukes are different. *Fasciola hepatica* and *Clonorchis sinensis* live not in the gut at all but in the bile ducts, the small tubes that carry bile from the liver to the intestine. They take up residence there and remain, sometimes for decades. *Fasciola* lives nine to thirteen years inside the host. *Clonorchis* has been documented to live thirty.

The damage they do is the slow architectural damage of decades of irritation. Adult flukes living in bile ducts cause chronic inflammation. The walls of the ducts thicken. They scar. Bile flow becomes impeded. Stones form in the gallbladder and within the ducts themselves. In heavy infections, the obstruction is severe enough to produce jaundice. The liver tissue, which has been handling the toxic byproducts of fluke metabolism continuously since the parasites first arrived, becomes progressively fibrotic. *Fasciola* migration through liver tissue — the journey the larvae take from the small intestine, through the abdominal cavity, into the liver itself — leaves tracks of necrotic damage that persist as scarring even after the flukes have moved into the bile ducts.

Long-term *Clonorchis* infection is associated with cholangiocarcinoma — bile duct cancer. The World Health Organization classifies the parasite as a carcinogen. Chronic inflammation of bile duct epithelium, sustained over decades, produces cellular changes that can become malignant. This is not theoretical. In regions where *Clonorchis* is endemic, bile duct cancer is far more common than it is in regions where the parasite is absent.

What this means for the person carrying liver flukes — usually without knowing — is that the liver, the body's central organ of detoxification, has been working under a chronic burden for as long as the flukes have been there. Everything the liver should be doing — clearing pharmaceutical metabolites, processing hormones, neutralizing environmental toxins, regulating cholesterol — has been done at a fraction of its full capacity. Energy that should have been available for these tasks has been spent instead on managing the chronic insult of the flukes.

The connection to the coffee enema protocol described in these pages is direct. Coffee enemas stimulate bile flow. They cause bile duct contraction. They are one of the few interventions that physically reach the location where liver flukes live. The green sludge that appears in the morning enema returns during a deep cleanse is not, simply, bile. It is decades of accumulated material being moved out of bile ducts that have been functioning under burden for as long as the host can remember. People are sometimes alarmed by what they see. They should not be. They are seeing what was, finally, being released.

What the Protozoa Take

Giardia does not invade tissue. It does not consume blood. It does something simpler and, in some ways, more devastating: it covers the surface of the small intestine like a carpet of clinging cells, and it prevents that surface from doing its work. Where *Giardia* attaches, nutrient absorption fails.

The villi, under the chronic mechanical pressure of *Giardia* coverage, flatten. The brush border enzymes that complete the digestion of food at the intestinal surface are disrupted. Fat malabsorption produces the fatty, foul-smelling stools that characterize *Giardia* infection. Lactose intolerance often develops or worsens. Vitamin B12 absorption fails. The small intestine, which had been doing the work of harvesting nutrients from food, becomes a passage that food moves through without yielding what it should.

The acute symptoms of *Giardia* infection — the explosive watery diarrhea, the bloating, the cramping — are well-known. What is less well-known is what *Giardia* leaves behind. Up to forty percent of people who have had a *Giardia* infection develop post-infectious irritable bowel syndrome, in which the gut continues to malfunction for months or years after the parasite itself has been cleared. The microbiome, disrupted by the infection, takes a long time to recover. The intestinal lining, damaged by the chronic mechanical pressure of the *Giardia* coverage, takes longer still. This is one of the reasons that rebuilding the microbiome after a deep cleanse is so important. The protocol does not end when the organisms are gone. It ends when the surfaces they damaged have healed.

Entamoeba histolytica does something different. The species name *histolytica* means "tissue-dissolving," and it is precise. The parasite secretes enzymes that dissolve the cells of the intestinal lining, and it consumes the dissolved tissue. The characteristic flask-shaped ulcers it leaves in the colon wall are visible in pathology specimens and are the clinical signature of invasive amebic infection. In severe cases the ulcers perforate the intestinal wall, and the parasites enter the bloodstream and travel to the liver, where they form abscesses — pockets of liquefied tissue that, on ultrasound, appear as dark voids in the body of the organ. From the liver they can spread to the lungs, occasionally to the brain.

In its non-invasive form, even *Entamoeba* causes persistent disruption — chronic low-grade intestinal inflammation, altered intestinal permeability, ongoing immune activation. It is one of the parasites whose effects can persist as a low chronic burden for years before the carrier seeks medical attention or, in many cases, before they ever notice that anything is wrong.

Cryptosporidium lives inside intestinal cells. It is a true intracellular parasite. It invades, reproduces, and bursts out to infect neighboring cells, leaving cellular destruction in its wake. In healthy adults, the infection is usually self-limiting — a week or two of profuse watery diarrhea, then resolution — but the damage to the intestinal lining persists after the organism is cleared. In immunocompromised individuals the infection can be devastating; in some untreated AIDS patients before the era of effective antiretroviral therapy, *Cryptosporidium* infections produced diarrhea of up to twenty liters per day, and people died of dehydration that no oral rehydration could keep pace with. The chlorine resistance of *Crypto* — its capacity to survive municipal water treatment — has made it the cause of large-scale waterborne outbreaks in cities across the developed world.

The Cumulative Picture

A single parasite alone might cause subtle effects. Two might compound. Multiple parasites across multiple families, carried for years and decades — and this is the situation of an enormous fraction of the human population — produce a body running at a fraction of its potential.

Consider what is happening, all at once, in such a body. The small intestine's absorptive surface is reduced by *Giardia* attachment in some areas, by *Strongyloides* villous atrophy in others, by tapeworm nutrient competition in still others. The large intestine carries the chronic inflammation of whipworm attachment sites and the small ulcerations of *Entamoeba* feeding. The bile ducts have been narrowing for a decade or two under fluke residence, their flow impaired. The liver has been carrying the toxic burden of fluke metabolism on top of every other detoxification it should have been doing. The microbiome has lost diversity from the chronic disruption of multiple parasites competing with the beneficial bacteria for resources. The immune system has been running, at low level, against all of these threats simultaneously, depleting the resources that should have been available for other defenses.

And the person living inside this body has felt — what? A chronic fatigue that has been there as long as they can remember. Digestion that has never quite been right. A mental clarity that arrives sometimes and recedes. A sleep that does not always restore. A skin that flares for reasons their dermatologist cannot explain. A mood that fluctuates more than they would like. They have come to think of this as their personality, their constitution, their normal. They have been told, perhaps, that they have irritable bowel syndrome, or fibromyalgia, or chronic fatigue syndrome, or some other diagnosis that names the cluster of symptoms without identifying the cause.

When the parasites are cleared — and the lining heals, and the microbiome rebalances, and the bile flows freely again, and the immune system can finally rest from a vigilance it had been holding for years — what returns is not a different person. It is the person who was always there underneath. The transformation that those who have done prolonged fasts describe in nearly mystical terms is, at its biological foundation, the lifting of a burden the carrier did not know they had been bearing.

Clarity they have never experienced. Energy that feels different in quality, not just quantity. Emotional stability that surprises them. A lightness that goes beyond the physical. None of this is mysterious. It is what a body without parasitic load feels like. Most people in the modern world have never felt it.

What has been described here is the cost of carrying these organisms. What follows is the work of setting them down.

*Figures referenced above: 7.1–7.16 **(online Figure Guide)*

Chapter 8

What This Protocol Cannot Reach

* * *

Before we go any further into the work of cleansing, there is something you need to understand. Something that must be said clearly, without softening, without ambiguity.

This protocol is designed for your gut. It is not designed for your brain. And the difference between those two things — between what lives in your intestines and what may live behind the bone of your skull — is the difference between work you can do at home, with herbs and water, and work that belongs in a hospital, with imaging and physicians and pharmaceutical antiparasitics. This chapter exists because that distinction matters more than almost anything else in this book.

The world of natural healing makes promises it cannot always keep. You have probably read claims that prolonged fasting clears brain parasites. You have probably read claims that clove tincture penetrates the blood-brain barrier and destroys cysts. You have probably read testimonials from people who say their headaches stopped, their fog lifted, their seizures resolved, all of it attributed to herbal cleansing. Some of those stories may be true. Some may be coincidence — symptoms resolving from other causes during the same period in which the cleanse happened. Some may be misattribution — gut work creating a systemic improvement that gets credited to brain clearance that never happened. And some, particularly the seizure stories, may describe people who got dangerously lucky.

The honest answer is that we do not know which is which. What we do know is that the medical literature on parasitic brain infections is clear, well-documented, and very different from what natural healing communities sometimes suggest. This chapter is here to make sure you understand that difference before you continue.

Which Parasites Reach the Brain

Most of the parasites discussed in this book live in the gut. They never see the brain. But some can reach it, and the ones that can deserve specific attention. The four most consequential are these:

• **Taenia solium** (the pork tapeworm, larval stage). When the eggs of *T. solium* are swallowed by a human, the larvae hatch in the small intestine and migrate through the bloodstream into the body's tissues — including the brain, where they form cysts. The condition is called neurocysticercosis. It is the leading infectious cause of acquired epilepsy in many parts of the world, documented across every continent including the United States. Confirmed cases happen in major American cities every year.

• **Toxoplasma gondii**. The protozoan most often acquired from cat feces or undercooked meat. It crosses the blood-brain barrier easily and forms tissue cysts that can persist for the rest of the host's life. Most people who carry it carry it without symptom, but in immunocompromised individuals the infection can reactivate. Estimates of human seroprevalence run from twenty percent in the United States to as high as eighty percent in some other countries.

• **Strongyloides stercoralis**, in disseminated hyperinfection cases, can carry larvae into the central nervous system. The cases are uncommon, but they occur, particularly in immunocompromised hosts.

• **Angiostrongylus cantonensis** (the rat lungworm). Causes eosinophilic meningitis. Acquired through contaminated produce or undercooked snails and slugs. Cases are increasingly reported in the southern United States and Hawaii.

These are not exotic conditions one reads about in tropical medicine textbooks. They are documented in regular medical practice. They are diagnosed and treated by physicians in major cities every year. The question, for any reader of this book, is not whether brain parasites exist. The question is whether the protocol you are about to undertake can address them.

What This Protocol Reaches

Let us be precise about what the herbs in this book actually do. The clove, black walnut, wormwood, berberine, oregano oil, mimosa pudica, and supporting herbs and extracts work primarily through the digestive tract and through systemic circulation after absorption.

What they reach reliably:

• The full length of the intestinal tract, directly.

• The bile ducts, through the morning coffee enema and through orally absorbed compounds.

• The liver tissue, through portal circulation.

• The bloodstream throughout the body.

• Migrating larvae moving through tissue in transit.

• Recently active organisms in muscle, in lung, in other peripheral tissues.

What they do not reach reliably:

• Mature parasitic cysts already established beyond the blood-brain barrier.

• Walled cysts of *Taenia solium* in brain tissue, which the parasite has constructed for long-term survival.

• Latent *Toxoplasma* cysts in brain parenchyma, which persist in a metabolically dormant state that even pharmaceutical antiparasitics struggle to penetrate.

• Calcified parasite remnants in brain tissue, which cannot be cleared by any protocol because they are no longer biologically active.

The blood-brain barrier exists for a reason. It evolved to keep things out of the brain — including, unfortunately, many of the compounds we might want to send in. Eugenol from clove does cross the blood-brain barrier in small amounts. Some compounds from black walnut and wormwood reach central nervous system tissue. But reaching therapeutic concentrations inside a mature parasite cyst — sealed within its own protective wall, embedded in nervous tissue — is a different problem entirely. Pharmaceutical antiparasitics designed specifically for this purpose, at high doses, with corticosteroid coverage, under hospital monitoring, sometimes fail to fully clear neurocysticercosis. Herbs at typical doses essentially do not. This is not a criticism of the herbs. It is a recognition of their actual capabilities and limitations.

Why This Matters Most

Here is the part that requires the most direct statement.

Killing parasites in the brain is dangerous in a way that killing them in the gut is not. When a parasite dies inside your intestine, its body is carried out through the digestive tract, mostly without you ever noticing. When a parasite dies inside brain tissue, something very different happens. The dying organism releases cellular contents into the surrounding tissue. The immune system mobilizes intensely against this debris. Local inflammation spikes. Blood vessels dilate. Tissue swells.

Your brain has no room to swell. It is surrounded by the bone of your skull. There is nowhere for the inflammation to go. Pressure rises inside the cranium, and what can follow is a cascade of consequences: seizures, severe headaches that do not respond to standard treatment, increased intracranial pressure, focal neurological deficits, stroke. In severe cases, death.

This is why hospital treatment of confirmed neurocysticercosis always includes corticosteroids alongside the antiparasitic medication — to control the inflammatory response from the dying parasites. People do not die from the parasites in their brain. They die from what happens when the parasites die.

If you have undiagnosed neurocysticercosis, and any portion of your protocol partially penetrates a brain cyst — enough to damage the larva, enough to trigger immune response — you could trigger exactly the inflammatory cascade that hospital protocols are designed to prevent. Without imaging to know what is actually in your brain. Without medical monitoring to catch trouble early. Without corticosteroids ready to suppress the inflammation. Without anti-seizure medication on hand if something goes wrong. This is not a target for self-directed treatment. This is, simply, a thing that should not be attempted at home.

Who Should Pause

The risk factors for parasitic brain infection are specific and identifiable. Most readers of this book do not have them. Some readers do. The latter group needs to know who they are before continuing.

Dietary history risk factors:

• Eating undercooked or raw pork at any point in life, in any country.

• Eating street food in regions where neurocysticercosis is endemic — Latin America, sub-Saharan Africa, parts of Asia, parts of Eastern Europe.

• Growing up in or having lived in such regions.

• Consuming unwashed produce that may have come into contact with pig feces.

Travel and occupational history risk factors:

• Extended time in endemic regions.

• Time spent in agricultural settings with poor sanitation, especially farms where pigs are kept.

• Work with pigs or in pork processing.

• Healthcare or laboratory work involving parasitic specimens.

Symptom risk factors (any of these warrant evaluation):

• Unexplained seizures, even brief, even years ago, even attributed at the time to some other cause.

• Severe headaches that come and go without clear pattern.

• Focal neurological symptoms — numbness, weakness, vision changes, balance issues.

• Episodes of confusion or mental status changes that resolved.

• Persistent unexplained vision changes.

Medical history risk factors that raise the stakes:

• Immunocompromised status from HIV, organ transplantation, immunosuppressive medication, or chemotherapy.

• Family members with documented parasitic brain infections (suggesting shared exposure).

• Previous diagnosis of any brain cyst or lesion of unclear origin.

Any one of these factors warrants medical evaluation before assuming this protocol is appropriate. Not all of them. **Any one.**

What Medical Evaluation Looks Like

If any of the above applies to you, the workup is well-established. A primary care physician can order most of it. An infectious disease specialist or neurologist will interpret the results.

The standard evaluation includes:

• **Brain MRI with gadolinium contrast.** The gold standard for identifying neurocysticercosis at any stage — active cysts, transitional cysts, calcified remnants. It can identify other brain parasitic conditions as well. Not invasive. Insurance often covers it when the clinical justification is reasonable.

• **EITB serology** for cysticercosis. The most reliable laboratory marker for *Taenia solium* exposure.

• **Toxoplasma IgG and IgM serology**, identifying past and current toxoplasmosis.

• **Strongyloides antibody testing**, where exposure history suggests it.

• **Eosinophil count** on a routine blood test, which can suggest tissue parasitism when elevated.

If something is found, treatment moves to specialists with experience in parasitic disease. Hospital-based protocols, with corticosteroid coverage and seizure prophylaxis, are the standard of care. The treatment is well-developed and, in most cases, effective. What is not effective, and what can be dangerous, is attempting to address brain parasites with herbs alone outside of medical supervision.

What This Protocol Is, and What It Is Not

The protocol in this book is a comprehensive cleansing system for the digestive tract. It is a method for clearing intestinal parasites and their eggs. It is a framework for liver and bile duct cleansing. It is a practice for restoring intestinal lining and microbiome. It is a path through prolonged water fasting with appropriate physiological support.

The protocol is not a treatment for confirmed parasitic brain infections. It is not a substitute for medical evaluation when brain involvement is suspected. It is not a replacement for hospital-based treatment of neurocysticercosis. It is not a way to address *Toxoplasma* cysts that have crossed into brain tissue. It is not a solution for any condition involving the central nervous system.

If you suspect brain involvement, your path is medical, not herbal. The same wisdom and caution that guides every part of this work also requires recognizing where its limits are.

A Conversation This Chapter Asks You to Have

If you have any of the risk factors described above and have not yet talked to a doctor about them, you need to.

The resistance to this is understandable. Many readers come to this book partly because conventional medicine has not served them well. The medical establishment can feel cold. It can feel dismissive of patient concerns that do not fit established diagnostic categories. It can feel oriented toward prescriptions rather than root causes. The impulse to handle one's own healing, after years of feeling unheard by physicians, is a real and reasonable impulse.

That impulse has limits. For confirmed parasitic brain infections, modern medicine has tools that traditional medicine does not have — imaging that can see what no herbalist or naturopath can see, pharmaceutical antiparasitics with proven efficacy against brain cysts, corticosteroids that prevent the inflammatory cascade from killing the patient, anti-seizure medication ready in case something goes wrong. This is one of the few places in this work where conventional medicine genuinely outperforms alternative approaches, and refusing the help that is on offer in such a case is not principled. It is, at best, a misunderstanding of where each tool belongs.

Going to a doctor about possible neurocysticercosis is not a betrayal of natural healing principles. It is the recognition that different problems require different tools. You can do every other part of this protocol with confidence and self-direction. You can heal your gut. You can clear your flukes. You can rebuild your microbiome. You can, in time, guide others through the same work. You can also recognize that one specific situation — possible parasitic brain involvement — sits outside the scope of what should be attempted without medical support. That recognition is wisdom, not weakness.

What to Do Right Now

If you are reading this and any of the warning categories above apply to you, the path is straightforward:

1. Schedule an appointment with your primary care physician before you begin the antiparasitic intensification of the fast.

2. Tell the physician about your dietary, travel, and exposure history. Tell them you are planning a prolonged fast with antiparasitic herbs.

3. Ask whether neurocysticercosis or other parasitic brain conditions should be ruled out first.

4. Request brain imaging with contrast if any risk factor exists. The MRI is the appropriate study.

5. Get baseline serological testing — cysticercosis antibody panel, *Toxoplasma* IgG and IgM, eosinophil count.

6. Wait for the results before beginning the antiparasitic intensification.

You can still do preparatory work during this period. You can adjust your diet. You can begin gentle hydration practices using water treated with ionic sulfated minerals. The aggressive antiparasitic phase should wait until brain involvement has been ruled out.

If something is found, work with specialists. Treatment of brain parasites belongs in a hospital setting, with experienced physicians, under careful monitoring. Once the brain situation is properly addressed under medical supervision, you may be able to return to the gut work later. The protocol in this book is not going anywhere.

If you have already started the protocol and now realize that a risk factor applies to you, pause the antiparasitic intensification. Continue gentle hydration with water treated with ionic sulfated minerals, and other mineral support. Schedule medical evaluation immediately. Do not stop reading this book — the gut work may still be appropriate for you, but only after the brain question has been properly answered.

A Final Word

The vast majority of people who pick up this book do not have brain parasites. Most readers will read this chapter, recognize that none of the risk factors apply to them, and continue with the protocol confident in its appropriate use. This chapter is here for the people who do have those risk factors, and for everyone else who needs to understand the limits of what this work does.

Knowing where a tool ends is part of using it well. Knowing what your protocol can reach, and what it cannot, is part of taking the work seriously. Knowing when to ask for help is part of healing wisely.

Take care of your gut. Get medical support for your brain. Do not confuse the two. The work we do in the chapters that follow is sacred and ancient and effective for what it is designed to address. For everything else, there are other tools, other practitioners, other paths.

Use the right tool for the right job. That is the foundation of every medicine that has ever worked.

Chapter 9

The Layers Within

* * *

If you have ever seen a core sample drawn from the floor of a lake, you have seen what time looks like when it is allowed to settle undisturbed. A long cylinder of mud, banded and striped from end to end. Each band is a year, or a decade, or a century. The pale layers were dry seasons. The dark were wet. The streaks of ash mark the year a volcano two thousand miles away put fire into the upper sky. The pollen frozen in one stratum tells what the trees around the lake were doing while a particular generation of children was learning to walk along its shore.

Geologists read these cores the way the rest of us read pages. The lake remembered. It had no choice. Whatever fell into it, drifted down through its waters, and came to rest on its floor became part of the record. The lake did not choose what to keep. The lake kept everything.

Your gut is such a place.

Most of us imagine the body as something that lives only in the present — a system that processes today's meal, fights today's infection, repairs today's damage, and then begins again tomorrow with a clean slate. This is not what the body does. The body remembers. The gut, in particular, is the most patient archive you carry. What has passed through it across the years has not simply passed. Some of it stayed. Some of it built. Some of it is still there.

Chapter 2 described the architecture of this place — the tube and its meadow of villi, the tight junctions that hold the locks, the inner ecosystem of bacteria older than your species. That was the geography. This chapter is about the geology. The way that geography accumulates time within itself. The strata that have built up across your years and that any honest cleanse must reckon with.

* * *

How a Body Becomes Layered

Consider what has actually happened inside the gut you are sitting with right now.

At the moment of your birth, your intestinal tract was, by most measures, sterile. Then your mother's body delivered the first microbial inheritance. The breath of the room delivered the second. Within hours, communities of bacteria were establishing themselves along the length of the tube, choosing their territories, beginning the partnership that would last as long as you did. By your first birthday, the rough shape of your microbiome was set. By your third, the architecture of your immune tolerance — what your body would and would not consider foreign — had been written largely by the bacterial communities of those early years.

Then, in most lives, the layers began.

An ear infection at four. A course of antibiotics that wiped out species your gut had spent years selecting and may not have ever fully replaced. A summer trip when a glass of water was something other than what you thought it was. A camping trip in your twenties where you drank from a stream and passed it off when the symptoms cleared in a week. A meal in another country, undercooked. A relationship that ended in a year of stress and the drinking that came with it. An autoimmune condition that arrived in your thirties without warning. A surgery. An anesthetic. A disrupted sleep cycle that lasted for years.

Each event left something. Some left bacterial extinctions — species that vanished from your inner ecology and did not return. Some left organisms that arrived and stayed. Some left damage to the lining itself, scar tissue or thinning where there had once been velvet. Some left biofilms — microbial fortresses constructed against future antibiotics, future stresses, future immune attacks, fortresses now occupying real estate that the body cannot easily reclaim. Some left eggs that hatched on schedules of their own and produced new generations that never met the original host event.

None of this announced itself at the time. The body's signals were vague. The fatigue felt like ordinary tiredness. The bloating felt like ordinary bloating. The food that no longer agreed with you was simply added to the list of things you no longer ate. And life moved on, and the layers compressed under the layers above them, and the gut you carry today is the cumulative weight of all of it.

This is what we mean when we speak of the layers within. Not the anatomical layers of the gut wall — those are the geography. The layers of time itself, sedimented inside the geography, year over year, decade over decade, until what you call your gut today is in fact a record of every gut you have ever had.

* * *

The Recent Layer

The topmost stratum is the most active and the most easily disturbed. This is the layer of the last year or two. Whatever you have been eating recently. Whatever you have been drinking. Whatever stress your nervous system has been carrying. The microbial communities established here are the youngest. The biofilms are the thinnest. Any parasites resident in this layer are still in their early establishment, often not yet reproducing at full rate, often still recoverable to herbal pressure within days.

When people report rapid early results from a fast — the clearer head within the first week, the lighter belly within the first three days, the energy returning before they had any reason to expect it — they are clearing the recent layer. The work is real, but the work is shallow. The gut has only just begun to remember what is below.

Most cleansing protocols never reach further than this. The popular three-day cleanse, the seasonal juice fast, the gentle herbal tincture — they address the recent layer and nothing beneath it. This is not nothing. The recent layer matters. But a body that contains only its recent layer is a body in perpetual surface treatment, removing what arrived this season and leaving everything older intact.

* * *

The Middle Layer

Beneath the recent is the layer of the last several years to the last decade. This is where the work of a serious protocol begins to make contact with what has been quietly waiting.

The middle layer is the layer of the established. Microbial communities that have been organizing for long enough to have built real architecture. Biofilms thick enough that the herbs of the surface protocol cannot penetrate them on the first pass, or the second. Parasitic adults that have been laying eggs for years — eggs that hatched and matured into new adults that are themselves now laying eggs. Damage to the intestinal lining that has had time to organize itself into something the body has accepted as the new baseline.

This is the layer where the body's signals begin to surface in ways that surprise the person doing the cleanse. Symptoms you had three years ago, briefly returning. Foods you tolerated until your late twenties, suddenly meaningful again. A skin condition you had once and forgot, reappearing for two days and then gone. These are not new problems. These are old problems that had been buried, and the protocol is excavating them.

The middle layer is also where the protocol begins to take real time. The first week was the recent. The middle layer responds to the second week and the third and the fourth. This is part of why the prolonged fast was always the prolonged fast — not because the body needed twenty-five days to do something a three-day fast could not. Because the layer below the surface needed twenty-five days to be reached at all.

* * *

The Deep Layer

Below the middle layer is what the body has been carrying for most of your life.

A single parasite from a single meal eaten at the age of six can still be present at forty. The Strongyloides described in Chapter 6 — the threadworm that reproduces internally without needing reinfection — is the most dramatic example, but it is not the only one. A pinworm exposure in childhood becomes a forty-year history of low-grade environmental reinfection. A protozoan picked up on a school trip lives quietly in the colon for decades, dividing slowly enough to escape both detection and clearance. A tapeworm from an undercooked meal at fifteen sheds eggs every day for twenty-five years.

The deep layer is also where the original microbial extinctions live. The bacterial species your three-year-old self carried, that did not survive the antibiotic at age four, that have not returned since. Species you might have inherited from generations of ancestors going back further than written record. Whether they will return at all is uncertain. Whether they would still know how to live in the gut you have given them is more uncertain still.

The deep layer does not respond to the first cleanse. It often does not respond fully to the second. It is not easily reached, and even when reached, is not easily moved. The deepest organisms have spent decades adapting to the specific conditions of your specific body. They have integrated themselves into the architecture. The body, in many cases, no longer recognizes them as foreign — the immune system has made peace with their presence because the cost of constant attack would have been too high.

Reaching this layer is the work of years, not weeks. It is the work of the cleanse you do, then the maintenance you do for a year afterward, then the second cleanse you do when something tells you it is time. The body releases its oldest residents the way a forest releases its oldest trees — slowly, with conditions, on its own schedule.

* * *

The Inherited Layer

And beneath even the deep layer is the layer that came from before you.

The microbial community you received at birth was not assembled for you. Your mother passed it forward, the way her mother had passed it forward to her, the way some of those bacterial lineages have been passed down through human bodies for tens of thousands of years and through pre-human bodies for tens of millions before that. Some of what lives in your gut today has lived in the guts of your direct maternal line for longer than the species you call your own has existed.

The dietary patterns you inherited are layered too. Cultural foods that your grandmother ate that taught your mother's gut what to expect, and then yours. The bread or the rice or the fermented vegetable that has been part of your family's food for generations carries microbial information that your body is, in a real sense, prepared for. The processed foods of the late twentieth century carry no such information for any of us.

Some of the parasites in this category, too. Helicobacter pylori, the bacterium that causes ulcers in some hosts and lives quietly in others, transmits within families and has done so for so long that strain analysis can trace human migration patterns out of Africa using H. pylori lineages alone. Whatever H. pylori you carry, you likely received from your mother, who likely received it from hers, in a chain of transmission that may go back longer than your family has known its own name.

The inherited layer is not something the cleanse fully addresses. It is not meant to. Some of what you inherited is partnership. Some of what you inherited is burden. Telling the difference requires more knowledge than any of us currently has. The cleanse works on the layers above this one. The inherited layer is the foundation on which the rest sits, and it deserves the respect of being left mostly alone.

* * *

The Excavation

Picture, now, the work of a cleanse in this frame.

You are not destroying anything. You are not waging war. The metaphors of combat that fill the wellness literature — cleansing as battle, parasites as enemies, the body as a battlefield — do not describe what is actually happening. What is actually happening is closer to archaeology. You are working through layers. The herbs are not weapons. They are tools — brushes, picks, the careful instruments of someone uncovering what is already there.

The recent layer comes up first because it is on top. It comes up easily, in days. As it clears, what was beneath begins to be reachable. The middle layer surfaces in the second and third weeks. As it clears, the deep layer becomes accessible — not all of it, not always all at once, but in pieces, in waves, in the strange returns that the body sometimes performs as it surfaces something it has been holding for thirty years.

This is why the protocol takes time. This is why the prolonged fast was always the prolonged fast. This is why people who do one cleanse and feel transformed often discover, two years later, that another cleanse is being asked of them — because the layer that surfaced this time was not visible last time, and could not have been.

It is also why the work is slow at the moments it should be slow. A faster excavation does not reach deeper. A faster excavation reaches the same depth and does more damage on the way. The herbs that work the deeper layers — the clove that reaches the eggs, the wormwood that reaches the larvae, the prolonged daily consistency that maintains lethal conditions long enough for the buried strata to surface — these are the slow tools. They are slow because the work is slow. The body that would let them be fast would also be a body that did not have the layered history they were designed to address.

What your body is asking of you is not speed. It is patience, and time, and a willingness to keep working when the work has stopped feeling like progress. The layer that surfaces in the fourth week was not reachable in the first. The body that emerges after the cleanse is not the body you started with. It is also not the body you were born with. It is something new — the body that has been excavated, layer by layer, and that knows itself a little better for having been allowed to surface what it had been carrying.

* * *

What This Chapter Has Asked You to See

You have a body that remembers.

Most of what is wrong with your gut, if anything is wrong, did not arrive yesterday. It was laid down in layers, slowly, by years of ordinary life, by exposures you did not know were exposures, by stresses you did not know were stresses, by foods that were never the foods your body had been preparing for. None of this is your fault. It is also not anyone else's fault. It is the cost of being alive in a body for as long as you have been, in the world you have lived in.

What follows in this book is the slow work of letting some of those layers go.

Not all of them. Not even most of them. The cleanse you are about to do will reach the recent layer cleanly, the middle layer with effort, and the deep layer in places, in pieces, on terms the body sets. The inherited layer will remain. The maintenance work after the cleanse will, over years, reach further. Some of what your body has been carrying will go with you to the end of your life, and that is not a failure. The body is not meant to be empty. The body is meant to be balanced. The cleanse is the work of restoring balance, not the work of erasing history.

The chapters ahead will describe the tools. The herbs. The hours. The fasting that does the deepest part of this work and the enemas that physically remove what the herbs have surfaced and the long quiet days during which the body does what only time and stillness allow it to do. All of it is in service of this one understanding: that you are layered, and that the work of taking care of yourself begins with knowing what is in the layers.

The lake remembered. The body remembers. What it does with what it has remembered — whether it carries the burden forward or whether it lets the older strata go — is the work of the chapters that follow.

This chapter contains no figures. The work it describes is internal and unseen.

Chapter 10

The Endocannabinoid System & Gut Health

A man stands at his kitchen counter in the early hours, before the house is up. The light through the window is gray, not yet warm. His shoulder is reminding him of itself in the way it has reminded him for years — a small ache that comes and goes by its own rhythms, here this morning, gone before lunch. He fills the kettle without thinking about any of this and sets it on the burner.

The mood that should have come up with the light has not quite come up with it. He has learned, over the years, to know this feeling not as a mood in itself but as the absence of his usual one — the sense of a body that did not finish, in the night, the work the night was for. The kettle begins to ring, and he thinks, as he reaches for it, that the hunger is also not where it should be. It will not arrive with the morning. It will gather sometime late, when the body has no real need for it, and when it speaks it will speak in a way that has nothing to do with food. He has watched this pattern for so long that it no longer surprises him.

For most of his life he thought of these as small separate failures of his own body. The shoulder. The mood. The hunger. He thought, as a person thinks, that he was getting older. He read what was being written about each of them, one by one, and the writing was honest about each thing in itself, and for many years he did not see them as one thing.

They are.

There is a quiet system in the body, woven through almost every other system the body has, whose work is to settle things. To bring pain that has done its job back below the place where the mind can feel it. To restore a mood, after a hard day, to the steady place a person knows as their own. To match hunger to what the body actually needs, on the morning that needs it. The system has been doing this work since before the man was born, and for most of his life he did not know it was there, because he did not need to.

It does not fail all at once. It thins, and grows slower, across years — until the pain that should resolve lingers into the next day and the day after, until the mood that should settle takes longer to settle, until the hunger drifts. None of this is the body breaking. The body is doing exactly what it has been asked to do, the way a body will. What is breaking is the quiet keeper inside it.

That keeper has a name. It is not a name most people know.

* * *

The keeper lives in every body. It is in the body of the woman who wakes a little before her alarm and lies in bed for a moment gathering herself. It is in the body of the boy at the breakfast table whose hunger arrived twenty minutes ago and is now the loudest thing in the room. It is in the body of the old man who, some years after losing his wife, has come to know that the grief which once felt as if it would never lift does lift, in its own time, and returns, and lifts again. The keeper has been at work in each of them. None of them have a name for it.

What the keeper does is steady work, and the steadying takes a few specific shapes that anyone with a body has felt.

It is the part of a person that, at the end of an ordinary evening, lets the day go. A body that has been upright and alert for sixteen hours will, when the keeper is well, soften toward sleep without being argued with. The day is allowed to recede. The mind quiets. Sleep arrives the way an evening tide arrives — not asked for, not negotiated, simply present. When the keeper is thinning, the day will not let go. A person lies in bed with the last hour still running, then another hour after that, and the sleep that finally comes is shallow and unfinished, the kind of sleep that does not leave the next morning rested.

It is the part of a person that, after a hard hour, finds the way back to the steady place. A stone is thrown into water; the water rises, opens, falls back, settles. A hard hour is the stone. The settling is the work of the keeper. When the keeper is well, hard hours pass through; when the keeper is tired, hard hours stay, and the steadiness that should have returned by evening is still missing the next morning.

It is the part of a person that hears the body's small reports and lets them go once they have been heard. The bumped elbow, the pulled muscle, the stubbed toe — each arrives to deliver a small message about a small injury, and each, when the message has been received, takes its leave. A keeper that has been overworked keeps the report running long after the message is delivered. The elbow that should have stopped hurting yesterday is still hurting today. The muscle that should have eased has not eased. A person begins, almost without noticing, to think of the pain as theirs to keep.

It is the part of a person that ties hunger to what the body has actually been doing. A long walk earns a meal; a quiet morning at a desk does not. When the keeper is well, hunger comes when the body has called for it. When the keeper falters, hunger arrives in the afternoon for reasons the afternoon did not produce, and what looks like appetite is something else wearing appetite's clothes.

It is the part of a person that, when something has gone wrong in the body, lets the alarm rise and then lets it fall. A scrape on a knee swells, reddens, hurts. Days later the redness is gone, the swelling is gone, and the body has finished the work of repair. The rising is the body's work. The falling is the keeper's. A keeper that is no longer reaching the falling-place leaves the body in a low simmering version of its alarm response — the joint that should have cooled has not cooled, the skin that should have settled has not settled, the body that has been trying for weeks to put down its alarm cannot find where it left it.

And it is the part of a person that holds the slow ordered rhythm of the gut. Food enters and is taken in, broken down, drawn across the long folded length of the small intestine. What remains is moved through the colon at the steady pace the body has kept since it was a small child. When the keeper is well, the rhythm holds. When the keeper falters, the rhythm falters with it: the gut speeds when it should slow, slows when it should move, forgets the timing it has known for decades. What was a quiet daily process becomes, slowly, the loudest thing in the room — a discomfort, then a pattern of discomfort, then a life rearranging itself around the gut, which is the wrong direction for any life to rearrange.

These are not separate functions of separate systems. They are one quiet attendance, doing one kind of steadying, in places that look like very different parts of being a person. The man at the kitchen counter, in the early hours, with the kettle ringing — what he is feeling, in three places at once, is the thinning of one keeper.

* * *

A keeper that has thinned has been asked for too much, for too long. That is the whole of it, said briefly. The longer answer lives in the small daily places where the asking happens, most of which a person never thinks of as asking too much, and most of which look, on any given day, like the ordinary shape of a modern life.

What asks too much, first, is a body that does not get to finish its night. Most of the repair work happens while a person sleeps. The hours when the body is still and the day is gone are when the small adjustments get made, the small balances restored, the work of bringing things back to where they should be completed before morning. A body that goes to bed late and rises early loses these hours, week after week, year after year. A body whose sleep is fractured by a phone, a child, a worry, a light, a screen across the room loses them differently — not all at once, but a piece at a time. A body that has trained itself to override the pull toward bed with caffeine in the late afternoon, or with the wakefulness of stress, or with the bright steady glow of a lit screen at midnight, has been asking the part of itself that does this work to do it with one hand tied behind its back. What it can do with what it is given, it does. What it cannot do is repair itself in hours it does not have.

What asks too much, also, is a stress that does not resolve. Stress in itself is not the problem. The body is built for the rising and the falling, the alarm and the standing-down. A sudden noise startles the body and, when the noise turns out to have been nothing, the body settles. The settling is the attendance inside it doing what it was made to do. What wears that attendance thin is the alarm that is never told it can stand down. The job that does not finish at five. The phone that does not stop. The argument that simmers across days. The grief that is held at arm's length because the days do not allow for grieving. A body designed for the rising and the falling will, when the falling never comes, stay at the rising-place, doing the work of rising, until it has nothing left to give.

What asks too much, also, is the steady arrival of food and substance that mimics or drowns out the body's own signals. The work of reading the body depends on the signals being honest — hunger that means hunger, fullness that means fullness, the body's own quiet language about what it needs and when. When the signals are noisy, the part that listens begins to lose its ear. Highly processed food, engineered to override the body's sense of enough, teaches the listening part that fullness is a moving target. Alcohol blunts the rising and the falling both. Cannabis, taken often, sits down in the very seat where the listening happens — the system inside the body that the cannabis plant is, in fact, named after. The body has its own version of what cannabis brings from outside: a network of molecules and receptors woven through almost every system the body has, called, in the literature, the endocannabinoid system. Endo, meaning within. The cannabis plant has been named after the system, not the system after the plant. When cannabis arrives often, the seat is taken by the louder occupant, and the endocannabinoid system's own quieter work happens less. Some medications, taken for years, do something similar. Each of these things has its place, and people reach for them for real reasons. Each also leaves the body's own language a little harder to hear, the morning after.

And there is the slower one, the one that names itself only by absence. Repair happens in the hours of the day when nothing is being asked of the body — when a person stares out a window for a minute, when the mind drifts at a stoplight, when a body sits in a chair without a screen, when the small unstructured spaces of an ordinary day let the part that does this work do what it does. A life that has filled those spaces, every one of them, with a stimulus or a task or a notification, has not given that part its daylight working hours. What it was meant to do, in small pieces, all day long, it cannot do at three in the morning instead.

These are not exotic burdens. They are the quiet weather of an ordinary life, and most lives carry some combination of them, in larger or smaller measure. The man at the kitchen counter has carried his combination for many years. The woman who lay in bed gathering herself before her alarm has carried hers. The old man who lost his wife has carried his. Each of them holds, inside their own body, an endocannabinoid system that has been doing more work than the years have given it a way to recover from. The keeper has had a name all along.

* * *

A system that has been thinned across years is not a system that is broken. It is a system that has not been given what it needs in order to recover, for as long as it has been asked to give. Recovery is its native condition. The same small daily places that thinned it, when changed, are the places that thicken it again.

A body that gets to finish its night will, given enough nights in succession, begin to find the keeper's work returning beneath it. The first nights of unfractured sleep do not feel particular; they feel like ordinary sleep, perhaps a little deeper than what the body had grown used to. After a week of them the morning ache that always lingered begins to go where aches are supposed to go. After a month, the mood that should have settled in the night settles in the night. The endocannabinoid system does its repair while the body is still. A body that is still long enough, often enough, gives it the hours it needs to do the repair.

A stress that has been allowed to resolve releases something the body has been holding for longer than it knew. The argument is finished. The job is set down. The grief, given its hours, begins to do what grief does, which is to thin. The endocannabinoid system was built for the falling that follows the rising, and when the falling is permitted, the system finds the work it was made to do is, after all, the work it can still do. The body remembers what settling feels like. The settling, once remembered, becomes available again.

A body whose signals are clean is a body whose endocannabinoid system can read them. Food that has not been engineered to override the sense of enough teaches the system, after some weeks, what enough feels like. The substance that was sitting in the system's seat, when it stops arriving, leaves the seat open. The body's own quiet language begins to be audible again, first in small things — a real hunger that arrives with the morning, a real fullness at the end of a meal — and then in larger ones. The system has been waiting to hear what it was made to hear.

And then there is stillness — the small unstructured spaces in a day that, if a person allows them, become the daylight working hours of the system. A walk without a phone. A meal without a screen. A moment, between one thing and the next, that is allowed to be a moment instead of a transition. None of these feel like medicine. They are not supposed to. They are the small daily acts of permission a body gives itself to be a body, and the system inside the body uses them as it was made to use them.

There is also the longer restoration. A body that is given the particular kind of rest that a prolonged fast provides receives something none of the smaller restorations can give it on their own. The whole of the digestive work pauses. The whole of the inflammatory low-level humming, in many bodies, quiets. The endocannabinoid system, which has been running its repair on whatever scattered hours it could find for years, is given days and then weeks of unbroken time. A great deal of what the body has been carrying, it begins to put down. The gut returning to its proper rhythm, the inflammation cooling, the mood steadying, the hunger becoming an honest signal again — all of these are forms of the endocannabinoid system finally being able to do its work. The prolonged fast is, among many other things, a vacation given to the keeper, after which the keeper returns to what it was before the years began to ask too much of it.

A man at his kitchen counter who begins, slowly, to give his body the things it has been asking for begins to find that the shoulder, on some mornings, does not ache. The mood, on some mornings, has come up with the light. The hunger, on some mornings, arrives with the morning. None of this happens all at once. The system has been thin for many years and it does not thicken in a week. But it thickens. It always thickens, when given what it needs.

* * *

A particular density of the endocannabinoid system's machinery lives in the gut. The receptors that the system uses to do its work are present throughout the body, but they are concentrated, in unusually high numbers, along the long folded length of the small intestine and the slow miles of the colon. The gut is, in this sense, one of the system's home territories. The slow rhythm of digestion the body has kept since childhood, the timing of food moving through, the careful partnership the gut maintains with the small living world of bacteria that lives in it — all of these are work the endocannabinoid system is helping to keep.

There is a continuous conversation between the gut and the rest of the body. A long nerve, the vagus, runs from the brain to the gut and back again, carrying messages in both directions all day. The gut tells the body what it has been given to digest, how the digesting is going, what the bacterial neighbors are reporting, what is happening at the layer where food meets the small intestine's wall. The body tells the gut what to expect, when to slow, when to move. The endocannabinoid system is one of the languages this conversation is conducted in. When the system is well, the conversation is in good order. When the system is thinned, the conversation goes a little wrong — the gut tells the body something the body cannot quite hear, the body tells the gut something the gut cannot quite read.

The gut wall is a single layer of cells, no thicker than a piece of tissue paper, that separates the inside of the body from the contents of the gut. That wall is patrolled, repaired, and held in good order by many small systems working together. The endocannabinoid system is one of the more important ones. It tells the cells of the wall when to tighten their joins with one another. It tells the immune cells positioned just behind the wall when to rise and when to stand down. It modulates how the wall responds to what it meets, on the side where food and bacteria and a thousand other things are passing through every hour of every day. A wall that has lost the steady help of the endocannabinoid system is a wall that is a little less able to hold what it was made to hold.

The bacterial neighbors who live along the gut wall are not separate from the endocannabinoid system's work either. A healthy community of bacteria sends signals across the wall that the system reads and responds to. A community that has been disturbed — by antibiotics, by poor food, by chronic inflammation, by the long simmer of a body that cannot stand down — sends different signals, and the system reads the difference. The two work together, each making the other's work easier when both are well, each making the other's work harder when one is failing. Restoring the endocannabinoid system in isolation from the bacterial community, or restoring the bacterial community in isolation from the endocannabinoid system, is harder than restoring them together.

Most of what is asked of a person, in service of the gut, is also something the endocannabinoid system has been waiting for someone to do. The fast that lets the gut rest is the same fast that lets the system rest. The food that does not lie to the gut is the same food that does not lie to the system. The stillness, the unfractured nights, the alarm allowed to stand down — all of it is the same work, in two languages, for one body.

* * *

It is a different morning. The same man is at the same counter, before the house is up, with the kettle on the burner. The light through the window is gray in the way it is gray every morning at this hour. His shoulder is, today, quiet. He notices the quietness only because he has noticed the ache so many other mornings. His mood has come up with the light. The hunger has not yet arrived; it will arrive later, with a meal, as it is supposed to.

For some months now he has been giving the body, in small ways, what the body had been asking for. He has gone to bed when his body began to ask him to. He has let, in the evenings, a stress that wanted to fall actually fall. He has eaten food whose signals he could trust. He has not, every minute of every day, asked something of himself. He has not, in any of this, been doing anything heroic. He has, in fact, been doing less than he had been doing before. The endocannabinoid system has noticed. It is doing more, now, with what it has been given.

The endocannabinoid system was woven into his body before he was born. It will be woven through it until the day he is no longer in it. Across the years between, it has been doing the quiet work of bringing things back, sometimes well, sometimes poorly, depending on what he has asked of it. The asking can change. When the asking changes, what the system can give back to him changes also. This has always been true. He simply did not, until late, know.

A body kept by the keeper is a body that the body's own small attendance is allowed to keep.

That is what the endocannabinoid system has been waiting, all along, to do.

Chart S — The Endocannabinoid System Across the Body

Six places in the body where the endocannabinoid system does its quiet work, in two columns: the way it shows up when the system is well, and the way it shows up when the system has thinned.

Body system	When the system is well	When the system is thinning
Sleep	The body softens toward sleep without being argued with. The mind quiets. Sleep is unfractured and the next morning is rested.	The day will not let go. Sleep takes longer to arrive, breaks across the night, and leaves the morning unfinished.
Mood	After a hard hour, the mood comes back to its own steady place the way water returns to its level after a stone is thrown.	Hard hours stay. The steadiness that should have returned by evening is still missing the next morning.
Pain	A small injury reports itself, the report is heard, and the pain takes its leave once the message has been received.	The pain that should have eased yesterday is still here today. A person begins to think of it as theirs to keep.
Hunger	Hunger arrives when the body has called for it and matches what the body has actually been doing.	Hunger arrives in the afternoon for reasons the afternoon did not produce. Appetite is something else wearing appetite's clothes.
Inflammation	When something has gone wrong, the alarm rises and then, the work being done, falls back to where it was before.	The alarm rises and stays risen. The joint, the skin, the gut keep simmering long after the original wrong has passed.
Gut motility	The slow ordered rhythm of the gut holds. Food enters, is taken in, is moved through at the steady pace the body has known for decades.	The rhythm falters. The gut speeds when it should slow, slows when it should move, forgets the timing it has known for years.

Chapter 11

Ketones — Your Brain's Preferred Fuel

* * *

For most of your life you have run on glucose. Every meal. Every snack. Every cup of something sweet. Glucose in, energy out, on a cycle so familiar your body runs it without a thought. Most modern adults have never spent more than a handful of consecutive hours in any state but this one. The wiring is so well-worn that the body, when asked to do anything else, treats the request as an emergency.

But glucose is not the only fuel your body knows how to use. It is simply the most convenient one — convenient because the modern food supply ensures it is always arriving, convenient because the digestive system can extract it from almost anything, convenient because it requires no metabolic adjustment to use. When that convenience disappears, when food stops arriving and the liver's emergency glucose stores empty, something else takes its place. Something so elegant and so efficient that many researchers now suspect it may actually be the *preferred* state rather than the backup. That something is ketones. What they are, what they do, and why their arrival in your bloodstream is one of the most consequential events of the entire fast — this is what follows.

The Moment Everything Shifts

Somewhere between **day two and day four** of your fast — depending on your metabolic history and activity level — something fundamental changes. Your liver empties its glucose stores. The supply runs out. The brain, which cannot run on fat directly, faces an apparent crisis.

Apparent. Because the body has a backup system that has been waiting, intact, since long before any human being knew what a calorie was. The system produces ketones, and once it begins running, the brain that thought it required glucose discovers it can run on something else entirely.

The process unfolds in four steps:

1. Glucose stores deplete. The liver's glycogen runs out within roughly 24 hours of the last meal in a moderately active person.

2. Fat begins to mobilize. Stored body fat releases fatty acids into the bloodstream.

3. The liver converts fatty acids to ketones. The liver takes the incoming fatty acids and produces ketone bodies, releasing them into the bloodstream.

4. Cells absorb and burn ketones. Every cell in the body that can use ketones — and most can — begins doing so.

You are not starving. You are running on a different fuel source, one your body has been carrying with it the entire time. The fat that the modern dietary culture treats as the enemy is, during a fast, exactly the strategic reserve your body evolved to depend on.

(Figure 10.1 — see the online Figure Guide)

The Three Ketone Bodies

Not all ketones are identical. The liver produces three distinct types, each with its own role and its own behavior in the body:

• **Beta-hydroxybutyrate (BHB)** — the primary ketone, approximately **78%** of total ketone production. Most abundant, most studied, travels freely in the bloodstream to all tissues, crosses the blood-brain barrier with notable ease. The ketone most directly linked to cognitive enhancement and neuroprotection. Directly activates endocannabinoid receptors. Has anti-inflammatory properties independent of its fuel function. This is the ketone measured in blood ketone testing.

• **Acetoacetate** — approximately **20%** of production. The first ketone the liver produces from fat breakdown. BHB is actually produced from acetoacetate. Used directly by the heart, kidneys, and brain for fuel, and by muscles during sustained activity.

• **Acetone** — the smallest fraction, approximately **2%**. Produced from the spontaneous breakdown of acetoacetate. Cannot be used for fuel — the body exhales it through the lungs. Responsible for the distinctive sweet, fruity breath of deep ketosis. The presence of acetone breath is one of the first signs your fast has successfully shifted into ketosis.

(Figure 10.2 — see the online Figure Guide)

How Your Body Uses Ketones

Different tissues use ketones with different efficiency and different preferences. Some take to ketones immediately. Some take longer to adapt. The hierarchy is worth knowing because it explains, organ by organ, why the fasted state feels so different from the fed one.

The brain. By far the largest consumer. The brain represents approximately 2% of body weight but consumes approximately 20% of total body energy. During prolonged fasting, as glucose disappears, the brain progressively shifts to ketone metabolism:

• Can derive up to **75%** of its energy from ketones during deep fasting.

• BHB crosses the blood-brain barrier **more efficiently** than glucose in many conditions.

• Neurons running on ketones produce **less oxidative stress** than those running on glucose.

• Mitochondrial function in brain cells improves on ketone fuel.

• The **prefrontal cortex** — responsible for focus, decision-making, clarity, and executive function — responds particularly well.

This is not theory. It is why you will experience — if you have not already — a quality of mental clarity during your fast that feels qualitatively different from anything food-fueled thinking produces. Sharper. Quieter. More present. The brain is operating on cleaner fuel, and the difference is felt rather than measured.

(Figure 10.3 — see the online Figure Guide)

The heart. The heart muscle runs continuously, every moment of every day, without rest. It needs the most reliable, efficient fuel available — and ketones suit it:

• The heart runs approximately **28% more efficiently** on ketones than on glucose.

• Cardiac mitochondria extract more ATP per unit of ketone than per unit of glucose.

• Ketones reduce **cardiac oxidative stress**.

• Heart rate typically slows and stabilizes during deep ketosis, a sign of improved efficiency.

• Many experienced fasters report a deep sense of cardiac calm — a steadiness in the chest that feels unmistakably physical.

(Figure 10.4 — see the online Figure Guide)

Skeletal muscles. One of the most important functions of ketosis during a prolonged fast is muscle preservation:

• Without ketones, the body would increasingly break down muscle protein for fuel.

• Ketones provide an alternative, sparing muscle from catabolism.

• Muscles can use ketones directly, reducing their demand on protein breakdown.

• Slow-twitch endurance muscle fibers are particularly efficient ketone users.

This muscle-sparing effect is one of the most important reasons to ensure your fast achieves and maintains deep ketosis. Not just for energy, but for the preservation of the body itself. The fasted state in deep ketosis is fundamentally different from simple starvation precisely because of this protection. The body in ketosis can sustain itself on its own fat reserves for far longer than the body in glucose-deprivation could ever sustain itself on muscle.

The kidneys. Kidneys are among the highest energy-consuming organs, filtering approximately 180 liters of blood daily. They use ketones to power this continuous filtration work, which reduces their metabolic burden during fasting and supports continued efficient toxin removal throughout the cleanse.

The lungs. Lung tissue uses ketones for cellular maintenance. The exhalation of acetone serves as a natural indicator of ketosis depth — deeper ketosis produces more pronounced acetone breath, which is why many fasters use breath as a simple real-time indicator of their metabolic state.

The gut lining. Particularly relevant to everything you are doing. Intestinal lining cells, called enterocytes, normally prefer **glutamine** as their primary fuel. During prolonged fasting, they adapt to ketones:

- Ketones support the continued function and repair of intestinal lining cells.
- This is why the gut lining can actively heal and regenerate during fasting rather than simply surviving it.
- Combined with L-Glutamine supplementation, you are providing the intestinal lining with fuel from two directions simultaneously.

The gut lining's capacity to regenerate during fasting depends on this adaptation. Without it, the lining would simply persist through the fast unchanged. With it, the lining can rebuild itself layer by layer in conditions of progressively reducing inflammation — the same rebuilding that the long arc of accumulated-layer clearance and lining renewal makes possible.

Ketones and the Brain — Going Deeper

The cognitive dimension of ketosis deserves more than a list of bullet points. The brain in ketosis is not simply the brain on a different fuel. It is, by nearly every measurable parameter, a brain operating in a different state.

The neurotransmitter balance shifts. Ketone metabolism increases **GABA**, the primary calming neurotransmitter, and reduces **glutamate**, the primary excitatory neurotransmitter. The result is a brain that is calmer yet more focused — less reactive, more clear. This GABA-to-glutamate shift is one of the reasons ketosis is being actively studied for the treatment of epilepsy, anxiety, and mood disorders. The therapeutic effect that some patients experience is not magic. It is neurochemistry.

Brain-derived neurotrophic factor — **BDNF** — increases significantly during ketosis. BDNF is sometimes called *fertilizer for the brain*. It promotes neuronal growth, neuronal repair, and the formation of new connections between neurons. Higher BDNF means enhanced neuroplasticity — the brain's ability to reorganize itself. This is why the fasting state is not just clear. It can feel genuinely changing at a cognitive and emotional level. The brain in deep fasting is in a more open state than it ordinarily is, and the things it does in that state — the patterns it lays down, the insights it produces, the emotional reprocessing it undertakes — can persist long after the fast ends.

Mitochondrial biogenesis accelerates. Ketosis stimulates the production of new mitochondria in brain cells. More mitochondria means more energy production capacity. The brain literally becomes more energetically capable during prolonged ketosis than it was at the start of the fast.

(Figure 10.5 — see the online Figure Guide)

(Figure 10.6 — see the online Figure Guide)

Coconut Oil, MCT, and Ketone Production

This is where your daily coconut oil addition becomes deeply relevant. Not all fats produce ketones with equal efficiency. **Medium-chain triglycerides** — MCTs — are uniquely suited to rapid ketone production:

• Unlike long-chain fats, MCTs are absorbed **directly into the portal vein** rather than into the lymphatic system.

• They travel immediately to the liver.

• They are converted to ketones rapidly and efficiently — within minutes of consumption.

• They do not require carnitine transport into mitochondria, unlike long-chain fats.

• They produce ketones even in the presence of some carbohydrates, unlike other fats.

Coconut oil is approximately **65% MCT** by composition, making it one of the richest natural MCT sources available. Adding coconut oil to your broth during early refeeding maintains ketone production during the transition phase, provides immediate brain fuel as glucose begins to return, and supports a gradual rather than abrupt transition out of ketosis. The cognitive clarity of the fasting state is preserved as long as possible during refeeding when MCTs are part of the early reintroduction.

(Figure 10.7 — see the online Figure Guide)

Measuring Your Ketosis

How do you know how deep your ketosis actually is? Three measurement methods are available:

• **Breath testing** measures acetone in exhaled breath. Non-invasive, with home devices widely available. A good indicator of trend, less precise than blood testing. The simplest real-time monitoring tool.

• **Urine testing** uses ketone strips and measures acetoacetate in urine. Less accurate in deep prolonged fasting — the kidneys become more efficient and excrete less. More useful in early ketosis than in deep fasting.

• **Blood testing** is the gold standard. A small finger-prick device, similar to glucose monitoring, measures BHB directly. The reference ranges are these:

• Nutritional ketosis: **0.5 to 3.0 mmol/L**

• Fasting ketosis: **3.0 to 8.0 mmol/L**

• Deep prolonged fasting: **8.0 to 10.0 mmol/L**

For a prolonged fast, blood testing gives you the most accurate picture of your metabolic state.

(Figure 10.8 — see the online Figure Guide)

The Euphoria Explained

The euphoric clarity of deep fasting is not a single phenomenon. It is the convergence of several things happening simultaneously, and the ketones described above are at the center of it. The full list:

• **BHB** activating endocannabinoid receptors directly.

• **Anandamide rising**, stimulated by both fasting and ketone production.

• **GABA increasing**, calming neural noise.

• **BDNF rising**, the brain entering a growth and repair state.

• **Inflammatory burden decreasing** as parasites and accumulated layers clear.

• **Mitochondrial efficiency improving** — more energy from less fuel.

• **Serotonin production normalizing** as the gut lining heals.

Each of these things is happening simultaneously. Together they produce a state that has no equivalent in ordinary waking life. Ancient traditions called it spiritual clarity. Modern neuroscience calls it optimized brain chemistry. Both are correct, and the same body produces the same state regardless of how its inhabitant chooses to describe it.

A Note on Electrolytes and Ketosis

Deep ketosis has one important metabolic side effect that requires attention. Ketone production causes the kidneys to excrete more sodium, and with sodium goes water and other electrolytes. This is the primary mechanism behind several phenomena you will experience or have already experienced during the fast:

• Increased urination in early fasting.

• The lightheadedness when changing positions.

• The importance of trace mineral replenishment throughout.

Maintaining electrolytes during ketosis is not just about comfort. It is about maintaining the conditions that allow ketosis to work safely. The deeper your ketosis, the more diligent your mineral replenishment needs to be. The pinch of salt in your morning water, the trace mineral solution, the magnesium in the evening — these are not optional accessories to the fast. They are the foundation that keeps the ketosis sustainable, and without them, the same metabolic state that produces clarity and healing can produce dangerous depletion instead. The detail of how to manage this is given more fully in the practical sections on trace minerals. What matters here is simply that the body in deep ketosis is working with a different mineral economy than the body in the fed state, and the protocol exists to keep that economy balanced.

What follows brings everything seen so far together — the parasites, the layers, the endocannabinoid system, the ketones — into the integrated biological picture of why prolonged fasting works the way it does. The architecture is what has been laid out here. What that architecture as a whole accomplishes, why every part of it depends on every other part, and why the duration of the fast is what it is, is what comes next.

*Figures referenced above: 10.1–10.8 **(online Figure Guide)*

Chapter 12

The Science of Why Prolonged Fasting Works

* * *

What you are about to read is a story. It is the story of one body, across forty days, doing the work that this book has been describing in pieces. The body is not anyone's in particular. It could be yours.

Until now, you have learned the parts. The architecture of the gut. The parasites that live within it. The layers of time that have settled into the tissues. The endocannabinoid system that has been quietly waiting. The ketones the body produces when food stops arriving. Each of those things has had its own chapter. Now they meet.

What follows is the science of how they meet. It is also the truth of what it feels like when they do. There is no honest way to describe a forty-day fast without describing both. The biology is not separate from the experience. The hunger that arrives in the middle of the second night is the same event as the metabolic switch beginning to throw. The grief that surfaces on day eleven for reasons you cannot name is the same event as the deep tissues releasing what they have been holding. The strange peace that arrives somewhere in the third week is not a gift. It is a measurement. It is the body telling you what it has finally let go of.

Read this chapter slowly. If you are considering this fast and what you read here makes you decide it is not for you, that is a useful chapter. The fast is not for everyone, and it is not for any reason. It is for one reason — the readiness to meet what is in your own body — and a reader who finishes this chapter and feels something other than that readiness has been served well by the chapter.

* * *

Before

Your last meal is a real meal. You eat it at a table or you eat it standing. You eat it with people you love or you eat it alone. You eat it knowing what it is, or you eat it without thinking, the way you have eaten ten thousand other meals before this one.

The body that finishes this meal does not know yet. The pancreas releases its insulin on schedule. The stomach begins its work. The small intestine — the meadow of villi from Chapter 2 — reaches up into the chyme and absorbs sugars and amino acids and fats into the bloodstream. The liver receives them, sorts them, sends some to storage, sends some onward. The cells of the body, every one of them, take in their share.

This is what your body has been doing every few hours for as long as you have been alive. The system is so familiar to you that you experience it as the absence of a system. You do not feel digestion happening. You feel fed. The fed state is the state you have lived in. It is the only state you know.

When the meal is over, you rinse the dish, or you do not. You sit for a while. You feel ordinary. Whatever you are about to do has not yet begun.

* * *

Hours 1 to 36

The first six hours pass without much. The meal is still being processed. Insulin is still elevated. The body has not yet noticed that nothing else is coming.

Hours six to twelve are when the conscious mind first checks in. You begin to notice that you are not eating. You think about what you would normally be eating. You realize that almost every part of your day is structured around meals — not just the eating itself, but the planning, the preparation, the cleaning up afterward, the conversations that happen while it is being eaten. You did not realize how much of your day was food until food was removed from it. The first emotion is not hunger. It is something closer to disorientation. You have not lost an organ. You have lost the rhythm by which the day organized itself.

Around hour eighteen, the liver finishes the last of its glycogen. This is the metabolic moment most people never experience because most people eat before it arrives. The blood glucose, no longer being refilled, drifts downward. The body activates its first backup — it begins releasing stored glucose from muscle tissue, and it begins gluconeogenesis, the process of converting amino acids into new glucose. These are stopgap measures. They will buy a day, perhaps two.

Somewhere between hour twenty-four and hour thirty-six, hunger arrives in waves. This is the first wave that most people who try to fast do not get past. It is not the polite hunger of having skipped lunch. It is hunger as a request from the body, repeated, escalating, accompanied by a low-grade panic that is not entirely emotional. Cortisol rises. Ghrelin — the primary hunger hormone — surges in approximately three-hour pulses, peaks, falls, and surges again. Each pulse carries with it not just the sensation of hunger but a kind of dread. The mind begins to negotiate. *Just one piece of fruit. Just a spoonful of broth. Just something.* The negotiation is real. The mind is running an ancient program. The body it lives in does not yet know that food is not coming, and it is mounting the responses that have kept your ancestors alive for two hundred thousand years.

The honest truth about this stretch is that it is harder than almost anyone tells you in advance. You will feel weak. You will feel cold. You may feel a kind of grief that has no obvious source. You may snap at someone for no reason. You may sit at a table while other people eat and feel a loneliness that is not quite loneliness but something older. You may, in the middle of the second night, lie awake at three in the morning convinced that this was a bad idea and that you should eat something in the morning and start again later, when the timing is better, when you are stronger, when the world cooperates more.

If you can stay through this stretch — if you can sit with the hunger, drink your salted water, accept that the panic is biology rather than truth — the body will move past it. The peak of ghrelin in a prolonged fast is not at thirty-six hours. It is at thirty-six hours. After that, ghrelin levels fall. They keep falling. By the end of the second day, hunger as a sensation has begun to recede. By the end of the third day, in most fasters, it is largely gone.

What that means is that the hardest part of a forty-day fast occurs in the first thirty-six hours. The body that survives the first night and a half emerges into a state most modern humans never experience. The hunger you have known your whole life — the hunger that comes between meals, between snacks, between the constant trickle of sugar into your blood — was not real hunger. It was a learned response to a learned eating schedule. Real hunger appears, peaks, and resolves on a timeline the body knows even when the conscious mind has forgotten it.

* * *

Days 2 to 4

Sometime in the second day, the body begins what Chapter 11 described in mechanism but cannot describe in feeling. The metabolic switch begins to throw.

Adipose tissue, which has been waiting through every meal of every day of your life as a reserve no one was asking it to be, finally receives the signal. Hormone-sensitive lipase activates. Stored triglycerides break down into fatty acids and glycerol. The fatty acids enter the bloodstream and travel to the liver. The liver, which has been a glucose factory for as long as you have been eating, retools. It begins producing ketone bodies. The first beta-hydroxybutyrate appears in your blood between hour forty-eight and hour seventy-two.

Your conscious mind does not know this is happening. What you experience is something different. You experience an unexpected steadiness. The hunger waves that defined the second night have begun to space out. The panic that came with them has lessened. You are still tired. You may still be cold. But the desperate quality of the first thirty-six hours has receded into something more sustainable.

This is also the period when the social architecture around food begins to make itself visible to you in ways it never has before. You skip a lunch with a colleague and they ask if you are okay. You smell coffee being made by someone else in the morning and find yourself paying attention to it the way you pay attention to music. You see an advertisement for a restaurant and discover that food advertising, which you previously experienced as background noise, is in fact addressed to a part of your brain you can now feel being addressed. You begin to understand how much of your culture is, in a strict sense, food culture. You did not know because you had been part of it. The fast removes you from it briefly, and from the outside you can see the shape of it.

There is grief in this. The grief is not that you cannot eat. The grief is the recognition that so much of your life has been organized around food that you do not entirely know who you are when food is removed. The dinner with your spouse. The breakfast on Sunday morning. The coffee you drink while you write. The wine you drink while you talk. The cake on a birthday. The bread broken at a meal that mattered. All of this is part of the architecture of your life, and the fast briefly dismantles it, and what is left is the version of you that has been there underneath the architecture all along.

Some readers — most readers, eventually — cry at some point during this stretch. Not for any single reason. Just that the body, no longer occupied with the constant low-grade work of digestion, has bandwidth to feel things it has not had time to feel. This is part of the fast working. It is not a side effect.

* * *

Days 5 to 7

Sometime around day five, the brain switches gears.

The neurons that have run on glucose for forty years begin running on ketones. Beta-hydroxybutyrate crosses the blood-brain barrier with greater efficiency than glucose ever did. The mitochondria of brain cells, which had been metabolizing sugar through processes that produce a steady drip of oxidative damage, begin metabolizing ketones through cleaner pathways. The brain, fueled differently, becomes a different brain.

What this feels like is hard to describe to someone who has not experienced it, and easy to describe to anyone who has. The mental noise quiets. The constant background chatter that you did not know was there until it stopped — the low hum of food-thoughts, blood-sugar fluctuations, mild dehydration, mild inflammation — fades into a clarity that is unmistakably new. Your thinking slows down and at the same time becomes more accurate. You write a sentence and it is the sentence you meant. You read a paragraph and it stays read. You sit with a difficult conversation and you do not flinch from it the way you might have a week ago.

The physiological reason is convergent. GABA, the calming neurotransmitter, is elevated. Glutamate, the excitatory one, is moderated. Brain-derived neurotrophic factor — BDNF, the molecule responsible for neuronal growth and repair — is rising. The endocannabinoid system, which Chapter 10 described as quietly waiting, begins to elevate anandamide, the molecule whose name comes from the Sanskrit word for bliss. None of this is metaphor. All of it is measurable. The clarity is not a feeling about a situation. It is the chemistry of a brain operating in a regime it almost never gets to operate in.

And the body itself is changing. Autophagy — the cellular self-cleaning process the body activates when food is no longer arriving — has been ramping up since day three and is now in full operation. The body, with no incoming protein to build new cells from, has begun disassembling and recycling its own damaged components. Misfolded proteins are being broken down for parts. Damaged mitochondria are being consumed and replaced. Cells that have been quietly malfunctioning for years are being identified and dissolved. What you are doing during these days is something the body has the capacity to do at no other time. You are giving it the conditions in which to repair itself at the molecular level, and it is taking the conditions and using them.

It is also the period during which the parasites in your gut, which have been thriving on a continuous food supply for as long as they have been there, lose access to that supply. The herbs of Chapter 19 begin to reach them through a body that is no longer overwhelmed with digestion. The biofilms thin. The first dying organisms begin to release their grip on the intestinal lining, and the lining — fueled now by ketones rather than glucose, supported by L-glutamine, no longer occupied with absorbing three meals a day — begins the active work of healing.

All of this is happening in the same body, in the same days, simultaneously. This is the convergence the chapter title was promising. Ketones, autophagy, the endocannabinoid system, the herbs, the gut lining, the parasites — all of these are not separate processes. They are the same process. Each one creates the conditions for the others. The body has entered a state in which all of them are working together, and it is the synchrony of their work that does what shorter cleanses cannot.

* * *

Days 8 to 14

And then the middle layer surfaces.

Chapter 9 described the layered nature of what has accumulated in your body across the years. The recent layer cleared in the first week. Now the layer below it begins to come up. What had been buried under more recent material becomes briefly visible, briefly active, and then — if the protocol holds — begins to clear.

What this looks like is unpredictable in detail and predictable in pattern. Symptoms you had three years ago return for two days and pass. A skin condition you forgot about reappears in a small patch and is gone by morning. An emotional pattern you used to have — a pattern of irritability or sadness or anxiety that you had stopped noticing because you had stopped being it — appears for an afternoon and clears. The body is releasing what it had been holding. None of this is the fast going wrong. It is the fast doing exactly what the long fast was always designed to do.

The social isolation, by now, is real. You have been not eating with people for over a week. The friend who invited you to dinner two weeks ago has stopped following up. The family member who supports you in principle has begun, in practice, to find your fast a little tedious to be around. You have learned, by this point, not to mention what you are doing unless someone asks, and you have learned that most people would prefer not to ask. You drink your salt water in a quiet kitchen while people you love eat real meals in another room or in another house, and you have started to notice things about your relationships you had never had reason to notice before.

There is a particular boredom to this stretch that is worth naming. The hours that used to be filled with meal preparation, eating, and cleanup are simply hours now. Three hours a day, in most lives, that no longer have an occupation. You may, depending on your habits, find yourself at a loss for what to do with them. Reading, walking, sitting. The fast forces a confrontation with empty time that the modern life is not designed for.

Most people, given three unscheduled hours, will fill them with their phone. The faster cannot fill them with food, and after a week they discover that the phone is not actually filling them either, and what is left is a quality of time that is unfamiliar and at first uncomfortable. Sit with this. The boredom is part of the work.

Days twelve through fourteen contain what most experienced fasters call the mid-fast trough. The early novelty of ketosis has passed. The end of the fast is still impossibly far away. The clarity that arrived around day six is still there, but you have grown used to it, and you are beginning to feel the sustained physical demands of being in this state. You may feel a flatness. You may feel a kind of homesickness for the person you were two weeks ago, when food was just food and life was just life. You may, at some point during these days, seriously consider ending the fast early. This is the point at which more fasters quit than at any other moment except the first thirty-six hours.

The honest answer to the question of why you should not quit is not motivational. It is biological. The deep work of the fast — the work that justifies the fast as a forty-day fast and not a fourteen-day fast — has not yet begun. What has happened so far has been the surface and the middle. The deep layer that Chapter 9 described is what the second half of the fast is for. If you stop now, you will have done meaningful work. You will not have done the work the protocol was designed for. The body has spent two weeks preparing itself to do the deep work, and it is ready, and it is waiting, and what comes next is what you have been preparing for.

* * *

Days 15 to 25

Something shifts in the third week.

The body, after two weeks in deep ketosis with autophagy in full operation, has reached a metabolic state most modern humans never reach. Blood ketones have risen into the range of eight to ten millimoles per liter. The brain has fully transitioned to ketone fuel. The endocannabinoid system is operating at elevated baseline. The immune system, no longer occupied with the constant small fires of digesting an industrial diet, has redirected its attention to the larger fires it had not had bandwidth for. Old infections begin to clear. Long-standing inflammation begins to subside. Joints that had hurt for a decade begin to move differently.

The deep parasites — the ones from Chapter 9, the ones from a single childhood exposure that have been quietly reproducing for twenty or thirty years — begin to release their hold. The biofilms that had protected them have thinned through fourteen consecutive days of herbal pressure. The intestinal lining, which had grown around them and accommodated them, is no longer hospitable. Eggs that had been laid and dormant begin to be reached by the clove. The accumulated parasitic ecosystem of decades begins, slowly, to come apart.

What you experience, alongside all of this, is a quality of stillness that is hard to describe. The hunger is fully gone. Food has, in some real sense, stopped existing for you. You walk past a bakery and smell bread and recognize it as something that another version of you used to want, and you observe the recognition without joining it. You drink your salt water without anticipation. You drink your water with attention. The relationship between you and food, which had been the central relationship of your life without your having ever thought of it as a relationship, has become something else. It has become quiet.

In this quietness, things surface.

A grief you have not visited in years arrives one afternoon and stays for an hour and leaves. A memory from childhood you had not recalled in decades returns with a clarity that is almost cinematic. A pattern in a relationship that you have not been able to see from inside it becomes visible from this distance the fast has placed you at. A decision you have been avoiding for years, sometimes for a long time, presents itself with an answer that feels obvious in a way it never has before.

This is not mystical. This is the default mode network of the brain, which had been occupied with the management of food and stimulation and social input, finally having the bandwidth to do its other job — the integration of memory, the long quiet processing of unfinished material, the synthesis of patterns the active mind was too busy to see. The fast does not give you access to anything that was not already there. It removes the noise that had been preventing access. What rises in the quiet is what your body had been carrying, waiting for the conditions in which to surface it.

Some of what surfaces is hard. Old hurts, old shames, old fears. Some of it is unexpectedly sweet. A capacity for joy you had not known was possible, present in small moments — the light through a window, a bird outside the kitchen, the texture of a piece of cloth between your fingers. The endocannabinoid system, fully active, is part of why these small moments carry a weight they did not carry before. The body, given enough time, returns to a baseline of perception that the modern over-stimulated nervous system has spent its life forgetting.

These are the days that make the fast worth the suffering of the first two weeks. They are not the goal of the fast — the parasites and the cleared layers are the goal — but they are the territory the goal opens into. Most people who complete a long fast describe these days as among the most important of their lives. Not because of euphoria. Because of contact. Contact with what they had been carrying. Contact with what they had been missing.

* * *

Days 26 to 40

The deepest territory of the fast is also the territory of its limits.

The body that has now been without food for nearly a month is doing things almost no human body in the modern world ever does. The depth of autophagy is unprecedented. The microbiome has been substantially restructured. The intestinal lining, fueled by ketones and L-glutamine for weeks, has rebuilt itself in ways that no shorter intervention could have produced. Inflammation markers have fallen to levels most fasters have never recorded in their adult life. Insulin sensitivity, growth hormone, mitochondrial efficiency — every metric of metabolic health is operating in a regime the modern diet has made nearly impossible to access.

And there are limits. Chapter 8 described what the protocol cannot reach. Those limits remain real. There are organisms in tissues that herbal pressure does not penetrate. There are damages that cannot be repaired in any single fast. There are layers — the inherited layer, the deepest layer, the layer of what your body received from before you — that this fast was not designed to address and should not try to. The wisdom of these days is not pushing for what the body cannot reach. It is letting the body do what it can do, while it is doing it, and trusting that what cannot be done now will be available to be done later, in another fast, in another year, in a body that has had the time between to integrate what this one accomplished.

The honest physical experience of these days is more demanding than the third week. You may notice fatigue you had not had earlier. You may sleep more. You may feel cold more easily. You may have less stamina for the things you could still do at day twenty. The body is still in a healing regime, but the body is also genuinely depleted of certain reserves that no fast can replace. This is the territory where the difference between a twenty-eight-day fast and a forty-day fast is not a small one. The body knows its own limit. Listening to that limit is part of the work. The author of this book has guided people through fasts of forty days. He has also ended fasts at thirty days, at thirty-five days, at thirty-eight days, when the body said it was done. The number on the calendar is not the goal. The completion of the work is the goal.

The emotional landscape of these days is often quieter than the third week's. The big surfacing has happened. What remains is integration. The patterns that became visible in the deep work are now becoming familiar. The version of you that has emerged through the fast is becoming the version of you you are. There is, in many fasters, a quality of acceptance during these final days that is different from the contact of the third week. The contact was the encounter. The acceptance is the absorption of what the encounter showed.

* * *

Refeeding

How you end the fast matters more than most fasters realize before they have ended one badly. The body that has been without food for thirty or forty days has adapted at every level to the absence of incoming nutrients. The digestive tract has reduced its enzyme production. The pancreas has reduced its insulin output. The gut microbiome has restructured itself to the conditions of the fast. To reintroduce food carelessly is to ask all of these systems to surge back into operation simultaneously, and it can produce — in extreme cases — the cascade known as refeeding syndrome, which can be life-threatening.

The refeeding chapters of this book describe the protocol in detail. What is worth noting here, in the synthesis, is that refeeding is not a separate event from the fast. It is part of the fast. The fast is not over until the body has been carefully returned to ordinary food. The first day of refeeding is bone broth in small amounts. The second day adds simple cooked vegetables. The third day adds proteins in carefully measured portions. The full return to a normal diet takes as many days as the fast itself was long, and during these days the body is doing work that is as important as anything that happened during the fast.

The emotional dimension of refeeding is its own territory. The first taste of real food after weeks of fasting is, for most people, an experience of intensity that no ordinary meal will ever match. A piece of cooked apple. A spoonful of bone broth with vegetables. A small portion of something simple. The flavor is not the flavor of food. It is the flavor of a body remembering food. Most fasters cry at this first meal. Many describe it as one of the most emotionally significant moments of their lives.

What you are returning to is not the same food culture you left. The bread that was bread before the fast tastes different now. The wine that was wine tastes louder. The processed foods that you ate without thinking are revealed as flavors your body experienced as assault but had been silent about. Many people, after a long fast, find that their relationship to food has shifted in ways that persist for years — some foods become unappetizing, some become precious, the emotional weight of meals changes. This is not a side effect of the fast. It is one of the things the fast was for.

* * *

After

The body that emerges from a successful prolonged fast is a different body, and is also the same body.

Different in the ways the chapters of this book have described. Cleared of layers that had accumulated for decades. Hosting a microbiome substantially closer to what it was before the modern diet disrupted it. Carrying an intestinal lining that has rebuilt itself. Operating with metabolic flexibility that had been trained out of it. Free, in many cases, of parasitic burdens that had been carried since childhood without ever being known.

Same in ways that are also worth naming. You are still you. The fast is not a transformation in the sense of becoming a different person. It is a clearing. The person you were under the layers is still the person you are. What has changed is how much of the layered material you are still carrying. The accumulated weight of ordinary life — the foods, the stresses, the small chronic burdens — has been temporarily lifted, and what remains is a clearer view of the person who was always there.

What you carry forward, beyond the cleared body, is an understanding. You know now what your body can do, given the right conditions. You know what hunger actually is. You know what real clarity feels like. You know what your relationship to food has been and what it could be. You know how much of your life had been organized around food and what life is like when it is briefly not. You know, in your body rather than in your mind, what the protocol you completed actually accomplished.

This understanding is the most durable thing the fast gives you. The cleared layers will accumulate again, slowly, across the years that follow. New exposures will arrive. New stresses will deposit their residues. The body that completed the fast will, over time, become a body that needs another fast. This is not failure. It is the nature of bodies in time. The first fast is not the only fast. It is the fast that taught you what fasting is and what it is for. The fasts that follow will be entered with a knowledge that the first fast did not have.

* * *

Why It Works

The synthesis the chapter title promised, in one paragraph, is this. The prolonged water fast works because every system the previous chapters described converges in a single sustained metabolic state that no shorter intervention can produce. The parasites lose their food supply at the same time the herbs reach them through a less obstructed gut, the same time the biofilms thin under sustained pressure, the same time the immune system is freed from its other work, the same time the gut lining is given the fuel and the time to rebuild itself, the same time the brain operates on a fuel that reduces inflammation rather than producing it, the same time the endocannabinoid system reaches a regulatory state that supports healing across every other system, the same time autophagy reaches the depth that allows cellular repair the body cannot do during ordinary life. None of these processes work alone. All of them work together. And the duration is what allows the deepest layers — the ones laid down across decades — to surface and clear in conditions that no shorter cleanse can sustain long enough to reach them.

The reason this protocol takes weeks rather than days is not that the work is slow. The work is fast, when the conditions are right. The reason is that the conditions take time to establish. The body must reach the metabolic state, must hold it, must reach the deeper state, must hold that, must reach the deepest state, must hold that, and only then can the layered material that has been accumulating for decades surface and be released. A three-day cleanse cannot reach this. A seven-day cleanse cannot reach this. Twenty-five days, thirty days, forty days — these are not arbitrary numbers. They are the durations the body needs to do what the body is capable of doing.

And this is also why the fast is honest about what it asks. It asks for the first thirty-six hours of hunger. It asks for the second-week trough. It asks for the social isolation, the boredom, the surfacing of what had been buried, the willingness to sit through stretches that do not feel like progress. None of this is incidental to the work. All of it is the work. The fast is not the suspension of life so that healing can happen. The fast is the form healing takes in a body that has been carrying what it has been carrying for as long as it has been carrying it.

What you have read in this chapter is one body's forty days. The fast you do, if you do one, will be your own. The biology will be the biology. The story will be yours.

This chapter contains no figures. The work it describes is happening inside a body that no figure could show.

Chapter 13

Trace Minerals, Hydration & Electrolytes

* * *

Water is life. But water alone, during a prolonged fast, is not enough. In fact, water alone — without what belongs alongside it — can quietly become dangerous.

The paradox seems counterintuitive at first. You are fasting. You are drinking water. Water is clean and pure and simple. More water must mean more cleansing. More water must mean better hydration. The body must be grateful for every additional glass that arrives.

It isn't, exactly. Drinking large amounts of pure water without adequate minerals does not cleanse more effectively. It depletes. The mechanism is simple, and once you understand it, the entire structure of the daily protocol stops feeling like overcaution and starts feeling like the careful balancing act it actually is.

What Water Actually Does in the Body

Water is the medium through which every biological process occurs. Nutrients dissolve in it and travel through it. Waste products dissolve in it and are eliminated through it. Electrical signals in the nervous system travel through it. Temperature is regulated through it. Every chemical reaction in every cell occurs in its presence.

But water does not work alone. For water to move correctly through the body — into cells, out of cells, through the kidneys, across membranes — it needs **electrolytes**. Electrolytes are minerals that carry an electrical charge when dissolved in water, and without them, water cannot do its job. With inadequate electrolytes present, water actually draws minerals out of cells through osmosis as it passes through. The water that should have been hydrating the body is instead, in this state, leaching the body of what little mineral content remains.

During a prolonged fast, where you are consuming water continuously and eating nothing, this mineral loss becomes critical. The pinch of salt in every glass is not a flavor adjustment. It is what makes the water functional rather than depleting.

The Electrolytes

Six electrolytes deserve specific attention during prolonged fasting. Each has its own role and its own consequences when it falls short.

Sodium — the primary regulator of fluid balance.

• Controls how much water stays in the bloodstream versus enters cells.

• Maintains blood pressure and blood volume.

• Essential for nerve signal transmission.

• The first electrolyte to become depleted during water fasting.

• Depletion causes headaches, dizziness, nausea, muscle weakness, confusion.

• Severe depletion — **hyponatremia** — can cause seizures and be life-threatening.

Water treated with ionic sulfated minerals, with a pinch of Himalayan salt in every glass, is not optional during a prolonged fast. It is the single most important mineral intervention you can make.

Potassium — the cellular electrolyte.

• Primary electrolyte inside cells; works in partnership with sodium outside cells.

• Essential for **cardiac rhythm** — the heart's electrical system depends on potassium.

• Regulates muscle contraction, including the heart muscle.

• Supports nerve function throughout the body.

• Depletion causes muscle cramps, weakness, heart palpitations, fatigue.

• Severe depletion — **cardiac arrhythmia** — is one of the most serious risks of prolonged fasting.

Magnesium — the master mineral.

• Required for over **600** enzymatic reactions in the body.

• Regulates both sodium and potassium transport.

• Essential for nerve function, muscle relaxation, and sleep.

• Supports the detoxification work of the liver.

• Depleted rapidly by stress, fasting, and enemas.

• Depletion causes muscle cramps, insomnia, anxiety, headaches, constipation.

• One of the most commonly deficient minerals even before fasting begins.

Calcium — the structural and signaling mineral.

• Beyond its role in bone health, calcium is essential for cellular signaling.

• Required for muscle contraction, including the heart.

• Works intimately with magnesium — the two must be balanced.

• Depletion during fasting contributes to muscle cramping and nervous system dysregulation.

Chloride — the partner of sodium.

• Works alongside sodium to maintain fluid balance.

• Essential component of stomach acid, relevant as digestion resumes during refeeding.

• Transported with sodium — adequate sodium intake generally ensures adequate chloride.

Phosphate — the refeeding mineral.

• Less critical during the fast itself.

• Becomes critically important during refeeding.

• **Refeeding syndrome** — the most dangerous complication of breaking a prolonged fast — is primarily driven by a sudden drop in phosphate.

• Understanding phosphate is essential for the refeeding chapters that follow.

Trace Minerals — Beyond Electrolytes

Electrolytes are the minerals needed in larger amounts. Trace minerals are needed in smaller amounts, but their importance is equally large. Trace minerals are coenzymes — the partners that activate enzymes throughout the body. Without them, the enzyme system that does the entire chemistry of being alive simply does not work.

During a prolonged fast, the trace mineral picture is challenging. You are consuming no food, therefore consuming no trace minerals through diet. You are drinking water continuously, flushing trace minerals through the kidneys. Every enema removes additional minerals through the colon wall. Every day, the deficit compounds. Without active replenishment, by the end of a long fast, the trace mineral pool would be running on fumes.

The key trace minerals during fasting and what they do:

Mineral

Primary Role During Fast

Zinc

Activates over 300 enzymes; immune function; intestinal lining repair

Selenium

Antioxidant enzyme activation; thyroid function; immune defense

Manganese

Protects intestinal cells from oxidative damage

Chromium

Blood sugar regulation; increasingly important as ketosis deepens

Molybdenum

Detoxification enzyme activation; critical as toxins mobilize

Iodine

Thyroid function; metabolic rate regulation

Copper

Energy production enzymes; iron metabolism

Silica

Connective tissue repair; intestinal lining integrity

A daily trace mineral solution — the kind that comes in concentrated drops added to water — is the single simplest way to keep this pool replenished without overcomplicating the protocol.

The Enema Factor

Every enema removes minerals. This is unavoidable, and it is not a reason to stop doing enemas. It is a reason to replenish consistently, on a schedule that matches the timing of the enemas themselves.

What each enema removes:

- Sodium and chloride, carried out with the water.
- Potassium, from intestinal secretions.
- Magnesium, particularly with plain water enemas.
- Trace minerals, in smaller amounts.

The replenishment window:

• Replenish within **30 minutes** of each enema.

• Do not wait until you feel symptoms — by then, depletion is already affecting you.

• Make replenishment as automatic as the enema itself. The two practices belong together.

This is why the daily protocol has mineral water immediately following each enema rather than at some later point. The timing is not arbitrary. It is matched to the rate at which the enemas remove what the minerals replace.

What Depletion Looks Like

Learning to read depletion signals early prevents them from becoming serious. The body announces mineral depletion in stages, and someone who can recognize the early stages can intervene before the later ones develop.

Early signals — easy to miss:

• Mild headache.

• Slight dizziness on standing.

• Muscle twitching, particularly in calves or eyelids.

• Mild fatigue increase beyond baseline fasting tiredness.

• Slight mood dip.

Moderate signals — take action now:

• Significant headache.

• Pronounced dizziness and lightheadedness.

• Muscle cramps, particularly in legs, feet, or hands.

• Heart palpitations — any awareness of your heartbeat is a signal worth heeding.

• Nausea outside the usual fasting pattern.

• Confusion or difficulty concentrating beyond normal fasting fog.

Serious signals — medical attention required:

• Severe muscle weakness.

• Irregular heartbeat.

• Confusion or disorientation.

• Inability to stand without significant dizziness.

• Severe nausea or vomiting.

• Any chest discomfort.

Discomfort is part of fasting. Depletion is not. Knowing the difference between the two — and acting on the signals before they progress — is one of the most important practical skills the prolonged faster develops.

The Complete Hydration Protocol

Here is exactly what to do, from waking to sleeping.

Time

Action

Waking

16 oz water treated with ionic sulfated minerals + Himalayan salt

Mid-morning

16 oz mineralized water

After morning enema

16 oz water + trace minerals immediately

Midday

8 oz coconut water or mineralized water + second trace minerals dose

Afternoon

16 oz mineralized water

After evening enema

16 oz water + trace minerals immediately

Evening

Epsom salt bath for transdermal magnesium

Before sleep

8 oz mineralized water + magnesium glycinate

Daily total: Minimum **96 to 128 oz** of fluid daily, all mineralized. More in warm weather or if sweating.

If lightheadedness occurs at any point, an additional pinch of salt in water immediately, before any other intervention. Salt is the fastest correction available.

(Figure 14.3 — see the online Figure Guide)

Water Quality Matters

Not all water is equal during a prolonged fast. The water you choose to use as the foundation of three months of consumption — preparation, fast, and refeeding combined — deserves attention.

Best options:

• **Reverse osmosis with remineralization.** Removes contaminants completely, then remineralization adds back beneficial minerals. The cleanest possible starting point with mineral support built in.

• **High-quality spring water.** Naturally contains trace minerals. Verify the source is tested and clean. Avoid plastic bottles where possible — plastics leach compounds during extended storage.

• **Filtered tap water.** Carbon filtration removes chlorine and many contaminants but does not remove all minerals or all contaminants. Acceptable with good filtration; add trace minerals.

Use with caution:

• **Distilled water.** Completely pure, stripped of all minerals. Without consistent mineral addition, can actually draw minerals from the body. If using distilled, trace mineral addition is absolutely non-negotiable.

• **Unfiltered tap water.** Chlorine directly harms beneficial bacteria, which is relevant even during fasting. May contain contaminants that add to the toxic burden you are trying to clear. Avoid where possible.

(Figure 14.1 — see the online Figure Guide)

Ionic Sulfated Minerals — The Recommended Base

Among the various forms in which trace minerals are sold for use in drinking water, the form recommended throughout this book is the ionic sulfated form. Where the prose says 'water treated with ionic sulfated minerals,' this is what is meant: a concentrated mineral solution, added by drops to drinking water, in which the minerals are present in their ionic state and bound with sulfate. The ionic sulfated form is more bioavailable than mineral sources sourced from sea-bed deposits. Sea-bed mineral products, sometimes called fulvic mineral solutions or ancient sea mineral concentrates, hold real value as supplementary mineral sources, but the ionic form moves into cells more readily and supports the kind of fast-and-recovery work this book describes more directly than the sea-bed sources do.

The recommendation is to use ionic sulfated minerals as the primary water treatment for all drinking water during the prep year and the fast itself, and as the base water for all enemas — with Himalayan sea salt added on top, at the prescribed concentration, for the evening salt water enema. The dose of mineral concentrate per glass of water is small — typically a few drops, the precise amount listed on the product instructions — and the taste of the water remains essentially unchanged. The body, however, receives a profile of trace minerals it would otherwise be running short of, throughout the duration of the fast.

Specific product recommendations and the precise dose ratios for drinking water and for the higher-concentration enema use are listed in the supplemental resources QR code at the back of this book.

For practitioners who prefer a light flavor with their drinking water, zero-sugar electrolyte packets containing the six essential minerals — typically sold in packets of six servings — are an acceptable alternative to plain Himalayan salt. The packets do not replace the ionic sulfated mineral concentrate, which remains the primary water treatment, but they can replace or supplement the Himalayan salt addition for those who find plain mineralized water difficult to drink in the volumes a prolonged fast requires. Specific products are listed in the supplemental resources QR code at the back of this book.

Himalayan Salt and Why It Matters

Not all salt is the same. The choice of salt during prolonged fasting is small but worth getting right.

Himalayan pink salt contains:

- Sodium chloride, the primary electrolyte.
- Up to **84 trace minerals** in small amounts, including many on the trace mineral list above.
- A naturally balanced mineral profile.
- No additives or anti-caking agents.

Table salt is primarily sodium chloride only, with trace minerals removed in processing and additives sometimes included. Not the preferred choice during fasting.

Celtic sea salt has a similar mineral profile to Himalayan and is a good alternative if Himalayan is unavailable. Higher moisture content means slightly different texture, but functionally similar.

The difference between these salts is not dramatic in any single glass of water, but during a prolonged fast where trace minerals are already depleted, every source of natural mineral diversity matters. Choose accordingly.

Coconut Water — Nature's Electrolyte Drink

When available, coconut water is one of the most valuable additions to the fasting hydration protocol. Natural coconut water contains:

- **Potassium**, in one of the richest natural concentrations available.
- **Sodium**, in natural balanced ratio with potassium.
- **Magnesium**, in smaller but meaningful amounts.
- **Calcium**, supporting cardiac and muscle function.
- **Natural enzymes**, supporting the body's enzyme systems.

Small amounts — 4 to 8 oz, once or twice daily — provide meaningful electrolyte support without significantly affecting the fasting state. The sugar content is low enough that ketosis is not interrupted, and the mineral content is high enough that the daily potassium burden is substantially eased.

The Epsom Salt Bath

Epsom salt is magnesium sulfate, and it has a quiet usefulness during a prolonged fast that has nothing to do with what happens in the digestive tract. The skin will absorb what the gut cannot afford to process.

The transdermal route:

- Magnesium passes through the skin directly into circulation.
- One of the most effective ways to replenish magnesium during fasting.
- Bypasses the digestive system entirely, which matters when digestion is paused.
- A 20-minute bath in 2 cups of Epsom salt in warm water provides meaningful magnesium replenishment.
- Particularly valuable in the evening, since magnesium supports sleep quality and overnight repair.

(Figure 14.2 — see the online Figure Guide)

Recognizing Adequate Hydration

How do you know you are getting this right? The body sends clear signals when the hydration and mineral protocol is working, and equally clear signals when it is not.

Signs of good hydration and mineral balance:

- Urine is pale yellow — not clear and not dark.
- Energy is consistent with the fasting baseline, not dropping unexpectedly.

• Muscle function feels stable — no cramping.

• Heart rhythm feels steady and calm.

• Mental clarity is at its fasting baseline.

• Lightheadedness on standing is mild and brief, resolving within seconds.

Signs that something needs attention:

• Urine is very dark — increase water immediately.

• Urine is completely clear — add more minerals.

• Persistent headache — add sodium.

• Muscle cramping — add magnesium and potassium.

• Heart awareness — add potassium; seek medical attention if it persists.

• Confusion — add sodium and seek medical attention if it does not quickly resolve.

The body, well-attended, will not let you fail in this area. The body, ignored, can deteriorate faster than the person fasting expects.

The Bottom Line

Your fast runs on water. Your water runs on minerals. Your minerals make everything else possible. Get this right and everything else is supported. Neglect it and nothing else can fully work.

The most sophisticated herbal protocol in the world cannot compensate for a depleted mineral foundation. The most carefully timed enema schedule cannot function optimally without adequate electrolytes. The deepest ketosis produces its most lasting benefits in a body that is properly mineralized.

Trace minerals are not a detail. They are the foundation beneath the foundation. The body that completes a forty-day fast in good condition is, almost without exception, a body that has been mineralized consistently and carefully throughout. The body that struggles or fails is, almost without exception, a body whose minerals were neglected or improvised. The choice is yours to make, every day, and the small daily discipline pays returns that compound across the duration of the work.

*Figures referenced above: 14.1–14.3 **(online Figure Guide)*

Chapter 14

Feeding the Brain During Fasting

* * *

Say it clearly from the start: the goal is never to fast as long as possible. The goal is to fast as efficiently as possible — and get out as soon as the work is done.

Most people think about prolonged fasting the wrong way. They imagine it as a kind of endurance test. A measure of willpower. A demonstration of how long the human body can be made to go without food. That is not what this is.

This protocol is a precision intervention, designed to accomplish specific biological goals in the shortest possible time. To clear accumulated layers. To eliminate parasitic load. To reset the microbiome. To heal the intestinal lining. To recalibrate the immune system. Every element of the protocol — the herbs, the enemas, the coffee, the clove oil, the additions described here — exists for one reason. To get the work done faster, so you can get out sooner, so you can begin rebuilding sooner.

The rebuilding is not what comes after the fast. The rebuilding begins the moment the conditions allow it.

Two Modes of Fasting

Not all fasting is the same. The protocol you are running uses two different modes, applied at different stages of the work, each suited to the particular biology of that stage.

Complete water fasting:

- Nothing but water and minerals.
- Maximum metabolic pressure on parasites and accumulated material.
- Maximum autophagic activity.
- Appropriate for the deepest cleansing phases.

Modified fasting:

- Small strategic additions — specific fats, specific nutrients.
- Maintains the core benefits of fasting.
- Begins nourishing the body, particularly the brain, without interrupting the cleanse.

• The intelligent bridge between complete fasting and refeeding.

The goal of this protocol is to move from complete fasting to modified fasting as soon as the biological conditions support it. Not to remain in complete fasting longer than necessary. The shift from one mode to the other is not a failure of will. It is the next stage of the protocol, applied at the moment the work is ready for it.

Why the Brain Needs Specific Attention

During a prolonged fast, the brain faces a unique challenge. Every other organ in the body can run directly on fat for fuel. The brain cannot.

The brain requires either glucose, which is unavailable during fasting, or ketones, which the liver produces from fat. During the transition into ketosis, the brain is adapting — shifting its metabolic machinery from one fuel system to another. This transition takes 2 to 4 days, and produces the cognitive symptoms most associated with early fasting:

• Brain fog.

• Difficulty concentrating.

• Mood instability.

• Headaches.

• Fatigue.

These symptoms are not signs that fasting is harming the brain. They are signs that the brain is changing its fuel source. Once ketosis is established, the symptoms resolve, and what replaces them — for most people — is a quality of mental clarity that is genuinely striking. The molecular shift has been laid out earlier; what follows is how to support it practically.

The transition must be supported. Once through it, the brain must be kept adequately fueled. This is not optional. The brain in deep fasting is doing some of the most consequential work of the entire protocol, and it does that work better when properly fueled than when running on fumes.

MCT Oil and Coconut Oil

Medium-chain triglycerides are unlike any other fat. Most dietary fats follow a long route to becoming energy — absorbed through the lymphatic system, transported through the bloodstream, stored or slowly released for fuel. MCTs take a shortcut:

• Absorbed **directly into the portal vein**.

• Travel immediately to the liver.

• Converted to ketones **within minutes**.

• Ketones cross the blood-brain barrier and reach neurons almost immediately.

From consumption to brain fuel, MCTs work faster than any other dietary fat. Coconut oil is approximately 65% MCT by composition, making it the most accessible and practical natural MCT source available. Pure MCT oil — refined from coconut or palm kernel oil — is even more concentrated and produces ketones more rapidly. Both are valuable. The choice between them is mostly one of preference and budget.

Does Adding Fat Break the Fast?

The honest answer requires nuance.

What adding small amounts of fat does:

• Provides ketone substrate, supporting brain function.

• Does not significantly raise insulin, the primary driver of metabolic shutdown.

• Does not halt autophagy at therapeutic doses.

• Does not reactivate the digestive system in a way that interrupts cleansing.

• Does not provide food for parasites, which require carbohydrates and proteins.

• Does not interrupt the migrating motor complex at small doses.

What adding small amounts of fat does not do:

• It does not constitute eating in any meaningful metabolic sense.

• It does not interrupt the core mechanisms that make prolonged fasting therapeutic.

A teaspoon of coconut oil or MCT oil is not a meal. It is a targeted neurological intervention. The dose is what matters here, and the threshold is reasonably well-established:

• Under **1 tablespoon** of pure fat — minimal metabolic disruption.

• Over **1 tablespoon** — begins to have more meaningful metabolic effects.

• The goal is the minimum effective dose — enough to support the brain, not enough to interrupt the cleanse.

When to Introduce MCT Support

Timing is everything. The wrong time to introduce fat is during the early transition, before ketosis has fully established. The right time is once the body has committed to fat metabolism on its own.

Days 1 to 3 — complete water fast.

• No fat additions during this phase.

• The metabolic shift into ketosis must happen without assistance.

• The body needs to fully deplete glucose stores and commit to fat metabolism.

• Adding fat here actually slows the transition.

Days 4 onward — once ketosis is established.

Signs of established ketosis:

• Sweet or fruity breath as acetone exhales.

• Reduced hunger as ketones suppress appetite signals.

• Beginning of mental clarity returning.

• Urine ketone strips showing positive reading.

Once these signs appear, small MCT or coconut oil additions are appropriate.

The progressive approach:

Days

Amount

Frequency

4 to 5

Half teaspoon MCT or coconut oil

Once daily, in warm water

6 to 10

1 teaspoon

Once or twice daily as tolerated

10 onward

Up to 1 tablespoon daily

Divided into 2 to 3 small doses

The Shift to Modified Fasting

As the cleansing protocol progresses — as parasite die-off cycles complete, as enema returns clarify, as body signals indicate that the deepest work is being done — the fast can begin transitioning from complete to modified.

The signs that modified fasting is appropriate:

• Enema returns becoming consistently cleaner.

• Gas and gurgling signals becoming less frequent and less urgent.

• Mental clarity reaching a sustained plateau.

• Energy stabilizing at a higher baseline.

• Tongue clearing and becoming pinker.

• Body odor neutralizing.

• The body's signals shifting from active cleansing to a quieter state.

Modified fasting looks like:

• Continued water and mineral protocol — unchanged.

• Continued herbal tincture protocol — unchanged.

• Continued enema protocol — unchanged.

• Small additions of:

• Coconut oil or MCT oil for brain fuel.

• Trace minerals and salt water for mineral and electrolyte support.

• Small amounts of fresh vegetable juice for gentle nutrient introduction.

• Ghee in warm water for butyrate to support intestinal lining.

None of these additions interrupt the cleansing work. All of them begin the rebuilding work. This is the intelligent fast. Not endurance. Efficiency.

Ghee — The Gut's First Rebuilding Food

Ghee deserves special mention. As the fast begins transitioning toward modified fasting, ghee is one of the first and most valuable additions you can make.

Why ghee specifically:

• Milk solids and lactose completely removed, leaving pure fat.

- Rich in **butyrate**, the primary fuel for intestinal lining cells.
- Butyrate begins rebuilding and strengthening tight junctions.
- Gentle on the liver, unlike many other fats.
- Stimulates bile production gently, beginning to reactivate bile flow.
- Contains fat-soluble vitamins — A, D, E, and K — that have been depleted during fasting.

The critical distinction:

- Ghee does not feed parasites.
- Ghee does not interrupt autophagy at small doses.
- Ghee does not significantly reactivate the digestive insulin response.
- Ghee begins the intestinal healing process from the inside.

Introduction protocol:

- Half teaspoon in warm water.
- Begin only when enema returns are showing consistent improvement.
- Increase to 1 teaspoon after 2 to 3 days if tolerating well.
- Watch for nausea — the gallbladder is reactivating, and too much too soon causes discomfort.

The Brain During Modified Fasting

As the fast shifts to modified, what happens cognitively? The mental clarity of deep ketosis — the quality already described — does not disappear with small fat additions. In fact, properly supported, it deepens.

Consistent ketone supply removes the fluctuations that can occur in pure water fasting. The brain receives steady fuel rather than the occasional dips that come with ketone variability. The addition of butyrate from ghee supports the gut-brain axis, the enteric nervous system, which influences cognitive function in ways that the brain in the head cannot fully replace. Mental clarity becomes not just present but stable and reliable.

This is the cognitive state in which the deepest insights of the fasting experience tend to arrive. Not in the fluctuating peaks of pure water fasting, where moments of clarity alternate with periods of fog. But in the steady clarity of an intelligently supported modified fast, where the conditions for sustained reflection have been created and maintained.

Cannabinoids and Brain Support

The endocannabinoid system support discussed in Chapter 10 becomes even more relevant during the modified fasting phase. As the fast shifts toward modified:

- **CBD** continues supporting anti-inflammatory processes as die-off completes.
- **CBG** begins its most important work — intestinal stem cell regeneration — as conditions improve.
- **Coconut oil as a carrier** for cannabinoids enhances their bioavailability. Fat-soluble compounds absorb better in the presence of fat.
- The combination of ketones and cannabinoids maintains the neurological state that makes the fasting experience so distinctive.

Taking CBD in coconut oil during the modified fasting phase gives you brain fuel and endocannabinoid system support simultaneously. One simple addition serving two critical functions.

The Mindset of the Intelligent Fast

Return to the principle stated at the start. You are not here to see how long you can endure. You are here to do five specific things:

1. Create the conditions that allow deep cleansing to occur.

2. Support that process with every available tool, to make it faster and more thorough.

3. Recognize when the conditions indicate the deepest work is done.

4. Begin rebuilding as soon as those conditions are met.

5. Exit the fast as soon as the work justifies it — not before, not a day longer than necessary.

The person who fasts intelligently for 25 days achieves more than the person who endures blindly for 40. The herbs accelerate the timeline. The enemas accelerate the timeline. The coffee enemas accelerate the timeline. The clove oil accelerates the timeline. The MCT and ghee additions accelerate the rebuilding. Everything in this protocol exists to compress the timeline. To get the work done. To get you out. To get you rebuilding. As fast as biology allows.

Daily Reference for Brain Support

Phase

Brain Support

Amount

Timing

Days 1 to 3

None — transition phase

—

—

Days 4 to 7

MCT or coconut oil

Half teaspoon

Once daily, morning

Days 8 to 14

MCT or coconut oil

1 teaspoon

Twice daily

Days 15 onward

MCT or coconut oil + ghee when signals indicate

1 teaspoon MCT + half teaspoon ghee in warm water

2 to 3 times daily

Modified fasting

MCT + ghee in warm water

As tolerated

Throughout day

(Figure 15.1 — see the online Figure Guide)

The Goal Said Simply

You are working toward a body that has been thoroughly cleansed. You are working toward a gut that has been genuinely renewed. You are working toward a microbiome ready to be rebuilt. And you want to get there as efficiently as possible.

Because what waits on the other side — the rebuilding, the refeeding, the renewal — is not the consolation prize after the fast. It is the destination the fast was always preparing you for.

*Figures referenced above: 15.1 **(online Figure Guide)*

Chapter 15

Reading Your Body's Signals

* * *

Your body has been speaking to you your whole life. Most of the time, drowned out by food and distraction and the constant noise of ordinary living, its voice was hard to hear. During a prolonged fast, that voice becomes unmistakable. This chapter teaches you how to listen.

Most people approach fasting by following a schedule. Day 1, do this. Day 14, do that. Day 30, do the other thing. Schedules are useful as starting points, but they are not what guides a thoughtful fast. The body does not follow a calendar. It follows its own intelligence. Your enema today is not driven primarily by what day of the fast it is. It is driven by what your body is telling you needs to happen today. Your decision to add ghee, to extend the fast, to begin breaking the fast — none of these should be made primarily by the calendar. They should be made by reading the signals your body is sending.

The body speaks through many channels simultaneously. Learning to read all of them gives you a complete picture. Reading only one or two means missing critical information. The major categories of signal you will work with throughout the fast are these:

- **Digestive signals** — gas, bloating, gurgling, pressure, nausea.
- **Energy signals** — fatigue patterns, energy fluctuations, sustained levels.
- **Mental signals** — clarity, fog, mood, emotional states.
- **Physical signals** — body temperature, lightheadedness, muscle function.
- **Sensory signals** — body odor, breath, tongue coating, skin changes.
- **Enema return signals** — what your body releases tells you what is happening inside.
- **Sleep signals** — quality, duration, dream activity.

Each channel carries unique information. Together they form a complete language. The chapter that follows is essentially a dictionary for that language, organized by category.

Digestive Signals

The most common signals during fasting come from the digestive system itself, and they are also the most informative for guiding daily decisions about enemas, herbs, and rest.

Gas and bloating. What it means depends on the pattern.

• *Building gas pressure with no food in the system:* Material in the intestinal walls is loosening and fermenting. Old layers releasing gas as they break down. A clear signal that an enema would help release the pressure. Often accompanied by visible abdominal distension.

• *Sudden gas release after a quiet period:* A new layer has just released. Often follows a period of no signals. May be accompanied by relief and lightness afterward.

• *Persistent low-grade bloating:* Ongoing fermentation activity from candida or biofilm breakdown. May indicate the herbal protocol is doing meaningful work. Often accompanies the deepest die-off phases.

Gurgling sounds. Audible intestinal movement.

• Indicates active peristalsis or migrating motor complex activity.

• Material is shifting through the small intestine.

• Generally a positive sign — the gut is working.

• Sudden loud gurgling may indicate a layer has just detached and is moving.

• Combined with abdominal pressure, often signals readiness for an enema.

Nausea. One of the most important signals to learn to interpret.

• *Mild nausea without other symptoms:* Often indicates **toxin reabsorption** — die-off material being reabsorbed from the colon back into the bloodstream. An enema relieves this nausea quickly by removing the source. A clear signal that the body is asking for clearing.

• *Nausea with headache:* Suggests significant toxin load. The combination indicates aggressive die-off or layer release. Coffee enema is particularly helpful — it supports the liver in processing the toxic load.

• *Nausea with anxiety or panic:* May indicate electrolyte depletion. Add minerals immediately. If it does not resolve within 30 minutes, seek medical attention.

Acid reflux and burping. These signals come from upper digestive tract activity.

• Burping during fasting often indicates upper intestinal gas working its way up.

• Acid reflux sensation suggests gas pressure from the small intestine pushing upward.

• Both signal a need to release pressure downward.

• An enema typically resolves the upward pressure by clearing the downward path.

Energy Signals

Each day during fasting has a characteristic energy pattern. Once you learn it, departures from the pattern become informative in their own right.

The typical pattern in established fasting:

- *Wake:* energy moderate, mind clear.
- *Mid-morning:* energy good, often peak mental clarity window.
- *Midday:* natural slight dip, common to all human metabolism.
- *Afternoon:* energy returns, often a productive period.
- *Evening:* natural wind-down, deeper relaxation than usual.
- *Night:* sleep arrives easily, often deeper than baseline.

Disruptions to this pattern signal something:

- *Sudden fatigue without clear reason:* often indicates active layer release. Toxic load increasing in the bloodstream temporarily. Body directing resources toward processing the release. Rest, hydrate, and listen — likely an enema is needed.

- *Sustained fatigue beyond normal:* may indicate electrolyte depletion. Could indicate insufficient mineral replenishment after enemas. Add trace minerals and salt; assess in 30 to 60 minutes.

- *Energy spike followed by crash:* often related to mineral fluctuations. Stabilize mineral intake by making it consistent throughout the day rather than concentrated at certain times.

- *Persistent low energy with mental clarity intact:* may indicate the body is in deep repair mode. Cellular renewal and tissue rebuilding consume significant resources. Often resolves naturally as the repair phase completes.

Mental Signals

The quality of your thinking is one of the most reliable indicators of where you are in the fast. The brain in deep ketosis communicates clearly when it is operating well, and equally clearly when something has shifted.

Mental clarity:

- *Sharpening clarity:* indicates ketosis is well established. The brain is running efficiently on ketones. A signal that the protocol is working. Use this clarity — it is one of the gifts of the fast.

- *Returning fog after a period of clarity:* almost always indicates a new toxin release. Layer breakdown is sending material into circulation. The fog is temporary, often resolving within hours. Hydrate, rest, and consider whether an enema is needed.

• *Persistent fog beyond the first week:* may indicate inadequate ketone production. Consider increasing MCT or coconut oil support. Could indicate insufficient mineral intake, particularly magnesium. Address mineralization before assuming the fog is normal.

Mood signals:

• *Sudden irritability:* often indicates blood sugar dropping or electrolyte depletion. Address minerals first before assuming psychological cause.

• *Unexpected sadness or grief:* emotional layers releasing, often without identifiable cause. The gut is releasing what was stored. Allow the emotion to move through without analysis. These releases are part of the cleansing, not interruptions to it.

• *Anxiety:* mild anxiety can indicate electrolyte issues. Persistent anxiety may indicate the negotiating mind from Chapter 26. Severe anxiety, particularly with physical symptoms, requires attention to minerals first and medical attention if not resolving.

• *Unexpected joy or peace:* often arrives in the deeper phases of fasting. Endocannabinoid system activation, ketosis, and cellular renewal converging. These states carry insights — capture them in writing while present.

Physical Signals

Body temperature. The fasting body runs cooler.

• Metabolic rate adjusts downward, particularly after week one.

• Cold hands and feet are normal during prolonged fasting.

• Wear layers; keep warm; do not underestimate this.

• Sudden warmth or fever-like sensations often indicate die-off — the immune system actively engaged.

• Persistent fever requires medical attention; distinguish carefully from die-off warmth.

Lightheadedness. The brain is asking for something — minerals, glucose, blood pressure, time. The severity tells you what:

• Mild lightheadedness on standing — common, usually indicates need for minerals.

• Lightheadedness sitting still — indicates more significant depletion.

• Lightheadedness with confusion — requires immediate attention.

• Lightheadedness with chest discomfort — medical attention.

Most lightheadedness is the body adjusting. Some is the body asking for help.

Muscle function:

• Mild weakness during prolonged fasting is normal, particularly in week one.

• Cramping indicates electrolyte depletion — add magnesium and potassium.

• Twitching often indicates magnesium deficiency.

• Significant weakness that does not resolve with minerals — medical attention.

Sensory Signals

Body odor. One of the most informative external signals.

• Body odor typically intensifies during the first two weeks.

• Indicates active toxin release through the skin.

• Strong odor changes may indicate specific releases — heavy metal mobilization, chemical residue clearing, parasite die-off.

• Body odor neutralizing in later weeks indicates the cleanse approaching completion.

Breath:

• *Sweet, fruity breath* (acetone) — indicates established ketosis.

• *Strong unpleasant breath* — indicates active gut fermentation or die-off.

• *Metallic taste or smell* — may indicate heavy metal mobilization.

• *Sour stomach acid breath* — indicates upper digestive activity.

• Breath neutralizing in later weeks parallels body odor — a clear progress indicator.

Tongue coating. The tongue is a mirror of gut activity.

• A coated tongue indicates active toxin release.

• Coating becoming thicker means more is releasing.

• Coating thinning and clearing indicates the cleanse progressing.

• *Yellow coating* suggests bile duct activity, common during liver fluke clearing.

• *White coating* suggests candida activity.

• A pink, clean tongue indicates the deeper work is largely complete.

(Figure 16.1 — see the online Figure Guide)

Skin. The largest organ of elimination.

• Skin breakouts are common during active die-off, particularly across the back, chest, and forehead.

• Skin sensitivity may temporarily increase.

• Itching can indicate liver-related toxin release.

• Skin clearing and improving indicates the cleanse progressing.

• The final phase often produces a noticeable luminosity — the result of cellular renewal reaching the skin.

Enema Return Signals

Perhaps the most direct visual feedback during the entire protocol. What comes out of the body during the morning and evening enemas tells, with little ambiguity, what work is being done.

Color and composition patterns:

• *Dark brown or black material:* old impacted fecal matter releasing. Common in the first week. Decreasing volume indicates progress.

• *Stringy or rubbery material:* mucoid plaque releasing. Often dark or olive-colored. May appear rope-like. Significant releases indicate deep layer clearance.

• *Green sludge:* bile release, particularly during coffee enemas. Indicates liver and bile duct activity. Increasing green indicates active fluke die-off and biliary clearing. Decreasing green over time indicates clearance progressing.

• *White or yellow stringy material:* often candida and biofilm release. Particularly common during weeks 2 to 3.

• *Small worm-like organisms:* visible parasites being expelled. Document what you see — note size, shape, color. Confirms organisms that were present.

• *Sandy or gritty material:* may indicate biliary sludge or small stones. Common during deep liver clearing phases.

• *Clear water with minimal debris:* indicates the current section is clean. A positive sign in the later weeks. Different from early-fast clear water, which simply indicates surface clearing.

The progression pattern:

Phase

Typical Returns

Week 1

Significant volume, dark material, surface clearing

Week 2

Mucoid material, candida releases, biofilm

Week 3

Older deeper layers, parasitic activity, varied releases

Week 4

Clearer returns with occasional deeper material

Week 5+

Mostly clear with rare debris

Sleep Signals

Sleep patterns during fasting:

• Sleep often becomes deeper in the first two weeks.

• Dreams may become extraordinarily vivid.

• Some people experience reduced sleep need — sleeping less but feeling more rested.

• Others sleep significantly more — the body using rest for cellular repair.

• Both are normal; listen to what your body needs.

Disruptions to sleep:

• Difficulty sleeping often indicates electrolyte depletion, particularly magnesium.

• Waking at consistent times may indicate organ system activity — the liver is typically active 1 to 3 AM in traditional Chinese medicine framing.

• Restless sleep with vivid disturbing dreams may indicate emotional layer release.

Putting It All Together

The skill is not reading any single signal. It is reading them together. Most decisions during the fast are best made on the basis of clusters of signals rather than any single observation, because the body rarely communicates one thing at a time. A typical cluster of signals tells a coherent story when read as a group.

Cluster 1 — Time for an enema:

• Building gas and bloating.

• Audible gurgling.

• Mild nausea.

• Slight headache.

• Sense of fullness or pressure.

The body is asking clearly: release this material.

Cluster 2 — Active die-off in progress:

• Sudden fatigue.

• Brain fog.

• Body odor intensifying.

• Tongue coating thickening.

• Mild flu-like sensations.

The body is processing significant load: support with hydration, minerals, rest.

Cluster 3 — Deep cleanse approaching completion:

• Sustained mental clarity.

• Stable energy.

• Body odor neutralizing.

• Tongue clearing.

• Enema returns consistently cleaner.

• Less frequent gas and gurgling.

The body is signaling that the deepest work is largely done. Modified fasting and gentle introduction of nutrients become appropriate.

The Most Important Signal of All

Above every individual signal, listen for one above all. The signal that something is wrong. Not uncomfortable. Not difficult. Genuinely wrong.

This signal is rarely subtle when it arrives. It carries a quality unlike any other fasting sensation. A sense that something fundamental is off. Symptoms that do not match the patterns described in this chapter. A feeling of genuine alarm rather than discomfort. Physical symptoms that escalate rather than resolve. Any combination of severe symptoms occurring together.

If this signal arrives, stop. Drink water treated with ionic sulfated minerals. Contact your medical support. Do not assume it will pass.

The fast is meant to challenge you. It is not meant to harm you. Knowing the difference is one of the most important skills any faster develops, and it is the skill that protects you from the rare situation that requires intervention.

A Daily Practice

Each evening, take five minutes to document the day's signals. The journal does not need to be elaborate. A simple template, filled in honestly, builds a record that becomes more useful with every entry.

A 7-Day Signal Log

Day *Date*	**Energy** *1–10, when it dipped*	**Mental clarity** *1–10, fog or sharp?*	**Mood** *one or two words*	**Digestive** *gas, bloating, gurgling, nausea*	**Body odor & breath** *intensity; sweet, sour, metallic*	**Tongue** *coating: thick/thin, color*	**Skin** *breakouts, itching, clarity*	**Enema returns** *color, consistency, debris*	**Sleep** *hours, quality 1–10, dreams*	**Anything unusual** *anything that doesn't fit above*
Day 1										
Day 2										
Day 3										
Day 4										
Day 5										
Day 6										
Day 7										

**A blank copy of this chart is at the back of the book, with other quick references — meant to be photocopied or photographed.*

This journal becomes invaluable. It reveals patterns you would otherwise miss. It documents your progress in measurable terms. It helps you communicate accurately with your medical support if something needs review. It becomes a record of what worked — which is useful for future fasts, your own and others', because guiding others through the work is something many practitioners eventually do.

Trust What Your Body Is Telling You

The body does not lie. It exaggerates sometimes. It panics occasionally. It expresses things in language that takes practice to interpret. But it does not lie.

Every signal carries information. Every piece of information matters. Every interpretation made with awareness brings you closer to understanding what your body actually needs. This skill, once developed, does not leave when the fast ends. You will read your body differently for the rest of your life. You will catch things earlier. You will respond more intelligently. You will live in your body with more awareness.

That is one of the lasting gifts of this work. Your body becomes legible to you. And once that happens, it stays legible.

*Figures referenced in this chapter: 16.1 **(online Figure Guide)*

Near-Blackouts and How to Save Yourself

The body of a person on Day 18 or Day 25 of a prolonged fast does not handle changes in position the way the body of a fed person does. Stand up too quickly from a chair, swing your legs off the bed and rise in one motion, push off the couch where you have been lying half-curled for an hour — and the blood that had been distributed throughout your body does not climb back to your brain fast enough to keep you upright. Your vision starts to sparkle. Your hearing thins. The room tilts. If you do nothing, the next thing that happens is the floor.

The technical name for this is orthostatic hypotension. The mechanism is worth understanding so that when it happens to you, you know what your body is doing and you know how to stop it. Blood is a dense fluid. Density seeks its lowest available point. When you stand, the blood that had been distributed evenly throughout the body settles downward into the legs and lower abdomen, where the lowest available point of the standing body is. In a fed, well-hydrated body, the autonomic nervous system catches this redistribution within a second — the heart beats faster, the blood vessels in the legs constrict, the blood pressure rebounds, and the brain stays fed with oxygen. The whole correction happens below your conscious notice.

On a long fast, several of those compensatory systems are running with less margin than usual. Blood volume is lower because you are running on less water and fewer salts than a fed body holds. The autonomic response is slower because the system is in conservation mode. Mineral status — especially magnesium and potassium — is lean. The result is that the compensation that normally happens in one second now takes three or four, and in those three or four seconds the brain is briefly under-perfused. You feel it as lightheadedness. If the under-perfusion goes deep enough or lasts long enough, the brain shuts down consciousness as a protective measure and you faint.

This is not a sign that the fast is failing. It is a sign that the body is doing exactly what bodies do when they are running on the conditions yours is running on. It happened to me five to ten times a day on the days when I was not paying attention. Most prolonged-fasting practitioners experience this at some frequency on the longer fasts. The honest position is that it is expected, it is manageable, and the only real danger is what you do in the seconds when it is happening.

On density, blood, and minerals

There is a deeper layer to this physiology that the practitioner who understands it will be able to feel in their own body across the fast. Blood is not just dense; it has a specific density that depends on what is dissolved in it. The minerals the body carries — sodium, potassium, magnesium, calcium, the others — are themselves denser than water. When the blood is well-mineralized, the fluid the heart is pumping has a density slightly higher than plain water. The vascular system, the kidneys, and the autonomic compensations the body uses to manage blood pressure are all calibrated for blood at that density.

When you drink plain water during a long fast without replacing minerals, the blood thins. The water joins the bloodstream, but the minerals that should have come with it do not. The blood you are now circulating is lower in density than the system was calibrated for. The kidneys notice and pull additional water out into urine to try to restore the balance, which lowers blood volume further. The mineral concentration in the remaining blood becomes more diluted, not less. The cells that need those minerals to function — the neurons in the brain, the muscle fibers in the heart, the smooth muscle in the vessels that constrict when you stand — get fewer of them per pulse of blood that reaches them. The autonomic compensation that normally happens in one second now takes three or four because the messengers it is using are not being delivered at the concentration the system expects.

This is the practitioner's framing for why mineral water and salted water prevent most orthostatic episodes during a long fast and why plain water makes them worse. The reader who has been told their whole life that water is what the body needs may have to recalibrate. On a normal-fed day, with food supplying minerals continuously, plain water is fine. On a fasted day, plain water without mineral replacement actively destabilizes the blood. The body responds to that destabilization by becoming less able to manage standing up, less able to keep the brain perfused with oxygen, less able to compensate for the demands of an ordinary movement. The kaleidoscope you see when you stand too fast on a long fast is often, at root, the result of blood that has been thinned past what the system can manage.

The correction is simple. Salt your morning water. Drink mineral-rich water through the day, not plain water. Use the electrolyte protocol described in Chapter 13. Magnesium-rich water at night supports both sleep and the smooth muscle that has to do the standing-up work the next morning. A practitioner who maintains blood density across a fast experiences fewer episodes; a practitioner who drinks plain water from the tap with nothing added experiences more, and the more does not become less with practice — it becomes the daily state.

The kaleidoscope — your early warning

There is a specific visual signature that announces a near-blackout is starting. Most people who grew up in the West have seen it before — most children have looked through a kaleidoscope, the small tube with mirrors and colored beads that produces shifting symmetrical patterns when you turn the end of it. The pattern your vision makes in the first seconds of a near-blackout looks like that. Sparkling. Rotating. Geometrically broken into wedges of light and dark that shift as you turn your head. Sometimes there is a halo of rainbow color around the edges. Sometimes the whole field becomes the pattern and the rest of the room disappears behind it.

This is your brain's hypoxia signal. The cells of the visual cortex are the first cells to register a drop in oxygen and they tell you about it through this characteristic pattern. The pattern is not random — it has been documented in fighter pilots experiencing G-induced loss of consciousness, in patients on cardiac bypass, in anyone whose brain has been briefly underfed with oxygen. When you see it, the brain is telling you that the next ten or fifteen seconds matter.

The five-second segments

From the moment the kaleidoscope starts, you have approximately fifteen seconds before you lose consciousness. The fifteen seconds break into three segments of five seconds each, and what you can do in each segment is different.

Seconds one through five: the kaleidoscope is starting. Vision is sparkling. You may feel tingling at the crown of the head or across the face. You can still see well enough to navigate. This is the window where the situation is most easily corrected. If you sit back down where you were, or bend forward at the waist to put your head below your heart, the blood returns to the brain within a breath or two and the episode is over. You can also brace your hands against a wall or the back of a chair and stay there for fifteen or twenty seconds, which is usually enough.

Seconds six through ten: vision is going dark. The kaleidoscope is being replaced by a closing tunnel — the edges of the visual field are black and the center is shrinking. You are still conscious but you can no longer see well enough to navigate. This is the window where you must get to the ground deliberately. Do not try to walk to a chair. Do not try to make it to the bed. Drop to your knees where you are. Hands on the floor. Head down. The fastest way to get blood to your brain is to put your brain below your heart, and the fastest way to do that is to be on your hands and knees on whatever surface is under you.

Seconds eleven through fifteen: consciousness is gone or going. The strange thing about this window is that the body often does not fall immediately. You may stand there, eyes open, a kind of muscular catalepsy holding you upright with no awareness inside the body driving it. The fall comes a second or two later, when the muscles release. If you are still standing when consciousness leaves, you fall with no protective reflexes, which is how people break wrists and skulls. This is why the protocol is to get to the ground in seconds six through ten — before consciousness is gone, while you can still choose.

The save-yourself protocol

Memorize this. Practice it once or twice when you are not fasting, so the body knows the motions before the brain has to summon them under stress.

Sparkling vision or tingling crown: bend forward at the waist. Hands on knees or hands on a chair. Head below the heart. Breathe. Five to ten seconds is usually enough.

If the symptoms intensify or do not resolve within those seconds: drop to your knees. Hands on the floor in front of you. Forehead almost to the floor or actually on the floor. Stay there a minute. Longer if needed.

Do not stand back up quickly. When the kaleidoscope has cleared and the room has returned, rise in stages. Sit up first. Wait ten seconds. Get to one knee. Wait ten seconds. Stand slowly with a hand on something stable.

If you cannot get yourself to the floor in time and you feel consciousness going: shout. Make noise. If anyone else is in the building, they will hear it and check on you. If you are alone, the shout at least announces to your own body that the situation is real, which sometimes triggers enough autonomic response to delay the fall by another second or two.

Prevention is easier than rescue

The honest truth about orthostatic episodes during a prolonged fast is that almost all of them are caused by some combination of moving too fast and blood that has been thinned past what the system can manage. Rising slowly from a lying position prevents most of them entirely. Sitting up for fifteen seconds before standing prevents most of the rest. Drinking salted and mineral-rich water through the day, not plain water, prevents most of the remainder. Lying with your legs slightly elevated when you rest, so the blood does not pool as deep, prevents the residual.

I will tell you to do all of this and I will also tell you that I did not do it. Twenty-eight days of fasting and I never learned to rise slowly. I got up and went. Five to ten near-blackouts a day, every day, for most of the fast. I am writing this on the day I broke that fast and I am telling you not to be the person I was. The body will forgive a great deal during a fast. It does not need to be tested at the edge of fainting every time you stand up. Slow movements cost nothing. Salted water costs almost nothing. Fast movements on a thinned bloodstream cost a little more each time.

On solo fasting and what is actually at stake

This is the part of the section that needs to be said directly, because the rest of the protocol assumes a thing the reader may not have fully reckoned with. Most people doing a prolonged fast are doing it alone. There is no nurse in the next room. There is no doctor on call. The Buchinger clinic in Germany has someone watching you twenty-four hours a day; the practitioner in their own home in Tennessee or California or Ohio does not.

This is closer to solo climbing than to medicine. The person on the wall has gear, has training, has done the route in their head a hundred times before they got to the rock — and when something goes wrong on the wall, the only person who can save them is the one who is on the wall. The doctor at the foot of the mountain will not arrive in time. The protocol the climber learned the year before is what saves them, if anything does. The fast is the same in this one specific way. The protocol you have read and the practice you have done before the fast began is what will save you when the kaleidoscope starts. Nobody else is coming. You are it.

The other side of this is what happens if you let it go too far. You faint. You fall. You hit your head. Someone finds you and calls an ambulance. The emergency room sees a person who has not eaten in twenty-five days, who has the heart rate and blood pressure of a person near collapse, who is producing ketones at levels that look pathological to a doctor trained on the fed metabolic state. The emergency room does not see what you see. They see a person who has been starving themselves and who has been found unconscious. They place you on a hold because that is the protocol when someone presents this way, and they put fluids and glucose into your arm without consulting you about phosphorus, magnesium, or thiamine — the three molecules that need to be in your bloodstream before glucose arrives, or refeeding syndrome will hit you on top of everything else.

That is the version of this story where you do not finish the fast on your own terms. You finish it in a hospital room being treated as an emergency by people who do not understand what you were doing. The version of this story where you finish on your own terms requires that you not let it go that far. The save-yourself protocol above is how you not let it go that far. Take it seriously. The cost of bending over for ten seconds when your vision starts to sparkle is nothing. The cost of not bending over is a hospital stay you did not want.

* * *

There is a clarity that comes in the deep middle of a long fast, and it is the most dangerous gift the work gives you.

By the third week the noise is gone. You wake in the morning and for a moment you do not remember you are fasting at all — there is only the clear room, the light, the work in front of you — until some discomfort moves through and reminds you what your body is doing. That forgetting is a sign the fast is working. It is also the place where people get lost.

The clarity can become a room you do not want to leave. The world outside the fast starts to look coarse against the quiet you have found. I have watched men decide, somewhere in that clarity, to keep going past what their body could carry, because coming out felt like coming down. Clarity is not the same as health. When the muscle begins to go — and you will feel it go, in the stairs, in the lift of a thing you used to lift without thought — that is your body telling you the cost has started to outrun the gift. Listen to that before you listen to the clarity.

Daily journaling is how you keep one hand on the ground. Each morning, before the clear room closes around you, write down where your body actually is: what is working, what is failing, what you lifted, what you could not. The page is the one place the fast cannot talk you out of the truth.

Know your number before you begin, and hold it loosely. With real preparation and the daily work done right, a person who sets out to fast forty days can usually finish around twenty-eight; a thirty-day fast usually lands near twenty-three. These are not targets to chase. They are the honest range of what a prepared body tends to give — so that when the clarity tells you to go further, you have a number in your pocket that was set by a clearer version of you, before the room got quiet.

Chapter 16

Lightheadedness and Euphoria

* * *

There are two kinds of lightness the body can feel, and the fasting body comes to know both of them.

The first is the lightness of standing up too quickly. The blood has not yet caught up. The head goes briefly empty. The room tilts, then steadies. A new thought sometimes arrives in that moment of tilt — sharp, unbidden, gone again as the body recovers. This is not euphoria. It is depletion, dressed for a moment in pleasant clothes. Drink the minerals. Sit a while. Stand again with care. The chapter before this one has already taught what to do.

The second kind of lightness is different. It does not flicker. It does not require a posture change to summon it. It arrives sometime in the second or third week, often when the practitioner is doing nothing in particular, and it does not leave. The body feels lighter in the way a room feels lighter when something heavy has been carried out of it and the door has been left open. Something has gone, and the going has changed the air.

This is the euphoria the long fasters speak of. Not the flicker. The state.

The flicker passes in seconds. The state holds across days.

What follows is what is in the way of the state. There are three things, and they are not the same thing called by three different names. They are three sources of the same weight, and the fast loosens each of them in its own way.

* * *

There is, first, what we have grown by feeding it.

A body is a kind of ground. What grows in it is what the ground was prepared for. The body that has eaten sugar for thirty years has become a particular kind of soil, and what grows in that soil is what the soil was made hospitable to. The candida thrives because the conditions for candida thriving have been laid in, year after year, meal after meal. The bacteria that ferment what should not be fermenting have been invited and re-invited a thousand times. Even the parasites that took up residence took up residence because the residence was built for them.

This is parasitic energy. Not energy that arrived by accident. Energy that arrived because we made the place where it could live. The body did not betray us. The body did exactly what bodies do — it grew what we kept giving it the conditions to grow.

The hook of a craving is not, mostly, the craving. It is the small organism that lives off what the craving brings in. The craving is the organism asking through us. The reach for the sweet thing is not entirely ours, has not been entirely ours for a long time, perhaps was never entirely ours.

When the food stops, the things that lived on the food begin to die. The dying is not pleasant. It comes through as fatigue, as flu-like sensations, as moods that pass through like weather. Each is a small ending. Each is one thing fewer asking through us. The euphoria that arrives in week three is partly this — the quiet of a body in which fewer voices are calling out, fewer organisms are demanding, fewer mouths are open to be fed. The body gets to be only the body again. That alone is most of what the lightness is.

* * *

There is, second, what was set in motion before.

Some of what we carry was not laid down by us in this season of our lives. It was laid down earlier — in childhood, in the years our memories do not fully reach, sometimes earlier than that. The hook on a particular pattern is sometimes so deep that no amount of present-tense effort can pull it. We feed the pattern not because we choose to but because the pattern was choosing for us before we had a choice in the matter.

This is karmic energy. The word carries a weight that other words do not. It names the thing honestly. Some of what runs us was set running before we got here, by us or by people we knew or by people we did not know. The pattern accumulates. The pattern is inherited. The pattern is older than the body it is currently using.

The fast does not erase what was set in motion. It does something stranger and gentler. It makes it visible.

In the fed state, the karmic pattern hides inside the daily noise of eating and digesting and craving and reaching. It is one signal among many, and it gets lost. In the fasted state, the noise drops away, and the pattern stands up out of the silence in its own outline. The practitioner sees it for what it is, sometimes for the first time in a life. *Oh. I have been doing this since I was nine. I did not know I was doing it. I did not know it was a thing being done.*

To see is most of the work. Once a pattern is seen clearly, it can be set down. Not always at once. Sometimes in stages. But seeing is the first stage and the longest stage, and the fast is what makes the seeing possible. The euphoria of week three is partly this — something that has been carried for decades is being set down, and the practitioner did not even know it was in their hands.

* * *

There is, third, what we draw to ourselves when we are low.

Vibrations match. This is not mysticism. Watch any room of people for an hour. The dispirited gather with the dispirited, not because they have decided to but because something in their atmospheres recognizes itself in the other. The tired person is not magnetic to the rested. The bitter person is not magnetic to the joyful. We attract what matches what we already are, and we are most likely to attract the matches we wish we could refuse when we ourselves are at our lowest.

This is the third energy, and it is not in the body. It is in the room. It comes through other people. The friend who only calls when they need something. The relative whose presence in a doorway lowers the temperature. The colleague whose every story is a complaint. We did not invent these people. We attracted them, or we were attracted to them, in seasons when our own state was low enough that the match made itself.

A long fast raises the state. Not all at once and not by magic. The body clearer, the patterns more visible, the inner voices fewer — the practitioner becomes, slowly, harder to match. The matches that used to land begin to slide. Friendships sometimes drift during a long fast. Phone calls go unreturned and feel, for the first time, easy not to return. People who fed on the practitioner's lower-vibration self find less to feed on, and they go elsewhere. This is not a tragedy. It is a release.

The space they leave behind is not empty for long. What enters in their place tends to be different in kind — quieter, more reciprocal, less demanding. Like calls to like in this direction too. The euphoria of the third week and after is partly this — the air around the practitioner has changed, and what walks into the changed air is changed in turn.

* * *

Three sources of weight. Three doors of release.

The pattern is the same in all three, and that is the worth of seeing them together. Something has been feeding on us. We participated in setting up the feeding, knowingly or unknowingly, in this lifetime or in something older or in the relational field around us. The fast pulls the food. The thing that was feeding loosens its grip. The grip loosens because the conditions for the grip are no longer being maintained.

This is what death and rebirth means in the practitioner's body. Not a single great dying. Many small ones. The candida dying. The pattern releasing. The match loosening. Each one a small ending. Each one room made for something that was waiting to come in.

The practitioner who completes a long fast does not arrive on the other side as the same person who started. Not because the fast performed magic. Because the fast removed what had been in the way, and what was in the way had been a great deal. The person who emerges is the person who was always there underneath — the one who could not be heard while so many other voices were doing the talking.

* * *

The lightness that arrives is the lightness of that person beginning to walk around in their own body again.

It does not flicker. It does not require a posture change. It arrives sometime in the second or third week, often when the practitioner is doing nothing in particular, and it does not leave when the fast ends. It carries forward into the months and years after. The practitioner who has felt it does not forget what it felt like, and does not, given a choice, return to the conditions that prevented it.

That is the deeper euphoria. It is not a feeling. It is a state of being less occupied by what is not us.

The fasted body knows. The mind, in time, learns to know also.

Chapter 17

The Enema Protocol

* * *

If the fast is the engine of this protocol, the enema is the exhaust system. Without it, everything the fast loosens — everything the herbs kill, everything the layers release — has nowhere to go. The material is reabsorbed back into the bloodstream and recycled into the very tissues you are trying to heal. The enema is not optional. It is what makes everything else work.

Most people approach enemas with reluctance. The cultural conditioning runs deep. Discomfort with the body. Squeamishness about the process. A sense that this is somehow undignified or unpleasant. Set those associations aside. What you are about to do is one of the oldest healing practices in human history. References to therapeutic enemas appear in medical texts from ancient Egypt, India, China, and Greece. Hippocrates prescribed them. So did doctors in colonial America. So do clinicians in functional medicine practices today. This is not a strange modern invention. It is a timeless tool that fell out of fashion when pharmaceutical alternatives appeared.

The body itself does not share the cultural reluctance. The body responds to thorough cleansing with deep relief. Approach this practice with respect, and the body responds in kind.

One thing to keep in mind before going further. The enema reaches only the large intestine. The small intestine, four times longer and the place most parasites prefer to live, clears by a different mechanism — covered in the chapter that follows.

Why Enemas Are Essential During Prolonged Fasting

Three reasons make enemas non-negotiable during this protocol.

First, peristalsis slows during fasting. In normal eating, the muscular contractions of the colon are stimulated by food entering the digestive tract. The arrival of new material signals downward movement. During fasting:

- No food entering means no peristalsis trigger.
- The colon's natural movement slows dramatically.
- Material that loosens from intestinal walls has no wave to carry it forward.

• Without intervention, that material can sit in the colon for days.

The enema mechanically replaces what peristalsis is no longer doing. It substitutes hydraulic pressure for the muscular pressure the body would ordinarily provide.

Second, reabsorption is the real risk. When parasites die, they release toxins. When biofilm breaks down, it releases trapped pathogens. When mucoid plaque dissolves, it releases years of accumulated material. When candida dies, it releases acetaldehyde and other byproducts. All of this material must leave the body. If it sits in the colon, it gets reabsorbed through the colon wall directly into the bloodstream. This reabsorption is the source of severe Herxheimer reactions, headaches, nausea, skin breakouts, mood disturbances, brain fog, and body odor. The enema interrupts the reabsorption cycle. It removes the toxic load before it can recirculate.

Third, the cleanse itself demands it. Without daily enemas:

• Cleansing slows dramatically.

• Each layer takes longer to fully release.

• Parasites die but their bodies are not expelled.

• The fast becomes significantly more uncomfortable.

• The total time required extends meaningfully.

With daily enemas — and on intensive days, twice-daily enemas — the entire timeline compresses. The work gets done faster. The discomfort is lessened. The exit from the fast arrives sooner. Every element of the philosophy from Chapter 14 depends on this practice.

What an Enema Actually Is

The mechanics are simple. An enema introduces fluid into the rectum and colon through the anus, typically using a bag, bucket, or bottle with a flexible tube. The fluid:

Before each enema, releasing trapped gas first allows the water to travel further and the work to reach deeper. See the Releasing Trapped Gas entry in the Working Tips section at the back of this book.

• Hydrates and softens accumulated material.

• Mechanically dislodges debris from the colon walls.

• Stimulates the colon to contract and release.

• Carries everything it has loosened out as it exits.

The volume — typically 32 to 48 ounces during a prolonged fast — fills the descending and transverse colon. With proper retention, fluid can reach the ascending colon and the ileocecal valve. With repeated use over time, the cumulative effect reaches deeper than any single session ever could.

(Figure 18.1 — see the online Figure Guide)

Equipment

Quality matters here. The equipment is used daily for weeks. Cheap or contaminated equipment defeats the purpose of the practice.

The enema bag or bucket. Look for:

- Stainless steel buckets or BPA-free silicone bags.
- Capacity of at least 2 quarts (64 ounces).
- Quality tubing — silicone preferred over PVC.
- Adjustable flow control clamp.

Avoid:

- Cheap rubber bags that may contain harmful compounds.
- Single-use disposable systems for repeated use.
- Equipment that cannot be thoroughly cleaned.

The tip:

- Smooth-tipped silicone or stainless steel — comfortable and easy to clean.
- Some practitioners prefer specialized colon tubes — softer and longer for deeper insertion.
- Avoid hard plastic tips.

Other supplies: Old towels (this gets messy). A clean comfortable space near the bathroom. Olive oil or coconut oil for lubrication. A timer for retention timing.

(Figure 18.2 — see the online Figure Guide)

The Basic Procedure

Once you have done this a few times, it becomes routine. The first session feels awkward; by the third or fourth, it feels like brushing teeth — a daily practice the body comes to welcome.

Preparation:

1. Clean all equipment thoroughly with hot water and a small amount of mild soap.

2. Prepare your enema solution — water, coffee, or salt water depending on the protocol.

3. Bring solution to body temperature: 98 to 100°F. Test on your wrist.

4. Hang the bag at hip height. Too high creates excessive pressure; too low slows flow significantly.

5. Open the clamp briefly to release air from the tubing; close before fluid escapes.

6. Lubricate the tip generously with olive oil or coconut oil.

The position. Several positions work; find what is most comfortable for you:

- **Left side lying** with knees drawn up. Most comfortable for many people; uses density to direct flow toward the descending colon.
- **Knee to chest:** kneeling with chest and shoulders on the floor. Allows deeper fluid penetration.
- **Back lying:** on a towel with knees bent. Accessible for some people who find side lying difficult.

Most experienced enema practitioners begin in left-side position and shift positions during retention to distribute the fluid throughout the colon.

The insertion:

- Insert the lubricated tip gently — 2 to 3 inches.
- Open the clamp slowly; begin with a slow flow.
- If cramping begins, close the clamp briefly, breathe deeply, resume slowly.
- Allow the full volume to enter at a comfortable pace.
- Take 5 to 10 minutes to fill. Rushing creates cramping and reduces retention quality.

The retention:

- Once the bag is empty, close the clamp and remove the tip carefully.
- Lie still and breathe deeply.
- Begin in left-side position.
- After 3 to 4 minutes, roll onto your back.
- After another 3 to 4 minutes, roll to right side.
- This rotation distributes fluid throughout the colon.

Retention times by enema type:

- **Coffee enema:** 12 to 15 minutes for full portal vein absorption.
- **Plain water enema:** 5 to 15 minutes.
- **Salt water enema:** 10 to 15 minutes.

Quality of relaxed retention matters more than absolute time. A tense ten minutes does less than a relaxed seven.

The release:

- When ready, go to the toilet.
- Allow the fluid and material to release naturally.
- Sometimes multiple releases occur over 20 to 30 minutes.
- Do not strain — let the colon do its work.
- Stay near the bathroom for the next hour.

Reading What You See

Chapter 15 covered enema return signals in detail. Pay attention to what you observe each time. This is real-time feedback about what is happening inside your body. The colors, textures, volumes, and patterns all carry information.

Experienced practitioners often photograph or document their returns. This reveals patterns over time, identifies what protocols are most effective, is useful for medical consultation if needed, and validates the work being done. This is not vanity. It is data.

The Two-Enema Daily Protocol

During active cleansing, twice-daily enemas serve different purposes.

Morning enema — coffee protocol. Discussed in detail in Chapter 18. The morning enema is the primary therapeutic enema:

- Coffee for portal vein absorption and bile duct stimulation.
- Removes overnight accumulation.
- Activates liver detoxification for the day ahead.
- Combined with clove oil for fluke targeting.

Timing:

- Within an hour of waking, after the morning herbs have had time to settle.
- Before any other supplements except trace minerals and L-Glutamine.
- Allows full day for residual effects.

Evening enema — salt water protocol. The evening enema serves complementary purposes:

• Clears die-off material accumulated through the day.

• Prevents overnight reabsorption of toxins.

• Soothes the intestinal lining after the day's activity.

• Salt water rather than coffee — gentler on the system before sleep.

Timing:

• 2 to 3 hours before sleep.

• After the last herbal tincture dose.

• Far enough from sleep that you can fully release before bed.

• Allows the body to rest cleanly through the night.

When to Add a Second or Third Enema

Even outside the standard twice-daily protocol, sometimes an additional enema becomes appropriate. The body usually signals clearly when this is the case.

Signs that an additional enema would help:

• Significant gas pressure that does not resolve.

• Persistent nausea suggesting toxin reabsorption.

• Unusual fatigue accompanying signs of die-off.

• Headache combined with abdominal discomfort.

• Body signaling clearly that something needs to come out.

Important boundaries:

• Maximum three enemas in 24 hours.

• Always replenish minerals between sessions.

• Stop if any enema produces unusual cramping or pain.

• Listen to the body — sometimes one enema is enough; sometimes more is needed.

Salt Water Enema Specifics

The evening companion to the morning coffee enema.

Ratio:

- 48 ounces water treated with ionic sulfated minerals.
- 1 to 2 teaspoons Himalayan salt.
- Stir until fully dissolved.
- Body temperature.

Why salt rather than plain water:

- Plain water draws minerals out of the colon wall through osmosis.
- Repeated plain water enemas can deplete mineral status.
- Salt creates an isotonic solution, preventing mineral loss.
- Salt has a gentle drawing effect on debris from the intestinal wall.
- Soothes and calms the intestinal lining.

Adding Therapeutic Compounds to Your Salt Water Enema

The salt water enema serves a different purpose than the morning coffee enema. Where coffee stimulates and activates, salt water soothes and clears. The additions that complement the salt water work focus on soothing the intestinal lining after the day's activity, providing a final antifungal sweep before sleep, mineral replenishment through direct absorption, and a final clearing of accumulated die-off.

Aloe vera juice — 4 ounces. The healer.

- Inner leaf aloe vera juice, not whole leaf.
- Soothes and supports intestinal lining repair.
- Mild antiparasitic and antifungal properties.
- Anti-inflammatory effects on irritated tissue.
- Supports healing of areas where parasites have been embedded.

Why evening rather than morning: the evening enema follows hours of cleansing activity. The intestinal lining benefits from soothing support overnight. Aloe combined with coffee can produce loose evacuation, which is better in the evening.

Magnesium chloride — half teaspoon. The relaxer.

- Powdered magnesium chloride dissolved in the salt water.
- Direct transdermal absorption through colon wall.

• Replenishes magnesium efficiently.

• Relaxes intestinal muscles.

• Supports sleep through magnesium's effect on the nervous system.

Particularly valuable because magnesium is rapidly depleted during fasting and enemas. Direct rectal absorption bypasses any digestive limitations. Supports overnight cellular repair processes. Improves sleep quality significantly.

Pau d'arco tincture — 1 teaspoon. The antifungal sweep.

• Strong antifungal, particularly effective against candida.

• Final sweep through the colon before sleep.

• Direct contact with biofilm communities.

• Systemic absorption extends antifungal effects throughout the night.

Particularly valuable during candida die-off phases, when white or yellow material appears in returns, throughout weeks 2 to 3 of the fast, and when tongue coating suggests active candida.

This combination supports healing and clearing while preparing the body for restorative sleep.

Plain Water Enemas

Sometimes a simple plain water enema is appropriate.

When to use:

• During preparation phase, the week before the fast begins.

• For people new to enemas — building tolerance and familiarity.

• Occasional sessions when salt is unavailable.

• When the body needs gentle clearing without therapeutic intensity.

Cautions:

• Repeated plain water enemas, without minerals, can deplete electrolytes.

• Always replenish minerals after plain water enemas.

• For prolonged daily use, salt water is preferred.

Common Concerns and How to Address Them

Cramping during fluid intake:

- Slow the flow — close the clamp briefly.
- Breathe deeply — relax the abdominal muscles.
- Accept a smaller volume if needed; better to retain less than to abandon the session.
- Often improves with practice.

Difficulty retaining the fluid:

- Begin with smaller volumes — 16 to 24 ounces — and work up over several days.
- Make sure fluid is at proper body temperature; too cold or too hot causes urgency.
- Start in left-side position — most comfortable for retention.
- Distract gently — read, listen to calm music — and allow the body to relax.

Pain or sharp discomfort:

- Stop immediately.
- Pain is not normal during enemas — discomfort yes, pain no.
- May indicate the tip is positioned incorrectly.
- May indicate hemorrhoids or other anatomical concerns.
- If pain persists or recurs, consult medical support.

Bleeding:

- Small amount of bright red blood usually indicates minor abrasion from the tip — resolves quickly.
- Larger amounts of blood or persistent bleeding — stop immediately and seek medical attention.
- Dark blood may indicate something more serious — medical evaluation needed.

Dizziness during or after:

- Often indicates fluid was too cold or position changes were too quick.
- Stay lying down longer.
- Replenish minerals immediately.
- If persistent, review hydration and electrolyte status.

The Replenishment Protocol

Every enema removes minerals. Every enema must be followed by replenishment.

Within 30 minutes of completion:

• 16 ounces water treated with ionic sulfated minerals.

• Pinch of Himalayan salt.

• For coffee enemas specifically, coconut water if available.

• For evening salt water enemas, magnesium glycinate before sleep.

This is not optional. This is not something to do later. This is part of the enema procedure itself, completed within the same hour.

Cleaning and Maintenance

Hygiene matters when this practice is daily.

After every session:

• Rinse all equipment thoroughly with hot water.

• Wash with mild soap — non-toxic preferred.

• Pay particular attention to the tip and tube interior.

• Hang to dry completely before next use.

Weekly deep clean:

• Hydrogen peroxide soak — equipment in dilute hydrogen peroxide solution for 10 minutes.

• Or boiling water rinse for stainless steel components.

• Replace silicone components if any sign of wear or staining.

Replacement schedule:

• Quality silicone tubing — every 6 to 12 months with daily use.

• Tips — every 3 to 6 months.

• Bag or bucket — annually or as condition warrants.

A Note on Privacy and Practice

This is a private practice. The setup, the time required, the immediate aftermath — all of it requires privacy and lack of interruption.

Practical considerations:

• Have a dedicated space if possible — a guest bathroom or private setup.

• Communicate clearly with household members about timing.

• Plan for 60 to 90 minutes uninterrupted from start to finish, including the full release time after retention.

Treat this practice with the dignity it deserves. Expect the same from everyone around you.

Optional Additions for Specific Situations

Beyond the standard morning and evening protocols, certain additions become valuable in specific circumstances. Each has its place; none of them belong in every session.

Apple cider vinegar — 1 to 2 tablespoons. For yeast and biofilm.

• Raw, unfiltered with the mother.

• Added to plain water enema, not coffee.

• Acidifies the colon environment briefly.

• Inhospitable to candida and certain bacteria.

• Helps disrupt biofilm structures.

Use during heavy candida phases, when biofilm seems particularly stubborn, or as occasional substitution for evening salt water. Avoid if the colon lining feels irritated, more than once or twice weekly, or in combination with coffee, which is too acidic together.

Garlic infusion — 2 to 3 cloves crushed. The broad-spectrum antimicrobial.

• Fresh organic garlic cloves crushed and steeped in warm water for 15 minutes.

• Strain thoroughly before adding to enema solution.

• Potent antimicrobial, antifungal, antiparasitic.

• Direct contact with all colon surfaces.

Use during aggressive parasite phases, when broad-spectrum action is needed, or as an occasional intensive intervention.

Cautions: strong odor and potential burning sensation. Start with 1 clove to test tolerance. Not for sensitive intestinal lining.

Probiotic liquid — 1 tablespoon. Late-stage rebuilding support.

- Liquid probiotic with multiple strains.
- Added to plain water or salt water — never coffee.
- Direct seeding of beneficial bacteria into the cleaned colon.
- Useful in the final days of the fast and during refeeding.

Use during the last few days before breaking the fast, the first few days of refeeding, and specifically for microbiome rebuilding.

Important: coffee inhibits probiotic activity — never combine. Body temperature solution — heat above 100°F kills probiotics. Not appropriate during heavy die-off phases.

Slippery elm — 2 tablespoons powdered. The deep soother.

- Mix slippery elm powder with warm water; strain through fine mesh.
- Add resulting mucilage to enema solution.
- Coats and soothes intestinal lining.
- Particularly valuable when lining feels irritated.

Use after particularly intensive die-off days, when evening enema produces unusual sensitivity, or during recovery from particularly aggressive protocols.

Ginger tea — 8 ounces strong infusion. The circulation enhancer.

- Strong ginger tea added to enema solution.
- Stimulates blood flow to colon wall.
- Mild warming effect.
- Anti-nausea properties.

Use during days with significant nausea, when circulation feels sluggish, or for cold-weather sessions when warming is welcome.

What Not to Add

Some compounds should never enter the colon. The list is short but worth being explicit about.

• **Hydrogen peroxide.** Despite some popular protocols recommending it, hydrogen peroxide damages the intestinal lining, disrupts the microbiome severely, and carries risk of serious adverse effects. The colon does not need oxygenation through this route.

• **Bleach or any disinfectant.** Should be obvious, but worth stating. Causes severe tissue damage. Has been promoted in dangerous fringe protocols. Never appropriate.

• **Essential oils not specifically food grade.** Diffuser oils contain compounds not meant for internal use. Many essential oils irritate tissue significantly. Only food-grade therapeutic oils, and only those specifically appropriate.

• **Soap or detergents.** Damages colon mucosa. Disrupts beneficial bacteria. No therapeutic benefit.

• **Excessive concentrations of anything.** More is not better with enema additions. The recommended amounts in these chapters are tested ranges. Exceeding them increases risk without increasing benefit.

Adjusting for Your Body's Response

Each person's body responds differently to specific additions. The general principle is to listen and adjust.

Reduce or eliminate an addition if you experience:

• Burning sensation during retention.

• Cramping that was not present with simpler solutions.

• Skin irritation around the rectum.

• Headache or systemic symptoms specifically following sessions with that addition.

• Persistent discomfort beyond normal enema sensations.

Continue the addition if you experience:

• Normal mild discomfort that resolves quickly.

• Increased volume of die-off material in returns.

• Improved energy or clarity following sessions.

• Reduced gas and bloating after sessions.

• Generally positive cumulative effects.

Listen to your body. Each addition is optional. The base coffee enema and salt water enema are fully therapeutic on their own. The additions amplify the work, but they do not create it.

Building Your Personal Protocol

Your protocol can evolve as the fast progresses. The intensity of additions should match the phase of the work.

Week 1 — foundation phase:

• Morning: basic coffee enema only — let the body adapt.

• Evening: basic salt water enema only.

Weeks 2 to 3 — active cleansing phase:

• Morning: coffee enema with clove oil, black walnut, milk thistle.

• Evening: salt water with aloe vera and magnesium chloride.

• Add pau d'arco when candida signs appear.

Weeks 4 onward — targeted phase:

• Morning: full coffee enema protocol.

• Evening: full salt water protocol.

• Specific situational additions based on body signals.

• Reduce overall additions as cleansing approaches completion.

Final days before breaking fast:

• Begin reducing antiparasitic additions.

• Begin introducing probiotic in evening enema.

• Lighter touch overall as body prepares to refeed.

Combinations That Work and Combinations to Avoid

Resist the temptation to add everything to every enema. The recommended morning and evening combinations are designed for compatibility. Compounds work synergistically rather than against each other. Total volume of additives stays within safe range. Different additions target different mechanisms.

Avoid these combinations:

• Coffee plus probiotic — coffee inhibits probiotic activity.

• Coffee plus apple cider vinegar — too acidic together.

• Multiple antifungals in same session — risk of excessive irritation.

• More than three additions in a single enema — diminishing returns.

Storage and Preparation Notes

Quality matters at every step.

• **Tinctures.** Store in dark glass bottles. Keep refrigerated after opening. Replace annually. Verify alcohol-based tinctures are appropriate for your situation.

• **Essential oils.** Food grade certification visible on label. Dark glass bottles only. Replace if appearance changes. Cool, dry storage.

• **Liquid herbs.** Aloe vera juice — refrigerate after opening. Inner leaf only; whole leaf can be irritating. Verify product has no added sugars or preservatives.

• **Powders.** Slippery elm: fresh powder is more effective than aged. Magnesium chloride: keep dry. Replace if any moisture or clumping appears.

The Cumulative Effect

Day one of enemas during a prolonged fast often produces modest results. The body is just beginning to mobilize what has been accumulating. The first enemas catch surface material — recent buildup, fecal residue, easy releases.

Day fifteen looks dramatically different. By the middle of the fast, the enemas are catching what the deeper work has loosened. Mucoid plaque from years past. Biofilm communities releasing. Parasites in various stages of die-off. Bile duct material from coffee enema work. Older, deeper, more substantial material than anything the early fast produced.

The cumulative effect is what matters. Day after day after day, each session reaching slightly deeper than the last. Each release supporting the next. The compound effect that makes prolonged daily enema practice fundamentally different from occasional use.

This is why the protocol works. Consistency over time. Letting the practice do its work.

Reframing the Practice

One last thought. For all the technical information in these pages, the daily enema is ultimately a simple act. A person. A bag of warm water. A quiet hour. And the willingness to participate consciously in their own healing.

That is all this is. A timeless practice, used by countless generations before you, available to anyone willing to overcome cultural conditioning and engage with their body directly. Approach it with that perspective. This is not strange. This is not undignified. This is one of the oldest forms of self-care humans have practiced, restored to its rightful place in your healing.

The body responds to thorough care with deep healing. This is one of the most thorough forms of care available.

*Figures referenced in this chapter: 18.1–18.2 **(online Figure Guide)*

Chapter 18

Coffee Enemas & Liver Cleansing

* * *

Of all the practices in this protocol, none generates more raised eyebrows than this one. Coffee. Through the rectum. Held for fifteen minutes. The cultural reaction is predictable. The biological reality is something else entirely. Coffee enemas have been used therapeutically for over a century, and they belong at the center of any serious cleansing protocol.

Coffee enemas are not new. References to them appear in the Merck Manual — the standard medical reference text — from the early 1900s until 1977. They were used routinely in hospitals, particularly for surgical patients and trauma cases. In the 1920s, German researchers documented their use for improving liver function and pain management. In the 1930s, Dr. Max Gerson made coffee enemas central to his approach to chronic disease, particularly cancer, and the Gerson Therapy continues to use them today. In the 1970s, they fell out of mainstream medical practice as pharmaceutical alternatives became dominant. But they never stopped working. Practitioners of integrative medicine, naturopathic medicine, functional medicine, and traditional healing systems have used coffee enemas continuously for the past century, because the physiological effects are genuine and reproducible. This is not a fringe practice. It is a forgotten one.

Why Coffee Enemas Reach Beyond the Colon

The enema is an effective instrument, but it is a short one. It reaches the colon — five feet of tissue at the lower end of the digestive tract — and there it stops. Beyond it, folded on itself in the body's deepest interior, lies the small intestine. Twenty-two feet of it. Four times longer than what the enema can reach. The place where most of what we eat is broken down, where most of what we absorb is taken up, and where most parasites, when they take up residence in a human body, prefer to live. None of that territory is touched by the fluid we administer through the rectum. The geometry simply does not allow it.

Which raises a question that does not at first announce itself, but settles in once you sit with the geometry. If the small intestine is four times longer than the large, and if it is — as the medical literature plainly states — the place most intestinal parasites prefer to live, then how does the small intestine get cleaned? The herbs reach it through the bloodstream. But herbs alone do not move debris. What moves the debris?

Two mechanisms, working in series. The first one has been working inside you all your life. You have probably never let it finish.

It is called the migrating motor complex, and it is the small intestine's own housekeeping system. The clinicians who study it actually call it the housekeeper, and the name is more accurate than scientific names usually are. Roughly every ninety to one hundred and twenty minutes, when the small intestine is empty, a wave of contractions begins high in the stomach and sweeps the entire length of the small bowel — twenty-two feet of folded, glistening tissue — pushing forward whatever the digestion has left behind. Sloughed cells. Stray bacteria. Fragments of biofilm. Anything that did not get absorbed. The wave moves all of it onward, toward the gateway between the small intestine and the large.

The wave was first observed in 1969, in dogs, by a researcher at the Mayo Clinic. It has been studied continuously since. It is well-established, well-mapped, and almost universally ignored in modern adult life.

The wave has one defining characteristic. The moment any food arrives in the stomach, the wave stops. It does not pause politely. It stops. It will not resume until the meal has cleared and an extended stretch of empty time has accumulated — usually two to three hours of nothing.

Now consider how a modern adult eats. Breakfast at seven. Coffee with cream at nine. A snack at eleven. Lunch at one. Something at three. Dinner at six. A handful of something at nine. Drinks with calories somewhere along the way. The housekeeping wave never starts. Or it starts and is interrupted, and starts again and is interrupted again, and never completes a single full sweep of the small bowel from the stomach to the gateway. For decades. For a lifetime, in many cases.

The body has been trying to clean itself, and we have not let it.

A prolonged fast changes everything about this. With no food entering the stomach for weeks at a time, the wave runs continuously. Cycle after cycle. Hour after hour. Day after day. Where ordinary life allows two or three completed cycles in a week, a thirty-day fast allows several hundred. The small intestine, finally, gets cleaned the way it was built to be cleaned.

This is one of the deepest things a prolonged fast accomplishes, and the practitioner does not have to do anything to make it happen. The fast itself is the only condition. Stop eating, and the housekeeper takes over. The body has been waiting for this.

* * *

The second mechanism is the coffee enema's gift, and it works in cooperation with the first.

When coffee is held in the colon, the caffeine and palmitates within it absorb through the hemorrhoidal veins, which empty directly into the hepatic portal system. The compounds travel up to the liver in concentrated form, faster and more directly than anything taken by mouth could reach it. There they dilate the bile ducts and stimulate the gallbladder to contract by roughly a third more than ordinary digestion would call for. Bile pours out of the gallbladder, down the common bile duct, into the small intestine.

Bile is the body's quiet janitor. It is golden-green, slightly viscous, alkaline. It carries away what the liver has spent the day processing — toxins, dead cellular material, the broken-down byproducts of medication and metabolism. It also alkalinizes whatever section of intestine it passes through, which matters because most parasites prefer the slight acidity of an unfasted gut. A flood of bile changes the chemistry under their feet.

And the bile does not sit. The housekeeping wave is already running, has been running for hours by the time the morning enema is administered. The wave catches the bile and what the bile has gathered, and carries the whole stream forward — through the jejunum, through the ileum, past the gateway, into the colon.

* * *

Two systems meeting in the middle of the body. The wave from above. The bile from the side. Both of them moving in the same direction. Both of them carrying what does not belong.

What was in the small intestine moves into the large intestine. The next morning's enema flushes the large intestine clean. The cycle resets. The next coffee enema triggers the next bile flood. The wave runs again.

Day after day, this happens. The cleaning is not a single event. It is a rhythm. The small intestine, twenty-two feet of folded tissue that no instrument from outside the body can reach, is cleaned by the body's own intelligence, given the conditions to do its work.

There is a kind of reverence that sometimes comes over a long-fasting practitioner, in the third or fourth week, when they begin to understand what is happening inside them without their having to make it happen. The body is doing the work. They are simply allowing it.

The temples of older traditions taught that the body itself was sacred ground. Not as metaphor. As architecture. A structure built to do exactly the work it is doing, when the conditions for that work are restored. The small intestine cleaning itself, cycle after patient cycle, while the practitioner sleeps and walks and prays and waits — this is the temple at work. The bile flowing on its golden schedule. The wave moving its quiet way through the long folded corridor. None of it asking permission. All of it asking only that we stop interrupting.

The protocol's job is to stop the interrupting. The body's job is everything else.

Why Coffee Specifically

The question is fair. Why coffee? What does coffee do that plain water does not? The answer involves three specific compounds, each with its own role.

Caffeine, through an unexpected route. When you drink coffee, caffeine reaches your bloodstream slowly through digestion. When caffeine is absorbed through the colon wall, it takes a different path:

- Absorbed directly into the **portal vein system**.
- The portal vein carries blood directly to the **liver** before circulation reaches the rest of the body.
- This means caffeine reaches the liver in **higher concentration** through the rectal route than through oral consumption.

• The liver responds with significant biological activity.

(Figure 18.3 — see the online Figure Guide)

Palmitic acid. A compound naturally present in coffee, palmitic acid does something specific when it reaches the liver:

• Stimulates the production of **glutathione S-transferase** by up to 700%.

• Glutathione is the body's master detoxification compound.

• This enzyme system is responsible for binding and eliminating toxins from the bloodstream.

• The result is a dramatic acceleration of the liver's detoxification capacity for several hours after the enema.

This is the single most important biochemical effect of the coffee enema. Without palmitic acid stimulating glutathione production, the practice would be merely interesting. With it, the practice becomes therapeutic.

Cafestol and kahweol. These compounds, found primarily in unfiltered coffee, also stimulate detoxification enzyme production and have anti-inflammatory effects on liver tissue.

Together, these three compounds make coffee uniquely suited to this therapeutic purpose. No other beverage produces these effects through the rectal route.

What Actually Happens During a Coffee Enema

Let us walk through the physiology, moment by moment.

Minutes 0 to 3 — insertion and distribution:

• The 48 ounces of coffee solution enters the colon.

• Distributes through the descending, transverse, and ascending colon.

• The colon walls absorb water immediately, a normal function.

• The first molecules of caffeine and palmitic acid enter the colon wall.

Minutes 3 to 8 — absorption begins:

• Coffee compounds cross the colon wall into the portal vein.

• Portal blood, now containing concentrated coffee compounds, travels directly to the liver.

• The liver receives a significant biochemical signal.

• Glutathione S-transferase production begins ramping up.

• Bile ducts begin to dilate in response to the stimulation.

Minutes 8 to 15 — peak therapeutic activity:

• Glutathione production at peak levels.

• Bile duct contraction begins — the gallbladder squeezing concentrated bile downward.

• Bile carries with it accumulated fluke debris, biliary sludge, and toxic compounds the liver has been processing.

• The liver's detoxification capacity is dramatically elevated.

• Caffeine in the system, but reaching the brain at lower levels than oral coffee, produces gentle alertness without the typical caffeine intensity.

Minutes 15 onward — release:

• The coffee solution and everything it has flushed exits the body.

• The liver continues working with elevated glutathione for several hours afterward.

• The bile duct flushing effect continues — bile flowing more freely throughout the day.

• The benefits of the enema extend well beyond the 15-minute session.

(Figure 18.4 — see the online Figure Guide)

The Green Sludge Phenomenon

If you have done coffee enemas for any length of time during a fast, you have probably seen it. Green material in the returns. Sometimes pale green. Sometimes dark green or even nearly black. Sometimes thick and ropy. Sometimes thin and stringy. This is bile.

Specifically, it is bile that has been stimulated to release from the gallbladder and bile ducts during the enema. In a healthy state, bile flows continuously and is bright green to greenish yellow. In a state of accumulated stress, bile becomes thicker as water is reabsorbed during prolonged sitting in the gallbladder; darker as oxidized compounds accumulate; sludgy as cholesterol and bilirubin crystallize; mixed with debris including dead fluke matter, biliary parasites, and toxic compounds the liver has been trying to eliminate.

Seeing green material in your returns is one of the most direct visual indicators that the coffee enema is doing meaningful work. The first few coffee enemas of a fast often produce dramatic green releases. This frequency typically decreases as the bile system clears. Continued occasional green releases throughout the fast indicate ongoing biliary work. By the end of the fast, green releases become rare, indicating the system has cleared significantly.

(Figure 18.5 — see the online Figure Guide)

Why Coffee Enemas Are Critical for Fluke Elimination

This is where coffee enemas become essential rather than merely beneficial. Liver flukes live in the bile ducts. The bile ducts are completely beyond the reach of normal enemas. Even drinking herbs that pass through the digestive tract reach the bile ducts only through systemic circulation. The coffee enema is the only intervention that directly stimulates bile duct flushing.

When the gallbladder contracts and bile ducts dilate, bile flows more vigorously through the entire biliary system. This flow:

• Carries dead fluke matter from the bile ducts into the small intestine.

• Flushes parasite eggs that have been deposited in bile duct walls.

• Mobilizes biliary sludge that has been protecting parasitic organisms.

• Forces release of compounds the liver has been holding.

This is why the coffee enema is non-negotiable for anyone seriously addressing fluke elimination. No other practice achieves this effect. The targeted fluke elimination protocol in Chapter 21 depends on it entirely.

Choosing the Right Coffee

Quality matters significantly here. The coffee that goes into a therapeutic enema is being absorbed directly into the portal vein and delivered straight to the liver. What you choose to put through your colon wall matters more than what you choose to drink.

Required characteristics:

• **Organic — non-negotiable.** Coffee is one of the most heavily pesticide-sprayed crops in the world. Conventional coffee absorbed through the colon wall delivers those pesticides directly into the portal circulation. This concentrated chemical exposure to the liver is exactly the opposite of what you are trying to accomplish.

• **Light to medium roast preferred.** Higher levels of palmitic acid in less roasted coffee. More cafestol and kahweol preserved. The therapeutic compounds are partially destroyed by extreme heat. Dark roast coffee is less effective for this purpose.

• **Specific therapeutic coffees.** Several brands sell coffee specifically for enema use, tend to be organic, light roast, and grown at high altitude. Higher altitude coffee tends to have higher concentrations of beneficial compounds. Look for brands marketed for therapeutic use; Gerson Institute approved coffees are a good benchmark.

Avoid:

• Decaffeinated coffee — defeats the purpose.

• Instant coffee — significantly reduced therapeutic compounds.

• Conventional grocery store coffee — pesticide load.

• Flavored coffees — additives serve no therapeutic purpose.

The Brewing Process

Proper brewing extracts the therapeutic compounds while keeping the solution gentle on the colon. The recipe and procedure below have been used essentially unchanged since the Gerson Therapy formalized them.

Equipment:

• Stainless steel or glass pot — never aluminum.

• Fine mesh strainer or coffee filter.

• 48-ounce capacity for the final solution.

Process:

1. Bring water to boil. 48 ounces water treated with ionic sulfated minerals in a pot, brought to full rolling boil.

2. Add coffee. 3 tablespoons organic ground coffee — the standard therapeutic ratio. Stir into boiling water and reduce heat slightly.

3. Simmer 15 minutes. This extraction time is important — shorter extracts less of the therapeutic compounds. Maintain gentle simmer, not aggressive boiling. Stir occasionally.

4. Strain thoroughly. All grounds must be removed. Use fine mesh strainer or coffee filter. Any grounds remaining will cause discomfort during retention.

5. Cool to body temperature. Add room-temperature water treated with ionic sulfated minerals if needed to bring to 48 ounces total. Test temperature on inner wrist before use — should feel comfortably warm. Too hot causes intestinal damage; too cold causes cramping and difficulty retaining.

6. Use immediately or refrigerate. Best used immediately. Can be refrigerated for up to 24 hours; rewarm to body temperature before use. Discard after 24 hours.

(Figure 18.6 — see the online Figure Guide)

The Standard Coffee Enema Procedure

Building on the basic enema procedure from Chapter 17, with coffee-specific considerations.

Preparation:

• Brew coffee solution as described above.

• Ensure all equipment is clean.

• Hang bag at hip height.

• Lubricate tip with olive oil or coconut oil.

Position. Begin in left-side lying position. This directs flow toward the descending colon and allows fluid to travel up through the transverse colon as volume increases.

Insertion. Slow insertion, 2 to 3 inches. Open clamp very slowly. Allow solution to enter at comfortable pace. 5 to 10 minutes for full volume.

Retention sequence:

Minutes

Position

0 to 4

Left side

4 to 8

Back, knees slightly bent

8 to 12

Right side

12 to 15

Return to left side or back

This rotation distributes solution throughout the colon, allows direct contact with all colon walls, maximizes portal vein absorption, and ensures bile duct stimulation.

Release. After 15 minutes, go to toilet. Allow full release — multiple cycles common. Stay near bathroom for 30 to 45 minutes. Document what you observe.

Adding Therapeutic Compounds to Your Coffee Enema

The coffee solution alone is therapeutic. The bile flow it triggers, the glutathione it stimulates, the bile-duct dilation it produces — all of this is real work. But the morning enema can do more. The additions that complement the coffee work focus on direct antiparasitic action, targeted egg destruction, and liver support during heavy detoxification. Three additions, each with its specific role. All added to fully cooled coffee solution before warming to body temperature.

Clove oil — 2 to 3 drops. The egg killer.

- Food-grade clove oil only.
- Added to fully cooled coffee solution before warming.
- Ensures eugenol distributes throughout the volume.
- Direct contact with any eggs deposited along the colon wall.
- Systemic absorption supports egg destruction in tissues beyond enema reach.

Why this combination works: coffee stimulates bile flow, flushing eggs from bile ducts. Clove oil destroys eggs in transit through the intestinal tract. Together they address eggs from both directions simultaneously.

Cautions: never exceed 3 drops in 48 ounces — clove oil is extremely potent. If burning sensation develops, reduce to 1 drop next session. Only food grade — never use diffuser oils internally.

Black walnut hull tincture — 1 teaspoon. The adult parasite killer.

- Direct antiparasitic action against adult worms living in or near the colon.
- Particularly effective against intestinal flukes, which the enema can reach.
- Systemic absorption extends antiparasitic effects beyond the colon.
- Combined with the coffee's biliary stimulation, flushes dead parasites efficiently.

Particularly valuable during active parasite die-off phases, when enema returns show visible parasitic material, and during the heaviest weeks of the antiparasitic protocol.

Milk thistle liquid extract — 1 teaspoon. The liver protector.

- Silymarin — the active compound — protects liver cells during heavy detoxification.
- Particularly important when significant fluke debris is being processed.
- Supports glutathione production alongside the coffee's effects.
- Reduces inflammation in liver tissue.

Particularly valuable on days when you anticipate heavy die-off, after the first noticeable green sludge appears in returns, throughout the fluke elimination phase, and when the liver feels tender or congested.

Together, clove oil and black walnut tincture form the parasite-killing core of the morning enema. Milk thistle is the protective companion. The full combination represents the most comprehensive single therapeutic intervention available through this protocol.

Frequency and Timing

During an active prolonged fast, coffee enemas are typically daily.

Standard protocol:

- One coffee enema daily, in the morning.
- Within an hour of waking, after the first dose of herbs.
- Followed by mineral replenishment immediately after.

Exception periods:

- Some intensive protocols use coffee enemas twice daily for short periods during heavy die-off.
- More than once daily should be approached with caution — caffeine levels can build up.
- Always replenish minerals more aggressively when increasing frequency.

Days off:

- Some practitioners take one day per week off coffee enemas.
- Allows the system to recalibrate.
- Salt water enema substitutes on days off.
- Optional rather than required.

Mineral Replenishment After Coffee Enemas

Coffee enemas can be more depleting than salt water enemas. The bile duct contraction releases concentrated bile, and with it significant electrolyte content. The colon absorbs the coffee solution, including its caffeine, which has mild diuretic effects.

Within 30 minutes of completion:

- 16 ounces water treated with ionic sulfated minerals.
- Generous pinch of Himalayan salt.
- 8 ounces coconut water if available.

This replenishment protocol is more important than usual after coffee enemas. The depletion is real, and the consequences of ignoring it compound day by day if uncorrected.

If you experience:

• *Heart palpitations:* reduce caffeine concentration next time, replenish potassium.

• *Headache:* increase sodium and water intake.

• *Anxiety or jitters:* caffeine sensitivity — reduce coffee amount.

• *Significant fatigue afterward:* increase mineral replenishment.

Caffeine Considerations

Coffee enemas deliver caffeine. This affects different people differently.

• **For coffee drinkers.** Generally well tolerated. Minimal jitters or sleep disruption when done in the morning. Most people experience gentle alertness rather than coffee buzz.

• **For non-coffee drinkers.** More likely to feel caffeine effects. Start with reduced amounts — 2 tablespoons coffee instead of 3. Build up over several sessions. Always do morning only — never evening for non-coffee drinkers.

• **For caffeine-sensitive individuals.** May still benefit from coffee enemas but at reduced concentration. Begin with 1 tablespoon coffee in 48 ounces water. Increase only as tolerated. Watch for sleep disruption and adjust.

• **Pregnancy and certain medical conditions.** Coffee enemas not appropriate during pregnancy. Consult medical support if any cardiac conditions, severe hypertension, or other contraindications. The general contraindications listed earlier apply to coffee enemas as well.

What Coffee Enemas Are Not

Some honest framing. Coffee enemas are not a replacement for medical treatment of any condition. Not a weight loss tool. Not a substitute for proper diet and lifestyle. Not effective for everyone in every circumstance. Not appropriate without proper medical supervision during prolonged fasting.

They are one tool among many in a comprehensive protocol. An effective tool, yes. A central tool for serious cleansing work, yes. But a tool, not a cure.

When to Pause Coffee Enemas

Even the most beneficial practice has its limits. Pause coffee enemas if you experience:

• Severe heart palpitations not resolving with mineral replenishment.

- Significant insomnia despite morning-only timing.
- Persistent headaches that worsen with each session.
- Any symptom that genuinely concerns you.
- Acute illness or fever.
- Unusual cramping that does not match normal enema sensations.

Switch to plain salt water enemas during pause periods. Resume coffee enemas only when symptoms have fully resolved.

A Personal Observation

This deserves to be said directly. Of everything in this protocol, the coffee enema is what most people skip. The cultural resistance is strongest here. The brewing process feels like extra effort. The combination of coffee and rectum produces internal resistance.

And yet, those who include coffee enemas consistently in their protocol report significantly different results than those who skip them. Faster overall progress. Cleaner enema returns. Better mental clarity through the fast. More efficient liver detoxification. Significantly better fluke clearance.

The discomfort with the practice is cultural. The benefits of the practice are biological. For anyone serious about deep cleansing, particularly anyone targeting fluke elimination, the coffee enema is not optional. It is the practice that makes the rest of the protocol significantly more effective.

A Final Reframe

Hear this clearly. Coffee enemas have a hundred years of clinical use behind them. The Merck Manual included them as standard practice for decades. Practitioners across multiple healing traditions use them today. They work because they engage the liver and bile ducts in ways no other practice does.

Approach this tool with the respect it deserves. Brew the coffee carefully. Use it consistently. Pay attention to what your body releases. And trust that the liver — the most metabolically complex organ in your body — knows what to do with the support you are offering it.

The Daily Enema Chart

	AM — Coffee Enema	PM — Salt Water Enema
Timing	Morning, on rising	2 to 3 hours before sleep
Base liquid	48 oz water with ionic sulfated minerals	48 oz water with ionic sulfated minerals
Coffee *	3 tbsp organic light-roast, simmered 15 min, strained	—
Salt *	—	1 to 2 tsp Himalayan salt, fully dissolved
Clove oil *	2 to 3 drops, food-grade only	—
Black walnut hull tincture *	1 teaspoon	—
Milk thistle extract **	1 teaspoon	—
Aloe vera juice **	—	4 oz, inner leaf only
Magnesium chloride **	—	½ teaspoon
Pau d'arco tincture **	—	1 teaspoon
Temperature	Body temperature	Body temperature
Hold time	12 to 15 minutes, with position rotation	10 to 15 minutes
Replenish after	16 oz water, trace minerals, pinch salt, coconut water if available	16 oz water with trace minerals; magnesium glycinate before sleep
Purpose	Egg killer, adult parasite killer, liver protector	Soother, relaxer, antifungal sweep

* **Essential.** The minimum that makes this enema therapeutic. Used from Week 1 onward.

** **Ideal.** The full protocol used in Weeks 2 onward. Adds liver protection and overnight support.

*** **Situational.** Optional additions used only when specific conditions apply — apple cider vinegar for yeast, garlic for aggressive parasite phases, slippery elm after irritation, ginger for nausea, probiotic for late stages. Catalogued in Chapter 17.

A blank copy of this chart is at the back, with other quick references — meant to be photocopied or photographed.

*Figures referenced above: 18.3–18.7 **(online Figure Guide)*

Chapter 19

The Herbal Antiparasitic Protocol

* * *

The enemas and flushes do the expelling. The herbs do the killing. This is the division of labor at the heart of this protocol, and understanding it changes how you approach every herb in this chapter.

You are not asking the herbs to flush. You are not asking them to clean. You are asking them to disable, weaken, and kill the organisms living inside you, so that everything else can carry the dead bodies out. That is what these herbs do. Each one in its own way. Each one targeting different organisms, different life stages, different locations in the body. The chapter that follows is the catalog of those tools — what they do, how they work together, and how to use them.

Most of the entries in this catalog are herbs in the strict sense — whole plants, or tinctures and capsules made from them. A few are not. Clove appears here both as a plant and as an essential oil. Berberine is an isolated alkaloid. Piperine is an extract of black pepper. Caprylic acid is a fatty acid found in coconut. They earn their place in this chapter because they do work the herbs alone cannot do, and the protocol uses all of them together. The word *herbal* is convenient shorthand. The reality is a small pharmacy of plant-derived medicines, refined by centuries of practice into the toolkit this chapter describes.

* * *

Why Herbs Rather Than Pharmaceuticals

The question deserves a direct answer. Conventional medicine has effective antiparasitic medications, and they work — sometimes very well. For an acute, confirmed infection with a known organism, they are often the right choice. But pharmaceutical antiparasitics carry limitations that herbs do not.

Most of them target a narrow range of organisms: you must already know what you are treating. They typically address one life stage — usually adults, rarely eggs. Their side-effect profiles are often as challenging as the infection itself. Their use periods are limited; most cannot be taken for the weeks of continuous coverage that full lifecycle clearance requires. They do not address biofilm, candida overgrowth, or the layered debris that protects parasites from anything trying to reach them. And because most parasitic infections are subclinical, pharmaceutical treatment is rarely offered without a clear diagnosis — which means the people who most need clearing are the people least likely to receive it.

Herbs do not have these limitations. They cover broad spectrums. Different herbs hit different life stages — eggs, larvae, adults — and the protocol layers them so the lifecycle is broken at every point. They are sustainable across the weeks of work this requires. They combine in ways pharmaceuticals cannot, with one herb's mechanism reinforcing another's. They disrupt biofilm and candida and the supporting environment, not just the organisms themselves. And they are appropriate for the reader to take in their own kitchen, on their own schedule, without a diagnosis.

This protocol uses herbs because the work it is doing is too long, too broad, and too multidimensional for pharmaceutical alternatives. The right tool for the right job — and for sustained antiparasitic work over weeks at a time, herbs are the right tool.

* * *

How Antiparasitic Herbs Actually Work

Different herbs work through different mechanisms. Understanding the mechanisms is what allows the practitioner to combine herbs intelligently rather than randomly. The major mechanisms in play in this protocol are these:

Direct toxicity — some herbs contain compounds directly toxic to parasites at concentrations that do not harm human cells. Black walnut hull, clove, and oregano work primarily this way.

Membrane disruption — some compounds dissolve or damage parasite cell membranes. Berberine and oregano oil work this way.

Reproductive interference — some herbs prevent parasites from reproducing without killing adults outright. Wormwood interferes with parasite reproductive cycles.

Paralysis — some herbs paralyze parasite muscle tissue so the organism cannot hold on to intestinal walls, allowing the body to expel it. Pumpkin seed and certain forms of mimosa pudica work this way.

Enzymatic disruption — some herbs inhibit critical parasite enzymes. Berberine works partly through this mechanism.

Biofilm disruption — some herbs break down the protective biofilm that shields parasites from everything else. Mimosa pudica seed is particularly effective here.

Egg destruction — few herbs penetrate the protective shell of parasite eggs. Clove is the standout, and the reason it has its own chapter.

Effective antiparasitic protocols combine herbs working through different mechanisms, creating coverage that no single herb provides alone. The classic triad below is the foundation; everything else builds on it.

* * *

The Classic Triad

Three herbs form the foundation of nearly every traditional antiparasitic protocol. Used together, they cover the complete parasite lifecycle. Their combination is older than any modern medical system, and it works because each herb covers what the others miss.

Black walnut hull — the adult killer. The unripe green hull of the black walnut, not the ripe brown hull, is one of the most potent antiparasitic herbs known. Its juglone content is directly toxic to adult worms across many species; its tannins disrupt parasite attachment to intestinal walls; and the iodine compounds it carries naturally add antimicrobial coverage that few other herbs match. Used by Native American tribes long before Europeans arrived on this continent. The dosing and full caution profile appear in the charts at the end of this chapter.

Wormwood — the larvae destroyer. *Artemisia absinthium* has been documented as an antiparasitic for over three thousand years — described in ancient Egyptian medical texts, threaded through European herbal traditions, and still in use across continents today. Its thujone content is what does most of the work, paired with sesquiterpene lactones that broaden the antimicrobial reach. Wormwood targets parasite larvae and juvenile organisms before they reach reproductive maturity — the life stage that most other antiparasitics miss. The 4-week maximum continuous use period is real. Respect it.

Clove — the egg killer. Clove receives its own chapter because what it does, nothing else does. Black walnut kills adults. Wormwood kills larvae. Clove kills eggs. Without clove, eggs survive the protocol and hatch into new generations. With clove, the lifecycle is broken at every stage. The full clove protocol is in Chapter 20.

The triad together: working through three different mechanisms, covering three different life stages, providing complete lifecycle coverage that no single herb achieves. Used in this combination for hundreds of years. The triad is the foundation. Everything else in this chapter builds on it.

* * *

Beyond the Triad — Specialized Support

Each of the herbs that follows adds specific capabilities the triad does not provide.

Berberine is an isolated alkaloid found in several plants — most notably Oregon grape root, goldenseal, and barberry. It is exceptional against giardia, effective against cryptosporidium, broad-spectrum against bacteria, and active against candida. It works through membrane disruption, enzymatic disruption, and biofilm breakdown — three mechanisms in one compound. Best taken between meals, where it can act directly on the gut without interference from food.

Oregano oil is the essential oil of *Origanum vulgare*, one of the most potent natural antimicrobials available. Its carvacrol and thymol content makes it exceptional against candida, broad-spectrum against pathogenic bacteria, and active against some protozoa. It is also a strong biofilm disrupter. Always diluted, always with food or a carrier oil — straight oregano oil irritates mucous membranes and will burn the throat. The 2-weeks-on / 1-week-off cycling protocol matters; continuous use erodes its effect.

Mimosa pudica seed does something no other herb in the protocol does. The seeds form a sticky, gel-like substance when they reach the digestive tract — a substance that physically grabs parasites from intestinal walls and acts as a mechanical scrubber through the small intestine. It binds heavy metals, adsorbs toxins, and pulls all of it out together. A different mechanism from any other herb in this chapter, and the reason mimosa pudica earns a place beside the chemical antiparasitics.

Pumpkin seed is one of the oldest antiparasitic remedies known. Its active compound, cucurbitacin, paralyzes parasite muscle tissue so the organism loses its grip and is expelled. Particularly effective against tapeworms. The traditional protocol — a cup of raw seeds chewed thoroughly on an empty stomach — is reserved for post-fast use; during the fast itself, the capsule form is appropriate.

* * *

Specific Herbs for Fluke Work

Three herbs deserve specific mention for their role in the fluke elimination work that intensifies in the middle weeks of the protocol.

Chanca piedra — the stone breaker. *Phyllanthus niruri*, used in South American herbal medicine for centuries. It clears bile duct sludge, helps move small biliary stones, improves bile flow, and reduces inflammation in liver tissue — all of which matter when flukes are being killed in numbers and the liver is processing the debris. Particularly important during weeks 3 and 4 of the fast, when fluke clearing is at its most intense.

Milk thistle — the liver protector. Its silymarin content protects liver cells and supports their regeneration. Milk thistle is not antiparasitic. It is what allows the liver to handle the load of antiparasitic work without becoming overwhelmed. Taken throughout the fluke clearing phase, and safe for long-term use afterward.

Dandelion root — the bile mover. A common plant whose root stimulates bile production and flow, supports the liver in processing released toxins, and provides a mild laxative effect that supports clearing. Available as tea, tincture, or capsule — the reader's choice. The work it does is the same in any form.

Pau d'arco earns a place beside the fluke herbs and again in candida work. The inner bark of the *Tabebuia* tree, used in Indigenous medicine across South America for centuries before it ever crossed the Atlantic. Its naphthoquinone content — lapachol the most studied — is directly toxic to fungal cells and active against certain protozoa, including cryptosporidium as a secondary herb. It supports immune function during the heavy work of late fluke clearing. The traditional preparation is a tea brewed from the bark; the modern tincture is what most readers will use, and it works.

* * *

Caprylic Acid — The Candida Disruptor

Caprylic acid is not an herb. It is a medium-chain fatty acid found naturally in coconut oil, in palm kernel oil, and in human breast milk. What earns it a place in this chapter is what it does to candida.

Candida albicans, in its overgrowth form, is one of the most persistent infections a fasting protocol confronts. The cell wall of candida is built on a lipid bilayer that ordinary water-soluble compounds cannot penetrate. Caprylic acid, being itself a lipid, dissolves into the candida cell wall and disrupts it from within. The candida cell loses integrity and dies. Few compounds in nature do this as cleanly.

Caprylic acid is reserved for situations where candida is the active concern — heavy white tongue coating, persistent sugar cravings during the fast, recurrent thrush, the constellation of symptoms that signals candida overgrowth has been a long-standing presence in the body. When those signals are present, caprylic acid joins the protocol; when they are not, it is not needed. It is a situational tool, sharply effective where it applies.

The dosing and cautions are in the chart. The one practical note that belongs in prose: start at the lower end of the dose range. Caprylic acid die-off can be severe in someone with heavy candida overgrowth, and ramping up gradually is safer than starting at the top of the range.

* * *

Piperine — The Amplifier

This is not an antiparasitic herb itself, but it makes every other herb work better. Piperine, the active alkaloid in black pepper, increases the absorption of other herbs by up to 2000% for some compounds. It inhibits the enzymes that would otherwise metabolize herbs before they can reach therapeutic concentrations, dramatically increasing the effective dose of every other herb in this protocol.

The rule is simple: **every oral herbal dose should be accompanied by piperine.** Five to ten milligrams of piperine extract, or a small pinch of freshly ground black pepper, alongside each herbal dose. Without it, you are taking a fraction of the dose you think you are taking. With it, the herbs reach the concentrations the protocol depends on.

This is the difference between a protocol that works and one that fails for reasons the practitioner never identifies.

* * *

The Daily Schedule

The herbs of this protocol are taken at specific times across the day, in patterns that respect the digestive cycle, the enema timing, and the body's overnight rest. The full schedule appears as Chart 3 at the end of this chapter, photographable as a daily reference.

The complete daily protocol that integrates these herbs with the enemas, flushes, and other practices is laid out as a unified schedule in Chapter 22.

* * *

Quality and Sourcing

The herbs in this chapter cannot work if they are not what they claim to be. Quality and sourcing matter as much as the dosing schedule.

What to look for in a tincture: organic certification, made from fresh plant material when possible, glass bottles rather than plastic, verified species (particularly important for wormwood, where misidentification is common), and a reputable company with quality control standards.

Cheap herbs are often ineffective herbs. This protocol depends on the herbs actually doing their work. Quality matters here as much as anywhere in the entire protocol. If the herb is wrong, or if the dose is dilute, or if the species is misidentified, no schedule of consumption can compensate.

* * *

A Final Thought on These Herbs

These plants have been part of human medicine for thousands of years. Black walnut, used by Native American tribes long before Europeans arrived. Wormwood, described in ancient Egyptian medical texts. Clove, referenced in Chinese medicine over two thousand years ago. Mimosa pudica, used in Ayurvedic medicine for millennia. Pau d'arco, brewed by the Indigenous peoples of the Amazon long before any pharmacy existed.

You are not using new untested compounds. You are using the accumulated wisdom of countless generations of healers, refined through trial, error, and observation across cultures and centuries. The herbs in this chapter work because they have always worked. The protocol that arranges them works because the arrangement reflects what generations of careful observation discovered about how they work best together.

The next chapter goes into the most important single herb in this protocol — clove — in the depth that its central role deserves.

* * *

Doses below assume single-herb tinctures. For combination tinctures, follow the bottle's recommendations. See Chapter 20 for the tincture-versus-oil distinction.

Chart 3: The Daily Herbal Schedule

Time	What You Take
Upon waking	• Clove tincture, 4–6 drops, with piperine • L-Glutamine, 5 g
Mid-morning *(after coffee enema)*	• Black walnut hull tincture, 1 teaspoon, with piperine • Wormwood tincture, 4–6 drops, with piperine • Mimosa pudica, 1–2 capsules, with substantial water
Midday	• Clove tincture, 4–6 drops, with piperine (second dose) • Berberine, 500 mg, with piperine • Oregano oil, 2–4 drops in water or carrier oil
Mid-afternoon	• Pau d'arco tincture, 4–6 drops, with piperine • Chanca piedra, 1 capsule • Dandelion root, 30 drops tincture • Milk thistle, 250 mg
Evening *(before salt water enema)*	• Wormwood tincture, second dose, with piperine • Mimosa pudica, second dose if appropriate
Night	• Clove tincture, 4–6 drops, with piperine (third and final dose) • Milk thistle, 250 mg • Magnesium glycinate

The complete daily protocol that integrates these herbs with the enemas, flushes, and other practices is laid out as a unified schedule in Chapter 22.

Chart 1: What It Is

Substance	Type	Tagline	Active Compounds	Primary Targets	Mechanism
Black walnut hull *	Whole-plant tincture (unripe green hull)	The adult killer	Juglone; tannins; naturally occurring iodine compounds	Adult tapeworms (especially); adult roundworms incl. hookworm and whipworm; adult intestinal flukes; Candida; various pathogenic bacteria	Direct toxicity
Wormwood *	Whole-plant tincture (*Artemisia absinthium*)	The larvae destroyer	Thujone (most active); artemisinin (in sweet wormwood); sesquiterpene lactones; bitter compounds	Parasite larvae across many species; juvenile parasites pre-reproduction; some adult roundworms; certain protozoa (incl. malaria parasites historically)	Reproductive interference; broad antimicrobial; moderate biofilm disruption
Clove *	Essential oil and tincture (*Syzygium aromaticum*)	The egg killer	Eugenol (primary)	Parasite eggs across species — the singular role nothing else fills; adult organisms; bacteria; fungi	Egg shell penetration; direct toxicity
Piperine *	Black pepper extract	The amplifier	Piperine (the active alkaloid of *Piper nigrum*)	Not antiparasitic itself — increases bioavailability of every other herb in the protocol	Inhibits drug-metabolizing enzymes; increases absorption up to 2000% for some compounds
Berberine **	Isolated alkaloid (from Oregon grape root, goldenseal, barberry)	The protozoa specialist	Berberine	Giardia (exceptionally effective); Cryptosporidium; broad-spectrum bacteria; Candida; some parasites	Membrane disruption; enzymatic disruption; significant biofilm activity
Oregano oil **	Essential oil (*Origanum vulgare*)	The membrane breaker	Carvacrol (primary); thymol (secondary)	Candida (exceptional); broad-spectrum bacteria; some protozoa	Membrane disruption; strong biofilm disruption

Substance	Type	Tagline	Active Compounds	Primary Targets	Mechanism
Mimosa pudica **	Seed	The mechanical scrubber	Mucilaginous compounds that gel in the gut	All worm species (mechanical removal); biofilm; heavy metals; toxins	Mechanical adsorption — physically grabs and removes
Chanca piedra **	Whole-plant tincture / capsule (*Phyllanthus niruri*)	The stone breaker	Phyllanthin and related lignans	Bile duct sludge and small biliary stones; supports liver during fluke clearing	Bile flow stimulation; anti-inflammatory in bile ducts
Milk thistle **	Standardized extract (*Silybum marianum*)	The liver protector	Silymarin (silibinin and related flavonolignans)	Not antiparasitic — protects liver cells during heavy detox phases	Hepatocyte membrane stabilization; supports liver regeneration
Dandelion root **	Whole-plant tincture / tea / capsule (*Taraxacum officinale*)	The bile mover	Sesquiterpene lactones; taraxasterol; inulin	Supports bile production and flow; mild laxative effect	Bile stimulation; supports liver in processing released toxins
Pau d'arco **	Inner bark tincture or tea (*Tabebuia* tree species)	The South American antifungal	Naphthoquinones (lapachol the most studied); beta-lapachone	Candida; certain protozoa incl. Cryptosporidium (as secondary); some bacteria	Direct toxicity to fungal cells; immune modulation
Pumpkin seed ***	Whole seed (*Cucurbita pepo*)	The paralyzer	Cucurbitacin	Tapeworms (particularly effective); roundworms; some flukes	Paralysis of parasite muscle tissue
Caprylic acid ***	Medium-chain fatty acid (from coconut oil)	The Candida disruptor	Caprylic acid (octanoic acid)	Candida albicans (primary); other yeasts	Membrane disruption — inserts into the fungal lipid bilayer

Doses below assume single-herb tinctures. For combination tinctures, follow the bottle's recommendations. See Chapter 20 for the tincture-versus-oil distinction.

Chart 2: How to Use

Substance	Standard Dose	Form & Delivery	When in Protocol	Take With	Cautions
Black walnut hull *	1 teaspoon tincture, 3× daily	Oral tincture; can also be added to enema solution	Full duration of antiparasitic protocol	Piperine (every dose)	Avoid during pregnancy; possible interactions with certain medications; nut-allergic individuals may react
Wormwood *	4–6 drops tincture, 3× daily	Oral tincture	Full duration, but **maximum 4 weeks continuous**	Piperine (every dose)	Do not exceed dosing — thujone toxic at high doses; avoid during pregnancy; may interact with seizure medications
Clove *	4–6 drops tincture, 3× daily (morning, midday, night)	Oral tincture (food-grade essential oil for enema use — see Chapter 18)	Full duration	Piperine (every dose)	See Chapter 20 for the full clove protocol
Piperine *	5–10 mg extract with every oral herbal dose; or a small pinch of freshly ground black pepper	Capsule or pinch of pepper †	Every oral dose, every day	Taken alongside the herb it amplifies	Generally well-tolerated; can increase absorption of pharmaceuticals (consult a practitioner if on medications)
Berberine **	500 mg, 2× daily	Capsule †	Active antiparasitic phases (Weeks 2 onward)	Piperine; best between meals	Can cause digestive upset in sensitive individuals; not appropriate during pregnancy; may interact with diabetes medications
Oregano oil **	2–4 drops liquid oil, 2× daily, diluted in water or carrier oil	Oral, diluted	**Cycling: 2 weeks on, 1 week off**	Always with food or carrier oil — straight oregano oil irritates mucous membranes	Always dilute properly; not appropriate during pregnancy

Substance	Standard Dose	Form & Delivery	When in Protocol	Take With	Cautions
Mimosa pudica **	1–2 capsules, 3× daily on empty stomach	Capsule †	Throughout active antiparasitic protocol	Substantial water — the seeds need water to form the gel	Generally well-tolerated; space apart from medications by 2 hours, as the gel can adsorb pharmaceuticals
Chanca piedra **	1–2 capsules, 2× daily	Capsule (also available as tincture or tea) †	Fluke clearing phases — particularly important Weeks 3 and 4	—	Generally well-tolerated; consult practitioner if on blood pressure or diabetes medications
Milk thistle **	250–500 mg, 2× daily	Capsule (standardized to silymarin content) †	Liver-intensive phases; continue throughout fluke clearing; safe long-term	—	Safe for long-term use; rare allergic reactions in those sensitive to ragweed family
Dandelion root **	1 cup tea, 2× daily; or 30 drops tincture, 2× daily; or 500 mg capsule, 2× daily	Tea, tincture, or capsule (reader's choice) †	Throughout fluke clearing	—	Avoid if obstructed bile ducts or gallstones; possible mild diuretic effect
Pau d'arco **	4–6 drops tincture, 2× daily	Tincture or tea	Routine fluke-phase support; intensifies for Candida or Cryptosporidium phases	Piperine	Avoid during pregnancy; can interact with blood thinners
Pumpkin seed ***	Post-fast: 1 cup raw seeds chewed thoroughly on empty stomach. During fast: capsule form per label	Raw seeds (post-fast) or capsule (during fast) †	Best used in combination with other antiparasitic herbs; full effect requires post-fast use	—	Generally very safe; minor digestive upset possible at high doses
Caprylic acid ***	500–1000 mg, 2× daily with food	Capsule †	Candida-active phases only	Food (improves tolerance)	Can cause die-off symptoms in heavy Candida overgrowth — start at lower end of dose range; rarely contraindicated

* **Essential.** The classic triad plus piperine. The minimum that makes the protocol work.

** **Ideal.** Broad-spectrum and liver-phase support. Used from the second week onward.

*** **Situational.** Used when specific conditions apply.

† **Capsule note.** During a water fast, the preferred practice is to open the capsule and mix the powder into a small amount of water rather than swallow the capsule whole. Two reasons: digestive activity slows during fasting, so the capsule shell may not dissolve reliably; and gelatin capsules are an animal product some readers prefer to avoid during the fast. Vegetable cellulose capsules avoid the second concern but not the first. For powders too bitter to mix with water (berberine, oregano-derived compounds), the capsule is acceptable as long as it is a vegetable-cellulose type.

A Quick Reference — Which Herbs for Which Parasites

The protocol uses the same core herbs for nearly everyone, and that is by design. The triad — black walnut, wormwood, clove — addresses the great majority of human parasitic infections, and the supporting herbs cover the rest. But the protocol is not undifferentiated. Specific organisms respond to specific herbs more strongly, and knowing which herb leads against which parasite is part of running the protocol intelligently.

The table below summarizes what the chapter has been describing, organism by organism. The primary herb is what does the most against the adult form. The secondary herb is what reinforces it. The egg killer addresses the reproductive stage. The enhancer is what the protocol pairs alongside to push absorption or extend reach. For most readers, every herb in this table is in the cabinet by the time the fast begins. The table shows how each herb earns its place there.

Parasite	Primary Herb	Secondary Herb	Egg Killer	Enhanced By
Roundworms	Black walnut hull	Wormwood	Clove	Piperine
Tapeworms	Black walnut hull	Pumpkin seed	Clove	Mimosa pudica
Hookworm	Black walnut hull	Wormwood	Clove	Piperine
Whipworm	Black walnut hull	Wormwood	Clove	Piperine
Pinworms	Black walnut hull	Wormwood	Clove	*See Chapter 23 — special case*
Intestinal flukes	Black walnut hull	Wormwood	Clove	Coffee enema
Liver flukes	Chanca piedra	Milk thistle	Clove	Coffee enema + dandelion
Giardia	Berberine	Oregano oil	—	Piperine
Cryptosporidium	Berberine	Pau d'arco	—	Black walnut
Candida	Oregano oil	Caprylic acid	—	Berberine

Two patterns are worth noticing. First, **black walnut hull and clove appear across nearly every line**. They are the foundation, and the protocol depends on them. Second, **the flukes — both intestinal and liver — show coffee enema in the enhancer column**. This is not optional language. It is the same point made earlier in this chapter, summarized into one cell. The flukes are not addressable by herbs alone. The coffee enema is what allows the herbs to reach them.

Chapter 20

The Clove Protocol

* * *

Of every herb in the previous chapter — every plant, every tincture, every traditional remedy — one stands apart. Not because it is the strongest overall. Not because it kills the most adult parasites. Not because it does the most for biofilm or candida. Clove stands apart because it does the one thing nothing else does. It penetrates the egg.

This is the issue at the heart of every parasite cleanse that fails. Most antiparasitic protocols work beautifully against adult worms, larvae, and active organisms in their feeding stage. These are all relatively easy targets. The adults are physically large and metabolically active. They take in toxic compounds along with their food. They die under the pressure of consistent herbal exposure. The eggs are different.

A parasite egg is essentially a fortress. Surrounded by a thick protective shell — the chorion — the contents inside are metabolically dormant. The egg does not feed, so it does not absorb compounds from its environment. The shell resists most chemicals, most enzymes, most natural herbal compounds. The egg sits there, protected, waiting for the right conditions to hatch. When you kill all the adults but leave the eggs, the eggs hatch days, weeks, or months later. New adults emerge. The cycle continues. The cleanse appears to have failed. The person becomes convinced they have been reinfected. They have not been reinfected. They simply never finished.

What Makes the Egg Shell So Resistant

The chorion is one of nature's most effective protective structures. It is composed of multiple layers:

• An outer layer designed to survive harsh environmental conditions.

• A lipid-rich middle layer that prevents water-soluble compounds from passing through.

• An inner layer that maintains the embryo's protected environment.

Most antiparasitic compounds simply cannot get through these layers. Water-based herbs cannot penetrate the lipid barrier. Most alcohol-based tinctures cannot maintain effective concentration at the egg surface. Pharmaceutical antiparasitics typically fail to address eggs entirely. This is the wall that defeats most cleansing protocols, and it is the wall that clove climbs.

Why Eugenol Works

Eugenol is the active compound in clove that breaks through where everything else fails. Three properties make eugenol uniquely suited for egg destruction.

• **It is lipophilic.** Eugenol dissolves in fats and oils. It can penetrate the lipid-rich middle layer of the egg shell — the layer that blocks most other antiparasitic compounds. The lipid barrier becomes an entry point rather than a wall.

• **It disrupts cellular membranes.** Once inside the egg, eugenol attacks the developing embryo's cell membranes. It disrupts cellular respiration at the most fundamental level. The developing organism cannot complete its development. The egg becomes nonviable.

• **It accumulates in the egg.** Repeated exposure builds eugenol concentration in the egg interior. Each exposure brings the egg closer to nonviability. Sustained exposure over time achieves what single doses cannot.

This combination of properties is rare in the natural world. Few other compounds can penetrate the egg shell while remaining safe for human consumption. Clove is the standout, and has been recognized as such across multiple traditional medicine systems for centuries — long before anyone knew the molecular mechanism.

How Long It Takes

Egg destruction is not instantaneous. The timelines below assume consistent three-times-daily oral dosing combined with the enema additions covered in Chapters 17 and 18.

Egg Type	Days of Consistent Clove Exposure
Pinworm eggs	2 to 3 days
Roundworm eggs	3 to 5 days
Tapeworm eggs	5 to 7 days
Intestinal fluke eggs	7 to 10 days
Liver fluke eggs in bile ducts	10 to 14 days
Liver fluke eggs in liver tissue	14 to 21 days
Protozoa cysts	3 to 5 days

Skipping doses extends the timeline. Inconsistent dosing reduces effectiveness. The eggs do not pause their development just because you forgot a dose. This is one of the few places in the entire protocol where the difference between consistency and near-consistency is large enough to determine whether the work succeeds or fails.

The Three-Times-Daily Imperative

This is the single most important practical detail in the entire clove protocol. Eugenol does not accumulate in the body long-term. It is metabolized and cleared within 6 to 8 hours of consumption. This means a single morning dose loses effectiveness by mid-afternoon. Two doses per day creates 8- to 12-hour gaps. During those gaps, eggs continue developing without sufficient eugenol pressure. Surviving eggs that were almost destroyed have time to recover and continue developing.

With three doses daily — morning, midday, and evening — eugenol levels remain therapeutically effective for the full 24 hours. There is no window during which eggs can resume development. Cumulative pressure builds consistently. The full timeline above is achievable.

This is non-negotiable for serious egg elimination. Three doses daily, without exception, for the duration of the egg elimination phase.

Forms of Clove

A note on terminology before the table. *Clove tincture* and *clove oil* are different preparations and they are not interchangeable. The tincture is an alcohol-based extract of clove buds — milder, often blended with other antiparasitic herbs in combination tinctures, and dosed according to the bottle. The oil is the concentrated essential oil pressed or distilled directly from clove buds — significantly stronger, food-grade certification required.

The two forms have different roles in this protocol. **Tincture goes orally; oil goes in the enema.** Clove oil *can* technically be taken orally at 1 drop diluted in carrier — and many integrative-medicine references list it that way — but in personal experience the oil is highly irritating to the throat even diluted, and the tincture covers the oral role more comfortably without sacrificing effectiveness. Reserve the concentrated oil for enema use, where 2 to 3 drops in 48 ounces of solution gives a low-concentration delivery that the gut tolerates well. Use the oil only in the morning coffee enema; do not add it to the evening salt water enema, as eugenol can accumulate and cause stomach problems if dosed twice daily.

Mixing these up is one of the few protocol errors that produces a meaningfully wrong dose. Read the bottle. Confirm which form you have.

Forms of Clove

Form	Description	Standard Dose	Best Use
Clove tincture *	Alcohol-based extract of clove buds. Available as single-herb (clove only) or combination antiparasitic (clove blended with black walnut, wormwood, and others).	Follow the bottle's recommendations. Single-herb clove tinctures typically dose in the 4-to-6-drop range three times daily. Combination antiparasitic tinctures dose much higher per use because clove is diluted across multiple herbs — often 20+ drops per dose.	Daily oral protocol. The everyday workhorse form.
Concentrated clove oil — food grade *	Pure essential oil pressed or distilled directly from clove buds. Significantly more concentrated than tincture. Food-grade certification required.	2 to 3 drops in 48 oz morning coffee enema solution only. Reserved for enema use; oral use is not recommended in this protocol — see terminology note above. Do not add to evening enema.	Morning coffee enema additions and intensification phases.
Whole clove buds ***	Dried clove flower buds — the spice familiar from cooking. Releases eugenol gradually as chewed or steeped.	Per traditional preparation (chewed, or steeped as tea).	Maintenance phase after the intensive protocol.
Clove powder *** †	Ground clove buds. Releases eugenol as it digests. Variable potency depending on freshness.	Per capsule label or recipe.	Convenient for capsule preparation.

* **Essential.** Used during the active egg elimination phase.

*** **Situational.** Used in maintenance or specific preparation contexts.

† **On capsule preparation during the fast.** When using clove powder in capsule form, the same guidance applies as for the herbs in Chapter 19: open the capsule and mix the powder into a small amount of water rather than swallow the capsule whole. See Chapter 19's full capsule note for reasoning.

Quality and Sourcing

Clove quality varies significantly. The herb that does the most singular work in this protocol cannot do that work if it is poor-quality.

For tincture:

• Organic certification essential — clove crops are heavily sprayed.

• Made from fresh or recently dried buds.

• Dark amber to brown color.

• Strong aromatic smell.

• Reputable producer.

For essential oil:

• Food-grade certification visible on label.

• Therapeutic grade preferred.

• Verified eugenol content.

• Cold pressed or steam distilled.

For whole cloves:

• Plump and oily looking, not dry and shriveled.

• Strong aroma — fresh cloves are intensely fragrant.

The Complete Daily Clove Protocol

Time	Dose
Upon waking	Clove tincture (per bottle) + piperine, in water
Morning coffee enema	Food-grade clove oil — 2 to 3 drops in coffee solution
Midday	Clove tincture (per bottle) + piperine — 6 to 8 hours after morning
Evening	Clove tincture (per bottle) + piperine — before evening enema

"Per bottle" means follow the dose recommended on your tincture's label. See "Forms of Clove" above for the distinction between single-herb and combination antiparasitic tinctures.

This protocol, done consistently for the duration of the egg elimination phase, achieves what no other intervention can match.

When to Increase the Protocol

Consider increasing when:

• Two weeks into the protocol with continued signs of parasitic activity.

• Liver fluke eggs not yet showing signs of clearing.

• Persistent gas, bloating, or other parasite-related symptoms.

• Body signals suggest deeper egg load than initially apparent.

How to intensify:

• Increase morning coffee enema clove oil — from 2 drops to 3 drops. Keep this as the only daily clove oil enema; do not add it to the evening enema. The eugenol in concentrated clove oil can accumulate and cause stomach problems if dosed twice daily, even via enema.

• Increase tincture dose per the bottle's instructions if the label allows higher dosing.

• Extend the protocol an additional 5 to 7 days rather than escalating further.

• Layer in supporting herbs from Chapter 19 — chanca piedra and milk thistle for liver-tissue work, berberine for protozoa.

• Then assess whether further intensification is needed.

When to ease back:

• Burning or irritation of mouth or stomach develops.

• Headaches specifically following clove doses.

• Egg elimination signs suggest the work is largely complete.

• Approaching the end of the antiparasitic phase.

Recognizing the Work Is Done

Signs that suggest the protocol is largely complete:

• Enema returns no longer showing parasitic material.

• Tongue coating cleared and stable.

• Body odor neutralized.

• Energy stable at higher baseline.

• Mental clarity sustained.

• Gas and gurgling minimal.

• General sense of internal cleanness.

The conservative approach. Continue the full protocol for the planned duration even when signs suggest completion. Eggs at the deepest tissue levels may take the full timeline. Stopping too early is the most common cause of incomplete results. Better to continue an extra week than to leave eggs viable.

Cautions and Considerations

Clove is generally safe, but it has specific considerations.

• **Mucous membrane irritation.** Concentrated clove oil can irritate the mouth. Always dilute essential oil in carrier. Reduce dose if any burning sensation develops.

• **Blood thinning.** Eugenol has mild anticoagulant effects. Caution if taking blood thinners. Discontinue 2 weeks before any planned surgery.

• **Liver enzyme effects.** High doses can affect liver enzyme metabolism. Monitor liver function if doing extended protocols.

• **Pregnancy and breastfeeding.** Avoid concentrated forms during pregnancy.

• **Drug interactions.** May interact with anticoagulants and diabetes medications. Discuss with medical support if taking any prescription medications.

Why Clove Has Been Used for So Long

This protocol uses clove because clove works. But clove has been used as an antiparasitic across cultures and centuries for the same reason. Traditional Chinese medicine documented its antiparasitic use over 2,000 years ago. Ayurvedic medicine has used clove for similar purposes for millennia. Medieval European herbalists used clove against intestinal worms. Various indigenous medicine systems worldwide independently identified its antiparasitic properties.

People did not know about eugenol or chorions or lipid penetration. They simply observed that clove worked when other things did not. The science has caught up to the tradition.

A Personal Reflection

If there is one practice in this entire protocol the author would refuse to skip, it is consistent clove dosing. Other practices accelerate the work. Other herbs target other organisms. Other tools clear other accumulations. But only clove addresses the eggs.

Without consistent clove protocol, eggs survive. Surviving eggs hatch. Hatching eggs produce new adults. New adults reproduce. The cycle continues. Months after a thorough cleanse without proper egg elimination, the parasitic load can return to nearly its starting level. Three doses daily. Without exception. For the duration the eggs require. This is the practice that turns a temporary cleanse into a complete one. This is what makes the difference between brief relief and lasting transformation. Clove stands alone for a reason. Use it accordingly.

Chapter 21

The Targeted Fluke Elimination Protocol

* * *

Of every parasite in this book, flukes are the ones most people never fully address. They live in places enemas cannot reach. They hide in tissues that herbs alone cannot penetrate. They survive for decades — quietly, persistently, generation after generation. Most antiparasitic protocols barely touch them.

This chapter is different. This chapter is the comprehensive integrated approach, combining every tool covered so far into one unified attack on the most stubborn parasite you carry. The protocol that follows is the convergence point of everything in the previous six chapters — the herbs, the enemas, the coffee, the clove, the timing — applied at full intensity to the one organism family that requires every tool at once to fully eliminate.

Why Flukes Require a Special Protocol

Flukes present unique challenges that no single intervention solves:

- They live in **bile ducts and liver tissue,** beyond the reach of enemas.
- They lay eggs in **multiple locations simultaneously** — bile ducts, liver tissue, intestinal walls.
- Their eggs have **exceptionally thick shells,** among the most resistant in human parasitology.
- Adult liver flukes survive **9 to 30 years,** accumulating decades of egg deposits.
- Their lifecycle includes **migration through liver tissue,** leaving eggs embedded throughout.
- Standard antiparasitic herbs **do not reach** liver tissue effectively.
- Most cleansing protocols **never address** them at all.

The solution is not a single stronger tool. The solution is the coordinated use of every tool, each addressing a different aspect of the fluke problem.

The Architecture of the Attack

Six different mechanisms working together address every aspect of fluke biology.

• **Killing adult flukes.** Black walnut hull tincture for direct toxicity. Wormwood tincture for secondary action. Berberine through biliary support. Oral systemic absorption to reach flukes in tissue beyond enema reach.

• **Destroying fluke eggs.** Clove tincture three times daily orally. Clove oil in coffee enema directly to the colon. Sustained eugenol exposure building concentration over time.

• **Flushing the bile ducts.** Daily morning coffee enema, the bottom-up sweep that clears what the herbs have loosened. Chanca piedra orally to soften biliary stones. Dandelion root to encourage bile flow. The pressure builds from below; the herbs press from above; the bile ducts give up what they have held.

• **Mechanical clearing.** Mimosa pudica seed — its sticky gel grabs flukes from intestinal walls. Twice-daily enemas for physical expulsion. Pumpkin seed (post-fast) to paralyze fluke muscle for easier removal.

• **Liver protection.** Milk thistle orally and in enemas. L-Glutamine to support liver cells. Trace minerals as coenzymes for liver enzymes. Coconut oil and MCT to support ketone production for cellular energy.

• **Biofilm disruption.** Berberine for strong biofilm disruption. Mimosa pudica for physical disruption. Black walnut for secondary biofilm activity.

The Daily Targeted Protocol

Time	Action
6:30–7:00 AM — Upon waking	16 oz water + trace minerals + Himalayan salt; L-Glutamine 5 g; aloe vera 2 oz; clove tincture (per bottle) + piperine
7:00–9:00 AM — Morning coffee enema	48 oz brewed organic coffee + 2 to 3 drops clove oil + 1 tsp black walnut tincture + 1 tsp milk thistle extract; 12 to 15 min retention
9:30 AM — Mid-morning	Black walnut 1 tsp + piperine; wormwood 4 to 6 drops + piperine; mimosa pudica 1 to 2 caps; CBD; Lion's Mane 500 mg; 1 tsp coconut/MCT oil
12:30 PM — Midday	Clove tincture (per bottle) + piperine; berberine 500 mg + piperine; oregano oil 2 to 4 drops in carrier
3:00 PM — Mid-afternoon	Pau d'arco 4 to 6 drops + piperine; chanca piedra 1 cap; dandelion root 30 drops; milk thistle 250 mg
6:30 PM — Pre-evening enema	Wormwood 4 to 6 drops + piperine (2nd dose); mimosa pudica 1 to 2 caps (2nd dose)
7:00–9:00 PM — Evening salt water enema	48 oz water + 1 to 2 tsp Himalayan salt + 4 oz aloe vera + ½ tsp magnesium chloride + 1 tsp pau d'arco; 10 to 15 min retention
8:30 PM — Evening	Clove tincture (per bottle) + piperine (3rd dose); milk thistle 250 mg; magnesium glycinate 300 to 400 mg; L-Glutamine 5 g; CBN

Coffee enemas and MCT/coconut oil enter the protocol on Day 8, after ketosis is fully established. See Chapter 22's phase chart for the phased start.

The complete schedule with all integrating practices is laid out in unified form in Chapter 22.

Duration of the Targeted Protocol

The duration of the targeted phase scales with the severity of the suspected fluke load.

• **Minimum duration:** 14 days of consistent daily protocol — addresses adult flukes and surface eggs.

• **Standard duration:** 21 days — addresses deeper egg deposits and allows multiple complete egg destruction cycles.

• **Extended duration for heavy fluke load:** 28 days or more — for those with significant suspected liver fluke history.

Signs you have completed the targeted phase:

• Green sludge in coffee enema returns has decreased significantly.

• Tongue coating cleared and stable.

• Right-sided abdominal sensation has resolved.

• Mental clarity is sustained.

• Energy is stable at higher baseline.

• General sense of internal cleanness.

Why Standard Protocols Often Fail With Flukes

Five reasons that most protocols fail to address flukes adequately:

• **No bile duct intervention.** Liver flukes live in bile ducts. Without coffee enemas, bile ducts are not flushed.

• **No egg destruction emphasis.** Most protocols focus on adults. Eggs survive any protocol that does not specifically address them.

• **Insufficient duration.** Many protocols run 7 to 14 days. Liver fluke eggs require 14 to 21 days minimum.

• **No liver support.** The liver bears enormous burden during fluke clearing. Without protection, liver function can become bottlenecked.

• **No biofilm disruption.** Flukes hide within biofilm communities. Without biofilm disruption, herbs cannot reach the organisms.

This protocol addresses every one of these failure modes simultaneously, which is why it is laid out as a unified system rather than a list of individual interventions.

What to Expect During the Protocol

Week	Enema Returns	Energy	Mental Clarity	Body Signs
Week 1	Significant green sludge	Energy fluctuations more pronounced	Reduced; flu-like symptoms possible as die-off accelerates	Right-sided abdominal sensation may increase temporarily; vivid dreams; emotional releases
Week 2	Green sludge often peaks then begins decreasing	Stabilizing at fluctuating but generally higher baseline	Improving in windows	Body odor neutralizing; tongue coating may shift before clearing
Week 3	Returns becoming progressively cleaner	More sustained	Reaching plateau	General sense of internal lightness developing; most fluke material has been cleared
Week 4 (if needed)	Final deep tissue eggs clearing	Maintenance level	Sustained	Confirmation that the work is complete

Common Mistakes to Avoid

• **Inconsistent clove dosing.** Missing morning, midday, or evening doses. Eugenol levels drop and eggs resume development.

• **Stopping too early.** Believing the work is done before deep eggs are cleared. Maintain full duration even when signs improve.

• **Inadequate mineral replenishment.** The intensive protocol depletes minerals significantly. Without replenishment, herbs become less effective.

• **Adding food too early.** Food during the active fluke phase reduces herb absorption.

Confirming the Work Is Complete

The protocol's completion is confirmed through three categories of evidence.

Visual signs in enema returns:

• Green sludge has decreased to occasional rather than consistent.

• Returns are predominantly clear with minimal debris.

• No visible parasitic material.

• No significant biofilm material.

Body signs:

- Right-sided abdominal sensation has fully resolved.
- Tongue is consistently pink and clean.
- Body odor is neutral.
- Breath is clean and not heavy.
- Energy is stable at the higher baseline.
- Mental clarity is sustained throughout the day.
- Sleep is deep and restorative.

Comprehensive testing:

- GI Map test conducted 4 to 6 weeks after protocol completion.
- Provides definitive confirmation through DNA detection.
- Establishes baseline for future monitoring.

The full testing and verification approach is covered in Chapter 34.Chapter 35Chapter 35

A Personal Reflection on This Work

Of all the work in this book, fluke elimination feels different. The flukes have been there for decades. They have caused damage you may not have recognized as damage. They have been a quiet drain on your liver, your bile ducts, your overall vitality. Removing them changes things.

People often describe the post-fluke clearing experience in distinctive terms. A lightness in the right side of the body where the liver lives. A sense of digestive ease that has been missing. Mental clarity with a particular quality. Energy that does not seem to belong to them. A feeling that something has been carried for a very long time — that they did not know they were carrying — that has now been set down.

That feeling is real. You really were carrying it. You really did not know. And it really has been set down. This is one of the moments where this work shows its full meaning.

Chapter 22

The Complete Daily Protocol

* * *

You have now learned every component. The fasting framework. The trace minerals. The brain support. The signals. The enemas. The coffee enema. The herbs. The clove protocol. The targeted fluke approach. Each chapter has covered its element in depth. This chapter brings them together — one day, start to finish, every practice, every herb, every supplement, every consideration, arranged in the order in which they actually occur.

This is the chapter you will refer to most often during the fast. Print it. Post it where you can see it. Refer to it throughout each day until the rhythm becomes automatic. Some days the schedule will flow exactly as written; some days your body will signal modifications — extra rest, additional enemas, modified timing. The schedule is the framework. Your body's signals refine it day by day.

The Complete Daily Schedule

6:30 AM — UPON WAKING

Hydration and foundation:

• 16 ounces water treated with ionic sulfated minerals

• Trace minerals — first dose

• Pinch Himalayan salt

• L-Glutamine — 5g in warm water

• 2 ounces aloe vera juice

First clove dose:

• Clove tincture — 4 to 6 drops with piperine

• In small amount of water

Brief journal entry:

• How did you sleep?

• Energy on waking — 1 to 10

- Mental clarity — 1 to 10
- Any unusual signals?

Wait 30 minutes before next step.

7:00 AM — MORNING COFFEE ENEMA

Solution preparation:

- Brew 3 tablespoons organic light-roast coffee in 48 ounces water treated with ionic sulfated minerals
- Simmer 15 minutes
- Strain completely
- Cool to body temperature

Add to cooled solution:

- 2 to 3 drops food-grade clove oil
- 1 teaspoon black walnut hull tincture
- 1 teaspoon milk thistle liquid extract

Procedure:

- Standard enema position rotation
- 12 to 15 minutes retention
- Full release at toilet

Immediate replenishment:

- 16 ounces water with trace minerals
- Generous pinch Himalayan salt
- 8 ounces coconut water if available

9:30 AM — MID-MORNING HERBS

Antiparasitic herbs:

- Black walnut hull tincture — 1 teaspoon with piperine
- Wormwood tincture — 4 to 6 drops with piperine
- Mimosa pudica — 1 to 2 capsules with substantial water

Brain support:

- 1 teaspoon coconut oil or MCT oil

• CBD oil — your regular dose

• Lion's Mane — 500mg

Mineral check:

• Continued mineralized water

• Trace minerals — second dose if not already taken

11:00 AM — HYDRATION AND CHECK-IN

• 16 ounces mineralized water with pinch of salt

• Brief body scan — what is your body telling you?

• Note any signals in your journal

12:30 PM — MIDDAY HERBS

Antiparasitic continuation:

• Clove tincture — 4 to 6 drops with piperine — second dose

• Berberine — 500mg with piperine

• Oregano oil — 2 to 4 drops in water with carrier oil

Continued hydration:

• 16 ounces mineralized water

• Pinch Himalayan salt

3:00 PM — MID-AFTERNOON

Liver and bile support:

• Pau d'arco tincture — 4 to 6 drops with piperine

• Chanca piedra — 1 capsule

• Dandelion root tincture — 30 drops

• Milk thistle — 250mg

Brain and ECS support:

• CBG oil if available

• 1 teaspoon coconut oil or MCT oil — second dose

Hydration:

• 8 ounces coconut water if available

• Or 16 ounces mineralized water

5:00 PM — LATE AFTERNOON

Hydration check:

• 16 ounces mineralized water

• Pinch Himalayan salt

• Trace minerals — third dose

Body assessment:

• How is energy?

• Any signs requiring attention?

• Should there be a second enema today?

6:30 PM — PRE-ENEMA HERBS

Final antiparasitic round:

• Wormwood tincture — 4 to 6 drops with piperine — second dose

• Mimosa pudica — 1 to 2 capsules with water — second dose

7:00 PM — EVENING SALT WATER ENEMA

Solution preparation:

• 48 ounces water treated with ionic sulfated minerals, with Himalayan sea salt at the prescribed concentration, at body temperature

• 1 to 2 teaspoons Himalayan salt — fully dissolved

Add:

• 4 ounces aloe vera juice

• Half teaspoon magnesium chloride

• 2 to 3 drops food-grade clove oil

• 1 teaspoon pau d'arco tincture

Procedure:

• Standard enema position rotation

• 10 to 15 minutes retention

• Full release at toilet

Immediate replenishment:

• 16 ounces water with trace minerals

• Pinch Himalayan salt

8:30 PM — EVENING WIND-DOWN

Final clove dose:

• Clove tincture — 4 to 6 drops with piperine — third and final dose

Liver protection overnight:

• Milk thistle — 250mg

Sleep support:

• Magnesium glycinate — 300 to 400mg

• L-Glutamine — 5g

• CBN if available

Brief evening journal:

• How was today overall?

• What did you notice in enema returns?

• What signals did your body send?

• Any insights or emotional releases?

10:00 PM — BEFORE SLEEP

• 8 ounces mineralized water

• Final pinch Himalayan salt

• Settle in for restorative sleep

The Master Daily Reference Chart

Time	Practice	Components
6:30–7:00 AM	Wake protocol	Water, trace minerals, salt, L-Glutamine, aloe, clove tincture
7:00–9:00 AM	Morning coffee enema	Coffee + clove oil + black walnut + milk thistle
9:30 AM	Mid-morning herbs	Black walnut + wormwood + mimosa pudica + CBD + MCT
11:00 AM	Hydration check	Mineralized water + assessment
12:30 PM	Midday herbs	Clove tincture + berberine + oregano oil
3:00 PM	Liver support	Pau d'arco + chanca piedra + dandelion + milk thistle + CBG + MCT
5:00 PM	Afternoon check	Mineralized water + assessment
6:30 PM	Pre-enema herbs	Wormwood + mimosa pudica
7:00–9:00 PM	Salt water enema	Salt + aloe + magnesium chloride + pau d'arco
8:30 PM	Evening protocol	Clove tincture + milk thistle + magnesium + L-Glutamine + CBN
10:00 PM	Before sleep	Final hydration

Coffee enemas and MCT/coconut oil enter the protocol on Day 8, after ketosis is fully established. See the phase chart below for the phased start.

What This Protocol Asks of You

Time commitment:

• The morning sequence — wake protocol through coffee enema and replenishment — takes approximately **2 hours**.

• The evening sequence takes approximately **1.5 hours**.

• Total dedicated protocol time daily — approximately **4 hours**.

Energy commitment:

• Especially in the first week, the protocol itself is tiring.

• Schedule should be cleared as much as possible during the fast.

• Plan around the protocol rather than fitting it into a normal schedule.

Financial commitment:

• Quality herbs and supplies are not inexpensive.

• Plan a budget before starting.

• Quality matters significantly — cheap herbs often deliver poor results.

Mental and emotional commitment:

• The protocol requires consistency and discipline.

• Some days you will not feel like doing all of it.

• Doing it anyway is part of the work.

This is not a casual undertaking. It is a sustained intentional practice for the duration of the fast.

Modifications for Different Phases

Phase	Days	Adjustments
Transition	Days 1 to 3	Skip MCT and coconut oil; let ketosis establish naturally. Reduce herbal doses to allow body to adjust. Lighter enemas — plain water or mild salt water acceptable. Do not begin coffee enemas. Establish the rhythm before full intensity.
Establishment	Days 4 to 7	Continue plain water enemas. Begin tincture-based herbal protocol at low doses. Body settling into deep ketosis. Do not begin coffee enemas or MCT yet — these enter at Day 8 to allow ketosis to fully establish without exogenous shortcuts.
Active cleansing	Days 8 to 21	Begin morning coffee enema with all therapeutic additions. Begin MCT and coconut oil support. Full herbal protocol. Both enemas with all therapeutic additions. This is the period of most intensive work — herbs at full doses.
Completion and exit	Days 22 onward	Continue full protocol while signs indicate ongoing work. Begin reducing antiparasitic intensity as signs of completion appear. Add ghee in warm water if signals support modified fasting. Prepare for refeeding.

The Rhythm Becomes Sacred

Something happens when you maintain this protocol consistently. The early days feel like effort. Setting timers. Checking schedules. Forcing yourself through resistance. By the second week, something shifts. The rhythm starts to feel natural. Your body begins anticipating each step. The protocol becomes less effort and more practice. By the third week, the rhythm has become sacred. The morning sequence is a ritual rather than a chore. The herbs and waters and enemas have become part of your daily life. Your body has organized itself around the protocol.

This is when the deepest work happens. When the practice has become rhythm. When the rhythm has become ritual. When the ritual has become simply how you live during this period of your life. That is the state in which transformation occurs, and the transformation is what every element of the schedule above has been building toward.

Half measures produce half results. The person who takes the herbs but skips the coffee enema has incomplete fluke clearing. The person who does the morning protocol but skips the evening enema lets toxins reabsorb overnight. Every element matters. Every element supports the goal. This is not a buffet to choose from. It is an integrated system designed to work together. Use it as designed, and it does the work it is designed to do.

Chapter 23

Pinworms — The Special Case

* * *

Of every parasite in this book, only one requires a chapter all to itself. Not because it is the most dangerous. Not because it is the most damaging. Not because it is the most stubborn. Simply because it is the most common, and because it does something none of the others do. It leaves your body. It lays eggs in your home. And it waits for you to swallow them again.

This is the one parasite that the protocol you have just learned cannot fully address by itself. This is why this chapter exists.

Most readers will not have expected a chapter focused on a single parasite this far into the book. The decision to include it was deliberate. Pinworms are, by global estimates, the most common parasitic infection in the developed world. They exist in households across every income level, every region, every level of cleanliness. They affect children most visibly, but they live in adults silently for decades. They are the parasite most likely to circulate through your home the fastest — between family members, across surfaces, in dust, in bedding, on doorknobs.

And the protocol in this book, as comprehensive as it is, does not fully eliminate them. The reason is not a flaw in the protocol. The reason is biology. Every other parasite this book addresses lives entirely inside you. Pinworms do not. They live partly inside you and partly in your environment, and the herbs and enemas that work so beautifully on the parasites in your gut have no reach into your bedsheets, your bathroom, or the dust on your floor.

That is why pinworms get their own chapter. A reader who completes the full forty-day protocol with perfect adherence and has pinworms — most often without knowing it — will finish the fast clear of pinworms in their gut. Within two weeks, they will have pinworms again. Not from new exposure. From their own home. This is the most common reason that thorough cleanse protocols appear to fail. They did not fail. The reader simply did not know they needed to attack on a second front. This chapter teaches that second front.

What They Are

Enterobius vermicularis. The small, white, threadlike worm that has lived alongside human beings for as long as we have records of human medicine. Adult pinworms are small. Females reach about half an inch in length. Males are smaller — a quarter inch at most. They are translucent white, almost glossy in appearance, and they move with surprising speed when removed from the body. They have been described in the medical writings of every civilization that has documented human anatomy at all. The Greeks knew them. The Romans knew them. The Chinese physicians of the medieval period described them in detail. They have been with us a long time.

Most people who carry them never know. In children, who tend to carry the heaviest loads, the classic sign is nighttime perianal itching that disrupts sleep. In adults, who often carry smaller numbers, symptoms are usually absent entirely. They simply live there, generation after generation, without ever announcing their presence. This is part of why they are so common. You cannot eliminate something you do not know you have. You cannot warn others to take precautions when you are unaware that you are a source.

By conservative estimates, more than two hundred million people worldwide currently carry them. By less conservative estimates, the number is twice that. Most are not children. Most are not living in conditions of poor hygiene. Most are people who would be surprised to learn that pinworms could possibly be in their bodies — and yet there they are, in homes across every continent, transmitting silently from person to person and from surface to surface.

The Lifecycle That Defeats Most Cleanses

Every parasite in this book has a lifecycle. Pinworms have one with a critical twist that distinguishes them from every other organism we have discussed.

The cycle begins when a person swallows microscopic pinworm eggs. The eggs are typically introduced through food, through hands, through dust, in quantities far too small to see. The eggs hatch in the small intestine. The larvae mature as they travel down through the digestive tract. By the time they reach the colon, about four to six weeks after the swallowed egg, they have become adult worms ready to reproduce.

Males and females mate in the colon. The males die shortly after. The females are left fertilized and gravid, full of eggs.

And then the females do something no other parasite in this book does. At night, typically in the deepest hours of sleep, the gravid females migrate down through the colon, out through the anus, onto the perianal skin. There they release their eggs. Ten thousand to fifteen thousand of them per female. On the skin around the anus. The female, exhausted from her long migration and her egg-laying, dies on the skin.

The eggs do not. Within four to six hours of being laid, the eggs become infective. They are ready to start the cycle again the moment they are swallowed.

This is where most cleanses fail. The eggs are no longer in the body where the herbs and enemas can reach them. They are everywhere they can be — and within twenty-four hours of a single egg-laying episode, the eggs are everywhere in the home:

- On the skin around the anus.

• On the fabric of the underwear and pajamas.

• On the bedsheets and pillowcase.

• On the hands, from unconscious scratching during sleep.

• Under the fingernails, where the scratching has placed them.

• On the bathroom doorknob touched after a sleepy visit.

• On the light switch turned off before going back to bed.

• On towels and washcloths.

• In the dust on the bedroom floor.

• In the air itself — pinworm eggs are so light that they become airborne when bedding is shaken.

When the host swallows even one — and they will, because the eggs are now on hands and food and surfaces — the cycle starts again. Pinworms do not need to reinfect from the outside world. They reinfect from inside the bedroom of their host.

Why the Current Protocol Is Not Enough

The herbs of this protocol work beautifully on pinworms inside the body. Clove tincture penetrates pinworm eggs as they pass through the gut. Black walnut hull and wormwood kill the adult worms. Mimosa pudica grabs them from the intestinal walls. The enemas flush them out. By the end of three weeks of full protocol, the gut is essentially pinworm-free.

But during those three weeks, every night, gravid females have been migrating out of the colon, laying eggs on the perianal skin, dying. Every morning, those eggs have been transferring to underwear, to sheets, to hands, to the bathroom. Every day, the eggs have been spreading through the home. When the fast ends, the body is clean. The environment is heavily contaminated. Within days of breaking the fast, the host swallows the first egg. Within four to six weeks, they have adult pinworms again.

Nothing about this is the practitioner's fault. It is simply how pinworms work. The protocol in this book was designed to address parasites in the gut. Pinworms exploit a gap that no internal protocol — herbal or pharmaceutical — can close on its own. The solution is to attack on multiple fronts simultaneously. That is what this chapter teaches.

The Three-Front War

To eliminate pinworms permanently requires attacking three places at once:

1. The body — herbal protocol plus pinworm-specific additions.

2. The environment — hygiene and cleaning practices that break the egg transmission cycle.

3. The household — coordinated treatment of every member living in the same home.

Miss any one front, and the cycle continues. Address all three for six weeks, and the cycle breaks.

Six weeks is not arbitrary. The pinworm lifecycle, from swallowed egg to egg-laying adult, takes four to six weeks. If the cycle is broken for less than that, there will always be a generation maturing in the gut that has not yet been touched by the protocol. Six weeks ensures that every generation present at the start of treatment has either been killed or has matured into adults that have themselves been killed. This is the discipline pinworm eradication requires. Most people fail not because they cannot do six weeks. They fail because they did not know that six weeks was the requirement.

The First Front — The Body

If you are running the full protocol described in this book, you are already doing most of what is needed for the body side. Continue everything you are already doing. The clove tincture three times daily is critical. The black walnut and wormwood are essential. The mimosa pudica supports the work. The enemas physically remove what the herbs kill.

Three additions improve pinworm-specific results:

• **Diatomaceous earth (food grade only).** Never use the type sold for swimming pool filtration — it is dangerous to ingest. The microscopic silica edges of food-grade diatomaceous earth physically damage pinworm exoskeletons and absorb moisture from their eggs, killing both. **Dose:** one tablespoon mixed in eight ounces of water, twice daily, on an empty stomach. Drink generous additional water with it, as the substance is dehydrating in its action. Continue for at least two weeks beyond the point where you no longer suspect pinworm activity.

• **Pumpkin seed (after the fast).** During an active water fast, chewed seeds break the fast — capsule or oil form is acceptable during fasting. After breaking the fast, raw pumpkin seeds become exceptionally effective. **Dose:** a quarter cup chewed thoroughly on an empty stomach in the morning, daily. The cucurbitacin in pumpkin seeds paralyzes pinworm musculature, releasing them from the intestinal walls.

• **Raw garlic (after the fast). Dose:** one to two cloves, crushed and allowed to sit for ten minutes (so the allicin compound can develop), then mixed with raw honey or absorbed into a small amount of olive oil. Take on an empty stomach in the morning. The allicin in fresh-crushed garlic is one of the most potent natural antimicrobials known to traditional medicine.

These three additions — diatomaceous earth during the fast, pumpkin seed and garlic after — significantly increase the body protocol's effectiveness against pinworms specifically.

The Second Front — The Environment

This is the part most people skip. This is also the part that determines whether the eradication succeeds or fails.

The environmental protocol exists for one purpose — to break the cycle of egg transmission from the body to the bedroom to the hands to the mouth back to the body. Without it, the herbs do their work and the environment refills the gut. With it, six weeks of consistent practice empties both the gut and the home.

Daily practices, every day for six weeks:

• **Shower in the morning, not at night.** Eggs laid on the perianal skin overnight are washed off in the morning, before they can transfer to daytime clothes and surfaces. Evening showers do nothing for pinworm eradication and may make matters worse by leaving the host clean before the female pinworms migrate out to lay their eggs.

• **Wash hands with hot soapy water** after every bathroom visit, before every meal, after handling bedding, after handling laundry, after scratching anywhere on the body.

• **Keep fingernails very short.** Pinworm eggs accumulate under fingernails, particularly after unconscious scratching during sleep, and long nails are pinworm reservoirs.

• **Stop nail biting and cuticle chewing completely** during the eradication window. The most direct route from environment back into body is through the mouth, and fingernails are where the eggs concentrate.

• **Wear underwear to bed.** The simple physical barrier between hand and perianal area during sleep prevents the worst of nighttime egg transfer to fingernails.

• **Change underwear and pajamas daily** — no exceptions.

Weekly practices, every week for six weeks:

• **Hot-wash all bedding** (minimum 130°F / 54°C). Eggs survive normal warm wash temperatures. They die in hot water. If your washer cannot reach this temperature, supplement with a high-heat dryer cycle of at least thirty minutes.

• **Hot-wash bath mats, towels, and washcloths.**

• **Vacuum bedrooms and high-traffic areas thoroughly.**

• **Damp-dust** (not dry-dust) bedroom and bathroom surfaces. Dry dusting just spreads eggs into the air.

• **Disinfect bathroom fixtures** (toilet seat, flush lever, faucet handles, doorknobs, light switches) with white vinegar or 70% alcohol.

• **Clean pet bedding.** Dogs and cats can mechanically transport pinworm eggs even though they do not host the parasite themselves.

One-time work at the start of the protocol:

• Wash all clothing in the home that has contacted skin.

• Wash all bedding throughout the house, not just the bedding of the person being treated. Eggs transfer between bedrooms through laundry baskets, hampers, and shared linen closets.

• Vacuum bedrooms, hallways, and high-traffic living areas thoroughly.

• Steam-clean bedroom carpets if possible. Eggs survive vacuuming alone.

• Damp-dust all surfaces in bedrooms and bathrooms.

• Wipe down all hard surfaces — bedroom furniture, bathroom fixtures, doorknobs, light switches, faucet handles, toilet seats and flush levers — with white vinegar or 70% alcohol.

• Empty the vacuum cleaner bag or canister outside the house immediately. A vacuum bag full of pinworm eggs sitting in a closet is itself an ongoing source of contamination.

• Replace toothbrushes. Bathroom dust settles on bristles, and a new toothbrush at the start of the protocol is a small investment with significant impact.

This level of environmental discipline seems extreme to most readers reading it for the first time. It is not extreme. It is what is required. The people who skip the environmental protocol do not eliminate pinworms. They temporarily reduce their pinworm load and then, within weeks, are reinfected from their own home. The discipline is not optional. It is the price of finishing the work.

The Third Front — The Household

If you live alone, this section does not apply to you. If you live with anyone, read it carefully.

Pinworms transfer between household members constantly. A partner who has even a few pinworms — even completely asymptomatic — is shedding eggs into the shared environment every night. A child carrying pinworms at school will bring eggs home daily. A roommate who does not believe pinworms are a concern will reinfect everyone within days of treatment ending. The household must be treated together, or the household will not be treated effectively at all.

Synchronized household treatment requires:

• **Every member runs an antiparasitic protocol simultaneously.** Adults can run the full protocol described in this book at appropriate doses. Children require pediatric herbalist guidance for safe dosing — do not improvise herb amounts for children.

• **All members start on the same day.** Staggered treatment fails.

• **All members complete the protocol on the same day.**

• **Every member follows the environmental protocol simultaneously** — morning showers, daily underwear and pajama changes, short fingernails, hand-washing hygiene, weekly hot-water bedding washes for everyone.

• **The shared environment receives one coordinated initial cleaning,** then weekly maintenance through the six-week window.

If anyone in the household refuses to participate, pinworms will not be eliminated. This is not pessimism. It is biology. If household participation cannot be achieved, the individual practitioner can still significantly reduce their own pinworm load through their personal protocol — but they should expect ongoing low-level reinfection until the household issue is addressed. This is one of the few places in this book where individual effort genuinely cannot overcome environmental factors. Pinworms exploit shared spaces. Eradication requires shared treatment.

The Six-Week Timeline

The six weeks of the eradication window have an internal structure that helps the practitioner know what to expect:

• **Week 1.** Original adults are dying under the herbal pressure. Eggs from earlier nights are still on surfaces. Possible new infections are still occurring from environmental eggs already present. The aggressive environmental cleanup is just beginning to reduce the load.

• **Week 2.** Most original adults have been eliminated. Eggs swallowed before treatment may now be larvae in the small intestine, working their way through the developmental cycle. Environmental load is reducing significantly through the daily and weekly cleaning practices.

• **Week 3.** New adults from environmental reinfection mature in the colon — and the herbal pressure kills them. The hygiene protocol is preventing further egg accumulation in the environment. The existing environmental eggs are aging toward non-viability.

• **Week 4.** Environmental egg load is substantially reduced. The cycle is nearly broken. Eggs typically lose viability within two to three weeks outside the host, and the environment is now turning over faster than it is being replenished.

• **Week 5.** Environmental eggs are becoming non-viable in significant numbers. Few new infections are occurring. The protocol is approaching completion.

• **Week 6.** The cycle should be fully broken if all three fronts have been maintained. From the seventh week onward, the maintenance phase begins, and the practitioner can verify the absence of pinworms through testing.

How to Verify

The test for pinworms is simple, free, and effective. It is called the adhesive tape test, sometimes the scotch tape test in older references.

Procedure:

1. In the morning, before bathing or wiping or any disturbance of the perianal area, press a piece of clear adhesive tape against the perianal skin.

2. Press firmly for two or three seconds.

3. Lift the tape and place it sticky-side-down on a piece of glass or a microscope slide.

4. Examine with a magnifying glass, or under a microscope if one is available.

Pinworm eggs are visible. They are flattened ovals about fifty micrometers long, asymmetric, with one side flatter than the other. Under magnification they look like tiny grains of rice.

Repeat the test on three consecutive mornings. Pinworms do not lay eggs every single night, and a single negative result does not confirm absence. Three consecutive negatives across three consecutive mornings is meaningful confirmation. If eggs appear at any point during the testing window, the cycle is not yet broken. Continue all three fronts for another two weeks before retesting.

For more definitive testing, a comprehensive stool analysis like the GI Map can detect *Enterobius* DNA, though it is less sensitive for pinworms specifically than the tape test, because pinworms lay their eggs externally rather than passing them in stool.

After the Eradication

Once pinworms are eliminated, they tend to stay eliminated. Reinfection requires swallowing pinworm eggs from a new source, and the most common new sources are identifiable:

- **Children in school environments.** Pinworms spread rapidly through classrooms, and a child who acquires them at school will bring them home.
- **Public bathrooms with poor hygiene.**
- **Contact with someone else's contaminated bedding or clothing.**
- **Travel to environments where hygiene is compromised.**

The long-term prevention practices are mostly common sense, but worth restating. Wash hands before eating. Keep fingernails short. Be cautious about shared bedding in unfamiliar places. Be aware that pinworms exist and can be picked up, particularly if you have children in school. If pinworm symptoms ever return — itching at night, restless sleep with nighttime scratching, visible white threads in stool — return to the three-front protocol immediately. Catching them early significantly shortens the eradication window the second time.

A Final Thought

Pinworms are humbling. They are the parasite that has lived alongside human beings since before recorded history. They infect roughly one in five children in the developed world. They quietly infect adults who would never imagine they could be hosts. They survive every cleanse that does not specifically address them. They circulate through families through ordinary hygiene gaps that nobody thinks twice about.

And they are addressed, in the end, by combining the herbs of the ancient practice with the modern understanding of how parasites actually transmit. The herbs alone are not enough. The hygiene alone is not enough. The household coordination alone is not enough. All three together, for six weeks, work.

The fact that pinworms require their own chapter in a book about prolonged fasting and parasite cleansing is a recognition of how unusual their lifecycle is. The fact that they are also among the most common parasites you carry is a recognition of how easily they hide in plain sight. This chapter exists because most people will need it, and most people will not know they need it.

If you suspect pinworms — even slightly — run the three-front protocol. If your family has experienced unexplained nighttime itching, particularly in children, run it. If you have completed full cleanses before and felt them not quite resolve, run it. The protocol works. But only when all three fronts are maintained.

Six weeks of discipline. Six weeks of household coordination. Six weeks of an environmental protocol that feels excessive until you understand why it exists. After that, pinworms are no longer part of your story. And that is no small thing.

Chapter 24

Parasite Elimination Timelines

* * *

There is a question that arrives, in some form, with nearly every reader who begins this protocol. How long. How long until the parasites are gone. How long until the lining begins to mend. How long until the work is finished and life can resume. The honest answer is that it depends, and what it depends on is the subject of this chapter.

Two readers can begin this protocol on the same day, follow the same schedule, take the same herbs, perform the same enemas — and finish at different times. The reason is not effort. The reason is starting condition. The body that arrives at this protocol with twelve years of careful eating finishes faster than the body that arrives carrying decades of standard Western diet. The body that has fasted before finishes faster than the body that has not. The body that includes the morning coffee enema finishes faster than the body that relies on herbs alone. The variables compound. The timelines respond.

What follows is not a promise. It is a map. The phases described below unfold in approximately this order in approximately these windows of time, depending on the conditions you bring to the work. Read the column that matches your situation. Use it as a frame for your expectations. Understand that your body will write its own version of this schedule, day by day, and that the value of these tables is not in their precision but in their pattern.

Why the Variables Matter

Five variables shape every parasite elimination timeline. Understanding them is the difference between expecting too much too soon and recognizing the work as it actually unfolds.

• **Whether you fast.** A body fasting and a body eating run on entirely different metabolic rules. Without food, the bowels enter a state where parasites lose their normal feeding environment, and the herbs reach the intestinal lining undiluted. With food, every herb is competing with digestion for absorption. Fasting compresses the timeline.

• **Whether you take antiparasitic herbs.** The herbs do the killing. Without them, fasting alone weakens parasites but rarely eliminates them. The herbs accelerate every phase that follows.

- **Whether you include the morning coffee enema.** This is the most important variable for liver fluke clearance. Without it, bile ducts are not flushed, and the parasites that live in the bile ducts remain largely untouched. The coffee enema is what allows the deeper layers of the work to begin.
- **Whether you have done this before.** A body that has cleared its primary parasitic load once carries less residual material the second time. The starting layers are thinner. The work goes faster. A second fast after a previous twenty-eight-day fast finishes in a fraction of the time of the first.
- **What your diet has been.** Twelve years of vegetarian eating produces a different intestinal environment than twelve years of standard Western eating. The microbiome is closer to what the protocol is trying to restore. The accumulated burden is lighter. The work begins at a more advanced starting point.

These variables compound. The reader fasting for the first time without herbs sits at one end of the spectrum. The reader fasting for the second time, with herbs, with the morning coffee enema, after years of clean eating, sits at the other end. Between them lies a wide range of timelines, all of them honest, all of them valid, all of them shaped by what the reader has brought to the work.

The Full Timeline Comparison

This table maps the major phases of the cleanse against the five most common reader scenarios. Each phase represents a real biological event — a population of parasites being addressed, a layer of accumulated material being released, a system beginning to recover. The day ranges are approximate. Your body may move through them slightly faster or slightly slower. The order of the phases, however, is consistent.

Phase	No Herbs / First Time	Herbs / First Time	Herbs + Coffee Enema / First Time	Herbs / Second Time After 28-Day Fast	Herbs + Coffee Enema / Second Time After 28-Day Fast + Vegetarian Diet
Surface clearing	Days 1–5	Days 1–3	Days 1–2	Days 1–2	Day 1
Candida die-off begins	Days 10–14	Days 7–10	Days 5–7	Days 5–7	Days 3–5
First parasite cycle cleared	Days 14–21	Days 10–14	Days 8–12	Days 7–10	Days 5–8
Biofilm disruption	Days 15–21	Days 10–14	Days 8–11	Days 8–12	Days 5–8
Intestinal fluke die-off begins	Days 18–25	Days 12–16	Days 9–13	Days 9–13	Days 6–9
Liver fluke bile duct flushing	Unlikely without coffee enema	Partial	Days 10–15	Days 10–14	Days 7–11
Fluke eggs targeted by clove	Days 21–28	Days 14–18	Days 12–16	Days 10–14	Days 7–11
Second parasite cycle	Days 21–28	Days 14–18	Days 12–15	Days 11–15	Days 8–12
Deep layer release	Days 22–30	Days 16–22	Days 13–18	Days 13–18	Days 9–14
Third parasite cycle	Days 28–35	Days 20–24	Days 16–20	Days 16–20	Days 11–16
Liver fluke clearance	Rarely achieved	Days 22–28	Days 18–24	Days 16–22	Days 12–18
Intestinal lining regenerating	Days 25–35	Days 18–24	Days 15–20	Days 15–21	Days 11–17
Fluke egg second cycle cleared	Rarely achieved	Days 24–30	Days 20–25	Days 18–24	Days 13–18
Estimated full cleanse	28–40 days	22–30 days	18–25 days	18–25 days	15–22 days

The first column is the longest path. It is included not to discourage but to be honest about what fasting alone can and cannot do. Fasting clears surface accumulation and weakens parasites, but it does not reliably eliminate the deeper organisms. The second column shows what herbs add. The third shows what the coffee enema adds on top of that. The fourth and fifth show what a body brings to the work the second time, especially when years of clean eating have prepared the ground.

Reading the Phases

Each phase in the table above represents a distinguishable event in the body. The signals are real, and learning to recognize them is part of how the reader knows the work is unfolding correctly.

• **Surface clearing.** The first wave. Easily mobilized debris from the upper colon and intestinal walls. Returns from the morning enema appear darker, more voluminous, more varied. Energy may dip briefly, then stabilize.

• **Candida die-off.** Yeast populations collapsing under fasting and herbal pressure. Often accompanied by transient brain fog, mild flu-like symptoms, white tongue coating that thickens before clearing. This phase passes within a few days when supported by trace minerals and adequate hydration.

• **First parasite cycle cleared.** The first generation of adult parasites — roundworms, tapeworms, smaller helminths — addressed by the herbs. Returns may show visible material. Energy often improves noticeably after this phase resolves.

• **Biofilm disruption.** The protective matrices that shelter parasitic communities are broken down by berberine, mimosa pudica, and black walnut. This phase exposes organisms that were previously hidden, often producing a temporary increase in die-off symptoms before signaling the deeper work to begin.

• **Intestinal fluke die-off begins.** The flukes living in the intestinal walls begin releasing their hold. The morning enema returns may show stringy, mucoid material. Right-sided abdominal sensation may intensify briefly.

• **Liver fluke bile duct flushing.** This phase is the one that does not happen without the morning coffee enema. The bile ducts release accumulated debris. Returns often show characteristic green sludge — the visible evidence that the deeper work is reaching the deepest layer.

• **Fluke eggs targeted by clove.** Sustained eugenol levels reach the eggs that other herbs cannot penetrate. This phase requires consistent three-times-daily clove dosing. Skipping doses lets eggs resume development. Consistency is what makes this phase work.

• **Second and third parasite cycles.** New generations of parasites that hatched during the protocol from eggs that were laid before clove reached them. Each cycle is smaller than the one before. By the third cycle, returns are noticeably cleaner.

• **Deep layer release.** The accumulated material that has been sitting in intestinal folds, often for years, begins to lift. This is sometimes accompanied by emotional releases, vivid dreams, a sense of internal lightness developing.

• **Liver fluke clearance.** The adult liver flukes — the most stubborn organisms in the human gut — finally addressed. This is the phase most protocols never reach. With the full stack, it becomes possible.

• **Intestinal lining regenerating.** The work shifts from clearing to rebuilding. Villi begin extending. Tight junctions begin reforming. The transformation described in the next chapter begins in earnest.

• **Fluke egg second cycle cleared.** The final eggs, the deepest deposits, the last residual generation. When this phase completes, the cleanse is complete.

Fluke-Specific Timelines

Flukes deserve their own table. They are the parasites most readers come to this protocol intending to address, and they are the parasites most likely to be missed by less comprehensive approaches. The following breakdown shows how each fluke phase responds to each level of intervention.

Fluke Type	No Herbs / No Coffee Enema	Herbs Only	Herbs + Coffee Enema First Time	Herbs + Coffee Enema Second Time + Vegetarian Diet
Intestinal flukes — adults	Rarely cleared	Days 12–18	Days 9–14	Days 6–10
Intestinal flukes — eggs	Never fully cleared	Days 18–25	Days 14–20	Days 10–15
Liver flukes — adults	Never without coffee enema	Partial only	Days 15–22	Days 10–16
Liver flukes — eggs	Never	Rarely	Days 20–26	Days 14–20
Bile duct clearance	Never	Partial	Days 12–18	Days 8–14

The first column is included as honest information. Fasting alone, however prolonged, does not address adult liver flukes or their eggs. The herbs reach the intestinal flukes but cannot reliably penetrate the bile ducts where liver flukes live. The coffee enema is what changes the equation. When the morning coffee enema is added to the herbal protocol, every fluke phase becomes addressable. When the protocol is undertaken a second time, by a body that has already cleared its primary load and has been eating clean food for years, the timelines compress further.

This is why the protocol is laid out as a system rather than a list of options. Each component reaches what the others cannot. Together, they reach everything.

The First Time and the Second Time

For readers who have completed a previous twenty-eight-day fast, this section addresses an important question. Does the second cleanse really go faster, and if so, why?

The answer is yes, and the reasons are biological.

- **The primary parasite load was addressed the first time.** What remains is residual — eggs that survived, deeper-tissue organisms that escaped the first pass, smaller populations that have re-established more slowly. The starting count is lower. The work to be done is less.
- **The intestinal lining is in better condition.** The villi have regenerated. The mucoid plaque has been cleared. The biofilm communities have been dismantled. Herbs reach their targets more efficiently because the lining no longer obstructs them.
- **The microbiome is healthier.** The first cleanse cleared the dysbiotic populations. The rebuilding phase that followed established more balanced bacterial communities. These communities cooperate with the protocol rather than resisting it.
- **The body remembers the rhythm.** The signals are familiar. The discipline is established. The reader knows what each sensation means. Fewer mistakes are made. The protocol runs more smoothly.
- **A clean diet between fasts compounds the advantage.** A reader who has eaten vegetarian or whole-food clean for years between fasts arrives at the second cleanse with a substantially lighter accumulated burden than the reader who has returned to standard eating. The starting layers are thinner. The clearing is faster.

The second fast is not a repetition of the first. It is a deeper continuation. What took thirty days the first time may take eighteen the second. What took forty days the first time may take twenty-two the second. The body that has been here before knows the way.

What These Numbers Are Not

A caution belongs here, near the end of this chapter, because the tables above can be read in ways that lead to disappointment.

These numbers are not promises. They are observed patterns. Some readers will move through the phases faster than the table suggests. Others will move through them more slowly. The tables describe the typical case, not every case.

These numbers are not finish lines. The clearing of parasites is not the same as the rebuilding of the gut. Even when the cleanse is complete in the sense described above, the deeper work of microbiome rebuilding and lining restoration continues for months. The estimated full cleanse window is the end of the elimination phase, not the end of the journey.

These numbers are not a substitute for paying attention to your body. The signals matter more than the schedule. If your body tells you a phase is still in progress when the table suggests it should be complete, trust your body. If your body tells you to slow down, slow down. If your body tells you you have arrived somewhere the table did not predict, the table is wrong, not your body.

The tables are a frame. The work is what fills the frame.

A Note on Patience

The reader who reaches this chapter is often the reader who is in the middle of the work, looking up to see how much is left. The honest answer is that the timeline you are on is the timeline your body has chosen for you. It is shaped by the variables you brought to the protocol and the consistency with which you are now executing it. The work cannot be rushed. The phases unfold in their own time. The clearing happens when the conditions for clearing are present.

What you can do is hold the conditions steady. Take the herbs on schedule. Perform the enemas as designed. Replenish the minerals. Attend to the signals. Trust the rhythm. The body that has been through this before knows what to do. The body that is going through it for the first time is learning, and the learning is part of the work.

Somewhere on the timeline above is the day your body will signal that the work is complete. You will know it when you arrive. Until then, the protocol continues, and the phases continue to unfold, and the body continues to do what it has been waiting all your life to do.

The Parasites Themselves

The tables above describe what happens to you. The tables that follow describe what happens to them. Every parasite in this book has a life cycle, and every life cycle has a duration. Egg to larva to adult. Hatching, migrating, maturing, reproducing, dying. The numbers vary by species. They vary by what the body has been given to work with. But the cycles are real, and they are the reason the protocol is structured the way it is. Understanding the cycle is understanding why the herbs are taken for the duration they are taken, why the fast lasts as long as it does, why the second time through finishes faster than the first.

What follows is a frame for the parasites themselves. Four families. Four tables. Each one shows how long the organism takes to complete its life cycle in a normal host, how long it survives in a fasting body without herbs, and how long it survives when the herbs are added. The numbers are biological, not promises. Read them as you would read tide charts. They describe what is typical. The body in front of you is what determines the rest.

Roundworms (Nematodes)

Roundworms are the most numerous parasites in human gut populations and the easiest to clear. They are the worms most readers picture when they hear the word — long, threadlike, mobile. Five species account for nearly all human roundworm infections. Their life cycles range from a few weeks to several months. Their adult lifespans are measured in years, but the herbs reach them quickly. With the triad running and the body in fasting state, every roundworm species in the table below is addressable inside two weeks.

Parasite	Egg	Larvae	Adult	Total Cycle	Starvation Only	With Herbal Tinctures
Ascaris	2–3 weeks to hatch	10–14 days migrating	Lives 1–2 years	3–4 weeks to mature	3–4 weeks	7–14 days
Whipworm	3 weeks to hatch	2–3 weeks developing	Lives 1–2 years	5–6 weeks to mature	4–5 weeks	10–14 days
Hookworm	Hatches in 1–2 days	5–10 days developing	Lives 1–2 years	5–6 weeks to mature	3–4 weeks	7–12 days
Pinworm	Hatches in 4–6 hours	No larvae stage	Lives 5–13 weeks	4–6 weeks to mature	2–3 weeks	5–10 days
Strongyloides	Hatches within hours	Can reinfect immediately	Lives months to years	2–4 weeks to mature	4–6 weeks	10–16 days

Tapeworms (Cestodes)

Tapeworms are the long-lived ones. The adults can persist for decades — twenty-five years for the beef and pork varieties, twenty for the fish — quietly absorbing nutrients across their length while the host has no idea they are there. The cycle from egg to adult is longer than for roundworms, and the protocol must run longer to address them. The herbs work, and the cycle collapses, but the timeline is in the two-to-three week range rather than the one-to-two week range. What matters most for tapeworms is duration. The protocol must continue past the point where the symptoms have eased.

Parasite	Egg	Larvae	Adult	Total Cycle	Starvation Only	With Herbal Tinctures
Beef tapeworm	Immediately infective	10–12 weeks in tissue	Lives up to 25 years	10–12 weeks to mature	4–6 weeks	14–21 days
Pork tapeworm	Immediately infective	8–10 weeks in tissue	Lives up to 25 years	8–10 weeks to mature	4–6 weeks	14–21 days
Fish tapeworm	2 weeks to hatch	Several weeks developing	Lives up to 20 years	3–6 weeks to mature	4–5 weeks	12–18 days
Dwarf tapeworm	Immediately infective	2 weeks developing	Lives several weeks	2–4 weeks to mature	2–3 weeks	7–12 days

Flukes (Trematodes)

Flukes are the protocol's hardest target. They are not in the gut where the herbs reach most easily. They live in the bile ducts, in the liver tissue itself, in places that herbs alone struggle to penetrate at therapeutic concentration. The Chinese liver fluke can live thirty years. The Fasciola can live thirteen. Their eggs are deeply embedded in tissue, and their adult forms hide behind layers of bile and biofilm that the standard herbal triad cannot fully reach. This is why the coffee enema appears in the column heading of the table below, where it appeared as an alternative in the previous tables. For flukes, the coffee enema is not optional. It is the difference between the cycle being addressable and the cycle being out of reach.

Parasite	Egg	Larvae	Adult	Total Cycle	Starvation Only	With Herbs + Coffee Enema
Intestinal fluke	3–7 weeks to hatch	Several weeks in snail host	Lives 2–3 years	6–8 weeks to mature	5–7 weeks	14–21 days
Liver fluke (Fasciola)	3–4 weeks to hatch	6–8 weeks developing	Lives 9–13 years	10–12 weeks to mature	Rarely cleared	18–28 days
Chinese liver fluke	1–2 weeks to hatch	Several weeks developing	Lives 20–30 years	4–6 weeks to mature	Rarely cleared	16–24 days
Heterophyes	1–2 weeks to hatch	4–6 weeks developing	Lives 1 year	4–6 weeks to mature	3–4 weeks	10–16 days

Protozoa

Protozoa are the smallest organisms in this group, and in some ways the most aggressive. They are single-celled. They divide rapidly — sometimes every eight hours, sometimes faster — and a single organism can become a population in a matter of days. What protects a body against them is not the speed of the kill but the speed of replacement. The protocol addresses protozoa fastest of all four families, often within the first week, because the herbs that work against them work against the dividing form directly. Berberine and oregano oil, in particular, are the protocol's protozoa specialists. The triad helps. These two finish the work.

Parasite	Cyst Stage	Active Stage	Replication Rate	Starvation Only	With Herbal Tinctures
Giardia	Immediately infective	Divides every 8–12 hours	Very rapid	2–3 weeks	5–10 days
Entamoeba	Immediately infective	Divides every 8 hours	Very rapid	2–4 weeks	7–12 days
Cryptosporidium	Immediately infective	Rapid intracellular	Extremely rapid	3–4 weeks	10–14 days
Blastocystis	Survives outside host	Divides every 12 hours	Moderate	2–3 weeks	5–8 days

Four families. Four timelines. The protocol is built to address all of them, and the duration of the protocol — the four to six weeks of herbs, the prolonged fast, the daily coffee enema — exists because of what the tables above show. Shorter interventions reach the protozoa and some of the roundworms. They miss the tapeworms. They almost entirely miss the flukes. The full protocol exists to reach what shorter ones cannot.

Figures referenced in this chapter: 25.1 (online Figure Guide)

Chapter 25

The Body's Quietest Conversation

There is a man, in his forties, who has spent twelve years living with a body that came back to him in pieces after a long fast. On an ordinary evening, at a friend's table, he eats a meal prepared with care — a stew of some kind, bread that the host had made that afternoon, wine in a glass with a pattern cut into it. He eats slowly, the way he has eaten for years, and at the end of the meal he thanks his host and walks home in the early autumn dark, thinking about the conversation rather than about the food.

It is sometime around midnight, lying in bed in the quiet of his own house, that he becomes aware of a small roughness somewhere along the long folded length of the small intestine — nothing that hurts, nothing that he would call a symptom, only a low note from a part of him that had been silent through dinner and is no longer silent now. The note is faint enough that a person not paying attention would miss it. He has spent twelve years paying attention.

In the early years he would have tried to work out what in the meal was responsible. The bread, perhaps. Or something the stew had been thickened with that he could not have known about. He would have lain awake running through the ingredients, building a small case, planning what he would or would not eat at this friend's table the next time he came. He no longer does any of this. The body has spoken in the only language it has. He has heard what it said. The speech and the hearing are, by now, almost the same gesture. He drinks a glass of water from the kitchen and returns to bed, and by the time the morning light has come into the bedroom the small roughness is no longer there.

The tissue that produced this report, this faint and accurate note from the long folded interior, has been at work in him for the whole of his life and has, for most of that life, not been heard from. It is a pink and intricate lining, the cells of which renew themselves every few days, and which lies along the twenty-some feet of the small intestine the way the lining of a deep cave runs along the walls of the cave — continuous, alive, in conversation with everything that passes through. When the man was a child it spoke to him, and he heard it, in the rough untrained way a child knows what does and does not sit well in his stomach. By the time he was twenty-five it had gone quiet, not because it had stopped speaking but because it had been speaking through a thickening haze of its own slow damage for so long that what arrived from it was no longer distinguishable from the ordinary background of being inside a body. He thought what he was hearing from his own gut was the gut itself. He had no way to know it was not.

What changed, twelve years ago, was a stretch of forty days during which nothing was asked of that lining at all. No food to admit or refuse. No decision to make about what was nourishing and what was harm. During those forty days the lining used the time, as a body will use time it has been given, to do what it had been postponing for the whole of his adult life. It made itself again. It had always been making itself, every cell of it replaced every few days since he was a small child, but the making had been laid down on top of the damage of the day before, and the day before that, and the years before that, so that what was being made was always shaped by what had not yet been allowed to heal. The forty days were the first stretch in his adult life when the making could happen without that shaping. By the end of those days, the tissue inside him was something it had not been since he was a boy.

In the years that followed, slowly, mostly without his noticing, it has continued to be that thing. The note he heard at midnight from the friend's stew, and the silence that returned by morning, are both of them the speech of a tissue that has come back into itself. They are not two different events. They are the same one, named twice. A lining that is well speaks both when it is troubled and when it is at ease, and the man, lying in his bed in the dark with the small roughness easing, is hearing both halves of the same sentence.

* * *

The bread the host had baked that afternoon was, by the time the man took his first bite of it, already in the early stages of being read. The work began in his mouth, where the saliva almost immediately started to break apart the long chains of starch into shorter pieces. It continued in the stomach, where an acid made of nothing more than salt, water, and a small concentration of hydrogen ions stripped away the larger structures and prepared what remained to be passed forward. By the time what had been bread reached the upper end of the small intestine, perhaps an hour after the meal, it was no longer recognizable as bread. It was a slow warm slurry, half-broken, still carrying the chemistry of the meal it had come from, arriving at the place where the real reading was about to happen.

The place where the reading was about to happen was the same pink intricate surface that, hours later, would speak from the man's bed. Spread out flat, that surface would carpet a tennis court. Folded into the small intestine, it lies in overlapping ridges and valleys and finger-like projections, so that what looks, on a scan, like a few feet of tubing is in fact an enormous interior landscape, every inch of which is doing work. The finger-like projections are called villi. Each villus is itself covered in smaller projections — microvilli — making the actual living edge between the body and the gut more like a coastline than a wall.

Every cell along this enormous folded coastline is, as the man sat at the friend's table, in the middle of a life measured in days. The cells of the lining renew themselves faster than almost any other tissue in the body. The skin takes weeks; the bone takes years; the lining of the small intestine takes between three and five days. New cells are being born, every hour of every day, in the shadowed crypts at the base of each villus, and they migrate slowly upward along the side of the villus toward its tip, doing the work of the surface as they go. At the tip they reach the end of their short life and are released into the gut to be carried away with what the body has finished using. The lining a person has at the end of any given week is, almost entirely, not the lining they had at the beginning of it.

What the cells are doing, while they live their short lives, is making a continuous decision about what to admit and what to turn away. That decision is the body's. Between every two adjacent cells of the surface is a join —

a tight junction, in the language of biology — that can tighten or loosen by very small amounts in response to what is arriving on the other side of the wall. When the joins are tight, only the small specific molecules the body has decided to take in are let through: the broken-down sugars from the bread, the amino acids from the stew, the minerals dissolved in the wine. Everything larger, everything not yet recognized as nourishment, stays on the gut side and is carried forward to be dealt with elsewhere or carried out.

The lining does not do this work alone. Above its surface, between the cells and the contents of the gut, lies a layer of mucus thick enough to hold a small ecology of its own. The bacterial community that has lived along the gut wall since the man was a small child lives in this mucus. Their presence and their signaling shape what the surface is and is not asked to do. Beneath, on the body side of the wall, lie immune cells positioned to receive what the surface reports and to act on it. The lining is, in this sense, less a wall than a meeting-place: the body's own cells above, in the mucus; the body's own cells below, in the immune tissue; and between them, the renewing layer that is continuously deciding what passes from one side to the other.

By the time the man had finished his stew and was walking home in the autumn dark, the bread he had eaten an hour before was, somewhere in the upper reaches of his small intestine, in the middle of being read by this surface and by all of its neighbors. The reading would continue, slowly, across the next several hours. Most of what arrived in that bread would be admitted, broken down further, drawn into the body to be used. A small portion of what arrived would, for reasons the surface was responsible for sensing, not be admitted. That small portion was the small roughness he would feel, sometime around midnight, settling into bed.

* * *

The man's lining was not always the lining that produced that small roughness with such accuracy. For most of his adult life before the fast it had been carrying damage of the kind that almost any modern adult body carries, accumulated slowly, in small daily increments, across years of asking the surface to read and decide about and pass judgment on things it was not built to handle in the quantities or combinations or frequencies in which the modern world delivers them.

The asking comes from many directions at once. Highly processed food, engineered to cross the surface faster and in greater volume than the lining was meant to admit, arrives meal after meal for years. Common medications — the over-the-counter pain relievers a person takes on the headaches of an ordinary week, the antibiotics taken for an infection that may have cleared on its own — pass through the gut and abrade or blunt the renewing surface as they go. The chronic stress of a life that does not allow its alarms to fall slows the lining's repair, day after day, the same way it slows every other repair the body wants to do. And the bacterial community above the surface, when it has been disturbed by any of these, sends signals that the surface reads differently than it would have read the signals of an undisturbed community.

What the damage looks like, mechanically, is a slow loosening of the joins between the cells of the surface. The tight junctions tighten and loosen, in a healthy lining, by very small amounts and in response to specific signals. In a lining that has been asked too much of for too long, the joins begin to loosen by larger amounts and in response to less specific signals. Things the body has not chosen to admit begin to cross the wall: fragments of food that should have stayed on the gut side, bacterial pieces that should have been kept out, molecules the immune cells beneath the wall are not expecting and do not know what to do with. This condition is sometimes called leaky gut, and the phrase is approximately accurate, though what is leaking is less the gut itself than the discipline of the joins between the cells.

The immune cells positioned just behind the wall, when they meet the things that should not have been there, do what immune cells do. They raise the body's response. The response is small if the breach is small and intermittent, larger if the breach is steady, and steady the way the body is now living: a low simmering alarm in the layer just behind the gut wall that has been on, in low form, for years. Many of what a person experiences as unrelated complaints — a mood that does not lift the way it used to, a joint that has been quietly inflamed for as long as they can remember, a skin condition that comes and goes by no logic they can find — are reports from a body whose immune system has been hearing, for a long time, things from across the gut wall that should not have been crossing it.

The lining is forgiving in one important sense. Even after years of damage, the cells continue to be born in the crypts, continue to migrate up the villus, continue to renew themselves on the schedule the body has kept since it was a small child. The damage does not stop the renewal. What the damage does is make every new layer of cells settle onto a surface that is already a little wrong, so that the new layer inherits the shape of the wrong, and the layer that follows inherits the shape of the layer that came before, until what is being made is something quite different from what would have been made on a clean substrate. This is why the damage persists across years of perfectly competent renewal. The renewal cannot, on its own, undo the shape of what it is being asked to renew on top of.

A lining that has been damaged in the slow ordinary way of a modern adult life will not, in the ordinary course of that life, repair the damage. The damage and the repair, in such a life, more or less keep pace with each other; the body maintains a steady state that is neither getting worse nor getting better, and a person comes to think of that steady state as simply how their body is. They do not think of it as something that could change.

* * *

What can change it, when nothing in the ordinary course of life will, is a stretch of time during which the lining is asked nothing. No food to admit or refuse. No decision to make about what is nourishing and what is harm. No flood of arrivals at the surface that the worn-down joins must try to sort, hour after hour, with the dulled attention of a tissue that has been working without rest for years.

The renewal does not stop when the eating stops. The cells continue to be born in the crypts; they continue to migrate up the villus; they continue to be released at the tip on the same three-to-five-day schedule the body has kept since before the man was born. What is different is that, for the first time in his adult life, the new cells are migrating into a surface that is not actively being damaged as they arrive. The wear that had been laid down across years of meals is no longer being laid down on top of itself. The next layer of cells settles into its place without inheriting a fresh shape of wrong from the layer above.

Above the surface, the mucus layer that had been thinned by the constant arrival of food and the constant need to defend against what the food carried begins to thicken. Inside that mucus, the bacterial community that had been driven for years toward the species that thrive in disturbance begins to shift slowly back toward the species that thrive in calm. And beneath the wall, the immune cells that had been on low alarm for years begin to receive less of what they had been reacting to and, in the absence of new arrivals, begin to come down off the alarm.

A person can do a great deal for the lining without ever fasting. They can eat food that was not engineered to abrade the surface, avoid the medications that blunt it, and quiet the stress that slows its repair. All of this helps, and all of this is part of the long-term care of a lining. But none of it offers the lining what an extended fast offers, which is not better arrivals at the surface but no arrivals at all. The cleaning that the lining does on itself, when nothing is asked of it, is different in kind from the cleaning it can do while continuing to work. There is a particular quality of repair that requires the work to stop entirely.

The forty days are a window. What happens inside the window is one thing, and the chapters that have already covered the fast itself have shown what that one thing looks like from the inside. What happens after the window closes — when the eating begins again, slowly, and the lining begins to meet food for the first time in its newly-renewed condition — is the long arc that the rest of this work is about.

* * *

The first food that arrives at a renewed lining is met differently than the food that arrived a hundred days before it. The arrivals are smaller, by careful design — the reintroduction of food after a long fast is a slow and deliberate thing — but the difference is not only one of volume. The surface itself is reading what it meets with a clarity it has not had in years. A spoonful of broth, the first real food a person takes after such a stretch, is met by a tissue capable of distinguishing things in it that, before the fast, would have been swept past in the ordinary noise of an overworked surface.

In the first days after the fast, the lining is doing work that is less about repair and more about re-learning. It tightens its joins around the small specific arrivals and lets them through. It signals to the immune cells beneath that what is arriving is known and safe. It begins, with each meal, to reestablish the rhythms of admit-and-refuse that had been blunted across the years before. A person in these first days often eats less than they expect to eat, is full sooner than they used to be, and notices flavors with a sharpness that surprises them.

Across the first weeks, the deeper work begins. The lining has been renewed, but the body around it is still carrying much of what years of damage left behind — the bacterial community is still rebalancing, the immune cells are still standing down, the body is still releasing what it had been holding. There is a moment, sometimes a private one, in the first or second week, where what the body has been holding comes out at last.

A person finds themselves, in a bathroom they did not expect to spend long in, in the company of what the lining has been keeping from the rest of them for a great many years.

Beneath all of this, the lining keeps doing its quiet work. Each new layer of cells now arrives onto a surface that is no longer carrying the damage of the previous meals. Each new layer carries forward, as a result, a slightly cleaner shape than the one before. The improvement is not visible from inside the experience. A person paying close attention may notice that, gradually, they are less reactive to foods they used to react to, less swollen at the end of meals, less subject to the small unease that had been the background of so many afternoons.

In the first months, the work moves below the surface of what a person consciously tracks. By now the bacterial community has completed much of its rebalancing, and the immune cells have fully come down off the chronic alarm of the years before. Above the surface, the mucus layer that had been thinned by years of overwork has thickened into a healthy depth. The lining now lives, for the first time in the man's adult life, in the conditions it was designed to live in. It has neighbors above it whose signaling it can read clearly. It has a defensive perimeter beneath it that is no longer firing. It has the quiet hours of an unstressed body in which to do its renewing work.

What happens in the years that follow — the years the man at the friend's table was twelve years into when the small roughness arrived — is a continuance of what began in the months. The lining keeps renewing, on its three-to-five-day schedule, in conditions that allow each renewal to settle cleanly onto the one before. The conditions are not perfect. A meal at a friend's table will sometimes carry something the lining cannot fully admit. A stressful season will sometimes thin the mucus a little. A course of medication, when one is needed, will sometimes abrade the surface. None of these returns the lining to the state it was in before the fast. The lining now has the capacity to absorb the small ordinary insults of being alive and to recover from them, the way a body that is well does, and to keep its baseline despite them.

And when, on an ordinary evening twelve years after the fast, something at a friend's table does not entirely agree, the lining reports. Not as it would have reported before — as a steady worsening of an already-worsened condition — but as the small clean note of a tissue that is well enough to know the difference between what does and does not belong, and to say so, faintly, to a body that is now in a position to hear.

* * *

The repair the fast makes possible is not, once begun, self-completing. It is a possibility opened in the body, and the body in the months that follow either takes the possibility further or gradually undoes it. Several of the things that can undo it are the same things that thinned the lining in the first place, returning, after the window has closed, to ask of the surface what it had asked before.

The most common is the return to the same food. A person who has spent forty days inside the quiet of an unfed body, who has watched their lining begin to remake itself, who has noticed in the first reintroduction meals a clarity they had not had in years, will sometimes, after a few weeks, return to the foods that had been damaging the surface before. They do this for honest reasons, most of them — the food is familiar, it is what their family eats, it is what is available at the airport and the convenience store and the meeting where lunch was provided. But the lining cannot distinguish between the convenient meal and the destructive one; it only reads what arrives. What returns to arriving, the surface returns to being damaged by.

The food is the most common return, but it is not the only one. The body whose immune cells came down off the simmering response during the fast can, if placed back into the long stress of an unresolving life, climb back onto the response within months; the lining lives inside the body that lives the life, and a life that does not permit its alarms to fall is a life inside which a healed lining will, slowly, begin to be worked on the way the previous lining was worked on. The medications a person takes by reflex do similar work over time. An over-the-counter pain reliever for the ordinary headache. A second one for the soreness that comes after a workout. A heartburn pill taken every evening for years. None of these are sinister; most of them, on the day they are taken, do exactly what the person reaching for them needed them to do. The cost is paid quietly, across the years, by the surface that has to keep doing its work while being abraded.

A lining that has been brought back to what it was meant to be has a considerable capacity to absorb small returns of the old asking. What it cannot absorb is the steady accumulation of them. A person who has done the work of a long fast, and who returns afterward to the life that produced the original damage, will find themselves, in some number of years, carrying a surface that looks more like the one they began with than the one the forty days produced. The fast is not, on its own, the work. The work is the slow long choosing of what to ask of the lining, day after day, in the years that follow.

* * *

It is some weeks after the evening at the friend's table. The man is at his own kitchen counter, in the early morning, making something simple — an egg, perhaps, with a little salt. He has been awake for half an hour. The house is quiet. He pays no particular attention to the cooking, or to the eating, or to the small decisions his body is making about what to do with the egg. None of these feel like decisions. They feel like the ordinary unnoticed business of being alive in a body.

He is not feeling, this morning, any small roughness anywhere along the long folded length of the small intestine. He is not feeling much of anything from his gut at all. This is not the silence of a tissue that has been overworked into mute background. It is the silence of a tissue that has nothing it needs to say.

The lining has been at this for twelve years. It has spoken when it had something to speak about, the small roughness of the friend's stew being one such speaking, and it has been quiet on the many ordinary mornings when nothing in particular needed to be reported. In both the speaking and the quiet it has been doing the same thing it has been doing since the man was a boy — reading what arrives, deciding what to admit, reporting to the rest of the body in the only language it has. The fast did not give the man a new lining. It gave him, for the first time in his adult life, the lining he had always had.

Chart T — The Arc of Repair After a Long Fast

A reference for what to expect across the months and years that follow a prolonged fast. The middle column tracks what is happening internally; the right column tracks what a person may experience and what is normal at each stage.

Time	What is happening inside	What a person may notice
First days	• Reintroduction begins with small amounts of simple food (broth, soft cooked vegetables). • Lining is reactivating digestion that has been paused for weeks. • Repair has not yet begun in earnest.	• Smaller appetite than expected; easily full. • Heightened sensitivity to flavor, salt, and sweetness. • Stools may be loose or irregular as digestion restarts.
First weeks	• Bacterial community begins to rebalance. • Immune cells beneath the lining come down off chronic alarm. • Body releases stored toxins and old undigested matter as eating resumes.	• Detox phase common in week one or two: looser stools, brief fatigue. • A heavier-than-usual evacuation event is possible. • Old food reactions begin to lessen.
First months	• Mucus layer rebuilds to full thickness. • Bacterial community completes most rebalancing. • New cells form on a clean substrate; each renewal cycle leaves the lining steadily improved.	• Reduced bloating after meals. • Foods that previously caused reactions may be tolerated. • Energy more stable; sleep quality often improves. • Skin may clear.
The years	• Lining renews every 3-5 days on a clean substrate. • Maintenance, not repair. • Capacity to absorb occasional insults (a poor meal, stressful week, needed medication) without reverting to chronic damage.	• Discomfort after a problem food is brief and clear, not dragging on for days. • Baseline digestion is reliable. • Rebuilding required only if life returns to chronic damage patterns.

Chapter 26

The Psychological Journey

* * *

The science tells you what is happening in your body. This chapter tells you what is happening in your mind. And the mind, it turns out, is where most fasts are won or lost. Not in the stomach. Not in the intestines. In the space between your ears, and in the stories you tell yourself there.

Forty days is a long time to spend inside your own head. The experience does not unfold evenly. It has phases — distinct ones, each with its own psychological texture, its own challenges, its own gifts. Learning to recognize which phase you are in transforms the experience from something that happens to you into something you navigate with awareness. That awareness is everything. The same biological work, conducted with awareness or without it, produces dramatically different experiences in the mind that is doing it. The body cannot be tricked. The mind, however, can be either an ally or an obstacle, and the difference is largely a matter of preparation.

Before we go further, a word of honesty. This chapter describes the psychological territory of prolonged fasting as reported by hundreds of people who have completed it, including the author. It is written to prepare you, not to alarm you. Every challenge described in these pages is navigable, and every one of them has been navigated, by ordinary people, many times.

But the chapter comes with an important caveat. The psychological experience of prolonged fasting is therapeutic only in the right context — approached from a place of genuine health-seeking, with appropriate medical context, with a stable relationship with one's own body. If at any point the content of this chapter resonates in a way that feels less like preparation and more like permission, please pause. Reach out to someone who can help you understand the difference. The Alliance for Eating Disorders Helpline is available at 1-866-662-1235. That number is not a formality. It is here because the work of fasting, when undertaken from the wrong place, can deepen patterns that need different kinds of support entirely.

The First Three Days

The first three days belong to the body. The mind wants to be philosophical about the fast — wants to settle into its meaning, wants to articulate its purpose, wants to begin the work of reflection that the practitioner has been anticipating. The body has other plans.

What the practitioner experiences in these days is real and physical. The hunger is insistent. It is not the polite hunger of a missed meal. It is the loud, urgent hunger of a system accustomed to regular feeding suddenly noticing that no feeding is coming. Headaches arrive, sometimes severe, as the brain transitions from glucose to ketone metabolism and the glucose-craving signaling pathways protest. Irritability rises — the body under metabolic stress communicates through mood, and the people around the faster will notice. Fatigue sets in as the system draws inward, conserving energy for the metabolic shift that is underway. Cravings come, not yet specific, just a generalized urgent wanting that pulses through awareness at unpredictable intervals.

The primary psychological challenge of these days is distinguishing genuine emergency from temporary discomfort. The body sends distress signals during this phase that feel urgent and important. The nervous system, accustomed to the regular arrival of food, registers the absence of food as a potential threat. To the mammal underneath the modern human, missing food for three days is the kind of thing that requires urgent action. The mammal does not know that the practitioner has chosen this. The mammal only knows that food is not arriving and that this is bad news.

Knowing precisely what is happening physiologically helps. Reminding yourself that this phase has a defined end — typically by day three or four — helps. Staying horizontal when possible, conserving energy, helps. Taking your trace minerals consistently, drinking your water, and staying connected to someone who has done this before — all of these help. What helps most, though, is simple recognition. The signals of these days are not commands. They are weather. They will pass. They have passed for everyone who has come before you, and they will pass for you.

The people who make it past day three almost always complete the fast. The first three days are the gatekeepers. Once they are behind you, the territory changes.

The Fourth Through Seventh Days

Something interesting happens as the physical hunger quiets. The mind rushes in to fill the space it left behind.

By day four or five, ketosis is establishing. Physical hunger has begun to soften — paradoxically, reliably. The cellular machinery has adapted to the new fuel source, and the loud signals that dominated the first three days have begun to fade. And exactly as this happens, exactly as the body's distress quiets, the mind becomes extraordinarily busy with food. Practitioners find themselves thinking about meals, about recipes, about flavors and textures, more constantly than they think about food in their ordinary lives. They watch cooking videos. They read menus. They browse recipes online with an attention that is almost compulsive. They become acutely, painfully aware of how much of their daily life had been organized around eating, and how much empty space exists in a day when that organization is removed.

This is the phase in which the meaning of food beyond nutrition becomes visible. The practitioner begins to see, perhaps for the first time, how much of their emotional life had been organized around eating. Food was not just fuel. It was comfort after a hard day. It was celebration of small good news. It was social connection, the structure around which time with loved ones organized itself. It was something to do when boredom arrived. It was reward, ritual, routine, marker of seasons and holidays and the rhythms of weeks. Removing food removes all of these things at once. What is left in their place is often uncomfortable, and almost always informative.

What the practitioner does with this discovery shapes the rest of the fast. The discomfort is the teaching. The boredom that arrives in the absence of meals is not empty time to be fled from. It is the space in which the practitioner can finally see what was being filled. Many people, doing prolonged fasting for the first time, are startled to realize how little of their relationship with food was about hunger and how much of it was about emotional regulation. The fast is, in this sense, a kind of psychological revelation that no amount of reading about emotional eating can produce. The eating has stopped. The patterns underneath the eating are still there, and they are now visible.

Journaling helps in this phase. Writing about what food meant beyond nutrition. Gentle movement helps — walks, stretching, time outside. Replacing food rituals with other rituals — herbal tea at the times you would have eaten, a meditation in the morning, a slow walk in the evening — gives the body something to do during the times it expected to receive food. Allowing the boredom without immediately fleeing from it is, perhaps, the most important practice. The boredom is information. It is showing you what your life had been organized around. Sit with it long enough to read what it has to say.

The Second Week

By the second week, the novelty of the fast has worn off. The end is still far away. And something unexpected arrives — a quiet grief.

This is often the most emotionally complex phase of the fast. What the practitioner feels, in the days from about eight through fourteen, is not always identifiable in the moment. There is a longing, but it is not always for food specifically. It is for the experience of eating. For the smell of cooking, the warmth and comfort that smell carries. For shared meals, for the social and relational dimensions of eating that have been part of human life since human life began. For the simple pleasure of taste, which the practitioner had taken for granted for an entire lifetime and is now consciously without.

Specific cravings often surface during this phase, and they are rarely random. The food a mother made when the practitioner was unwell as a child. The meal associated with a particular relationship — sometimes a relationship long ended. The taste connected to a time of safety, a place of belonging, a moment when the world felt simpler. These cravings carry emotional information. They are not, in most cases, about the food itself. They are about what the food was carrying — comfort, memory, connection, love, the texture of a particular time.

Pay attention to what comes up. The detailed sensory memories that surface during this phase are telling you something about what eating has been doing for you, beyond nourishment, for years. Most adults have layered emotional meaning onto specific foods so completely that they no longer notice they are doing it. The fast strips away the food and reveals the meaning beneath, and the meaning, exposed, is often the source of the longing more than the food itself.

Dreams about food are common in this phase, and they are sometimes remarkably vivid. People dream of full tables, of feasts, of meals shared with people who are no longer alive. The dreams are often emotional rather than gustatory in their substance — what the dreamer wakes remembering is not the taste but the warmth, not the food but the person who served it.

Allow the grief without judgment. It is real, and it is valid. Write about the specific cravings and what memories or feelings they carry. Find non-food ways to meet the underlying need — connection, warmth, rest, the comfort of being held by people who love you. Remember that the longing is not the same as the need. Longing can be felt fully, met partially, and survived. The discovery of this distinction is one of the more important teachings of the second week.

The Third Week

By the third week, the mind has changed tactics. The raw emotional longing of the second week gives way to something more sophisticated. Rational. Reasonable-sounding. Entirely convincing.

This is the negotiating mind, and it is the most psychologically dangerous phase of the entire fast. The internal voice begins producing arguments. *I have already proven my point. I can stop now. Just a small amount of broth. That's practically still fasting. My body is clearly telling me something. I should listen. I have done fifteen days. That's a great deal, by any standard. The research says the main benefits are achieved by day ten anyway. Why am I still doing this?*

Each argument sounds reasonable. Each is the mind trying to return to comfort, dressed up as wisdom. The practitioner, hearing these arguments inside their own head, in their own voice, is often unable at first to recognize them as the negotiating mind. They sound like sound thinking. They sound like good sense. They sound like the considered conclusions of a mature person assessing their situation honestly.

They are not. They are the same mind that wanted to skip the fast on day one, now armed with two weeks of fasting experience and dressed in the clothing of mature self-care. The arguments have evolved. The function has not changed. The function is to end the discomfort. The discomfort is the work. To end the work is to end the fast before it has accomplished what it can accomplish.

The critical skill of the third week is learning to hear the negotiating mind without obeying it. Not suppressing it — suppression rarely works for long. Not arguing with it — argument tends to give it more attention than it deserves. Simply recognizing it for what it is. *Oh. Hello. The negotiating mind has arrived. This is the day fifteen voice.* The recognition itself is most of the practice. Once the voice is named, it loses much of its power.

It is no longer the practitioner's own conclusions. It is a familiar visitor, doing what it does, and the practitioner can choose, calmly, whether to follow its suggestions or to continue the work.

What also happens in this phase is significant, and it is part of why this phase is so worth completing. Mental clarity begins arriving in unmistakable windows. The brain, fully adapted to ketones and operating with elevated endocannabinoid tone, produces moments of focus and calm that the practitioner has not experienced in years. The first genuinely transcendent moments of the fast often arrive in the third week — moments of stillness so complete that the practitioner finds themselves outside of time, watching their own life from a vantage point they had not known existed. The relationship with food shifts. It begins losing its emotional charge. The practitioner notices, sometimes with surprise, that they have not thought about food for several hours, and that when they do think about it, it carries less of the longing that defined the second week.

There is a sense of capability that arrives in this phase. The practitioner has done fifteen days. They begin to suspect they can do anything. The negotiating mind and the clarity arrive together. This phase contains both the greatest risk of stopping and the greatest rewards for continuing. The work of the third week is to remain anchored in the original intention — to return, again and again, to the answer to the question of why this fast is worth the difficulty — and to allow the clarity to arrive without letting the negotiating mind drown it out.

The Fourth Week

Something shifts in the fourth week. It is difficult to describe in purely psychological terms, because by this point the experience has moved beyond the purely psychological into territory that different traditions have named differently.

What practitioners describe, across many backgrounds and many traditions, is consistent enough to deserve attention. A deepening of stillness, in which the mental noise that characterized earlier phases quiets significantly. Heightened sensitivity — colors become more vivid, sounds more distinct, emotions closer to the surface and easier to feel. Detachment from ordinary concerns — things that felt important before the fast often feel distant and small from this new vantage point. Spontaneous emotional releases that no longer have obvious objects — crying without a clear reason, laughter arising unexpectedly, grief moving through without anything specific to grieve.

A sense of connection to something larger than the ordinary self. Different practitioners describe this differently. Religious practitioners describe it in the language of their tradition. Secular practitioners describe it in the language of mystery, or oneness, or simply the felt sense that the boundary between self and world has thinned. Whatever the language, the experience is reported with such consistency across so many traditions that to dismiss it as imagination would require dismissing thousands of years of human testimony from cultures that did not communicate with one another. The experience is real, in the sense that the practitioner has it. Whether it points to something beyond the practitioner is a question this book does not need to settle.

There is also clarity, sometimes, about things that had been unclear before — relationships, decisions, life direction. The mind, freed from its constant work of digesting food and managing the daily emotional regulation that food had been carrying, has resources available for reflection that it did not have access to in the fed state. People sometimes report that questions they had been carrying for years resolve during the fourth week. Not always with answers. Sometimes with the recognition that the question itself was wrongly framed.

Not everyone experiences this phase as transcendent. For some, it arrives instead as a flatness, a depression, an existential questioning that the earlier phases did not have. *Why am I doing this. What is any of this for.* Anger sometimes arrives — at people who are eating normally, at the fast itself, at the body for taking so long. A deep loneliness sometimes arrives, because the fast puts the practitioner outside the ordinary shared human experience temporarily, and that outside-ness can feel alienating before it begins to feel liberating.

Both the transcendence and the shadow are real. Both are part of the same territory. Neither lasts forever. The practitioner who feels the transcendence should journal it, because the insights of this phase can fade after the fast ends and the writing becomes a record to return to. The practitioner who feels the shadow should remember that this is normal — it does not mean something is wrong — and should lean into gentle spiritual or contemplative practice, prayer, meditation, time in nature, the company of people who can hold space for what is moving through. The fourth week should not be navigated alone if it can be helped. Connection with a guide, with someone who has walked this territory before, is valuable in any phase but particularly here.

Day thirty is coming, and with it a shift. Whatever the fourth week has held — light or shadow or some weave of both — it gives way to the final week, and the final week has its own character.

The Final Days

The home stretch carries its own unique psychology. The practitioner is close to the end. Closeness brings its own complications.

There is anticipation. The mind begins moving toward the first meal with single-minded focus. Detailed fantasies develop about what will be eaten, how it will taste, what the first bite will feel like. A countdown mentality sets in that can make each remaining day feel longer than the last. The excitement is genuine and earned — the practitioner has done the work, the work is nearly complete, the reward is approaching.

There is also, paradoxically, a reluctance that many experienced fasters report and that first-time fasters often find unexpected. The clean state that has been achieved feels precious and fragile. Food begins to feel like a threat to something the practitioner has worked hard to build. Some people feel genuinely afraid to eat again — afraid of contaminating what has been cleared, afraid of returning to patterns they have spent six weeks dismantling, afraid of losing the clarity they have only recently found.

Both the anticipation and the reluctance are normal. Both require conscious navigation. The vulnerability of these days is real. The body and the mind are at their most sensitive. Emotions run very close to the surface.

Small things can feel disproportionately large. This sensitivity is not weakness. It is the system in a state of deep openness, and the practitioner should treat it with gentleness and protection.

Begin planning the refeeding process carefully during these days. Having a clear protocol reduces anxiety about breaking the fast. Allow both the excitement and the reluctance without letting either drive the decision. Do not break the fast reactively, in response to either overwhelming excitement or overwhelming fear. Break it intentionally, on your timeline, with full awareness, according to the plan you have prepared. The chapters that follow describe how. Stay with the work that remains. The end is close. The way you end matters.

The Emotional Releases

Throughout all phases of the fast, but particularly in weeks three and four, emotional material surfaces unexpectedly. This phenomenon deserves its own consideration, because it is one of the least anticipated and most consequential aspects of prolonged fasting for many practitioners.

The gut, as we have discussed, contains over five hundred million neurons and produces the majority of the body's serotonin. Research increasingly supports what many traditions have known for millennia — the body stores unprocessed experience. Not metaphorically. The trauma, the grief, the unprocessed emotion that a person carries through life has physiological correlates. It lives in the nervous system, in the gut wall, in the patterns of muscular tension, in the chronic activation of stress pathways. It is not only psychological. It is somatic.

When the gut clears, this stored material can surface. People report crying about losses they thought they had processed years ago. Anger arising about situations long past, sometimes situations they had stopped thinking about decades ago. Grief for people, relationships, versions of themselves they had let go of. Joy that arrives unexpectedly, sourceless, sometimes during the most physically uncomfortable phases of the fast. Fear that passes through like weather, sometimes nameless, sometimes attached to specific old memories.

The instinct of most adults, when difficult emotion surfaces, is to suppress it, redirect it, or analyze it away. None of these is the right response in this context. Do not try to stop these releases. Do not try to analyze them in the moment. Allow them to move. They are not signs that something is wrong. They are signs that something long held is finally being released. The gut and the mind are cleaning house together, and the cleaning is part of the medicine. The practitioner who suppresses the emotional content of the fast extracts only half of what the fast can offer.

Most of these releases pass quickly when allowed to. A wave of grief that, if resisted, might last for days passes through in twenty minutes when simply felt. The practitioner emerges on the other side lighter. Something that had been carried, often for many years, has been set down. The setting down does not require analysis. It requires only the willingness to let what is moving move.

The Role of Intention

More than almost any other factor, intention determines the experience of a prolonged fast. The same forty days, undertaken with a clear and deeply personal reason, are entirely different from the same forty days undertaken without one.

People who fast with a clear and deeply personal *why* navigate the difficult phases more effectively. They interpret challenges as part of the process rather than as signs to stop. They extract more meaning from the experience. They are more likely to complete the full protocol. None of this is mysterious. The mind responds to purpose. Purpose creates the framework within which discomfort becomes meaningful, and meaningful discomfort is profoundly different from meaningless discomfort, even when the physical sensations are identical.

Before beginning any prolonged fast, write your intention. Not a vague goal. A specific, personal, deeply felt answer to the question of why this fast is worth the difficulty it will require. Write it as if you are making a promise to yourself. Then keep the writing somewhere you can return to it when the fast becomes hard. Read it on day three when the body is rebelling. Read it on day fifteen when the negotiating mind arrives. Read it on day twenty-eight when the shadow descends. Read it on day thirty-five when the anticipation of the end pulls you toward eating before you should.

Your intention is your anchor. In the storms that come, and storms will come, it is what keeps you from drifting. It is not a guarantee that you will complete the fast. It is the foundation of being able to.

A Note on Who Should Not Use This Chapter as a Guide

This chapter describes the psychological experience of fasting from a place of health. It is not a guide for everyone. If you recognize in these pages not a description of temporary challenge but a reflection of a familiar relationship with food and your body — please pause. The feelings described here — the sense of control, the clarity that comes with restriction, the pride in endurance — can be genuinely therapeutic in the right context. In the wrong context, they can feed something that was already hungry in a different way, and the work of fasting can become a different kind of harm dressed up as healing.

You deserve support that meets you where you actually are. The Alliance for Eating Disorders Helpline is at 1-866-662-1235. The number is here for the people who need it. If there is any uncertainty about whether the wrong context applies to you, please call. The conversation costs nothing. The wrong path, undertaken without recognition, can cost a great deal.

What Waits on the Other Side

For those who navigate this journey from a place of genuine health-seeking, what waits on the other side is rare. Not just a cleaner gut. Not just better numbers on a blood test. Something harder to measure and more important to acknowledge.

A different relationship with hunger. A different relationship with pleasure. A different relationship with need. The person who breaks a forty-day fast is not the same person who began it — not because the fast changed them from the outside, but because it created the conditions for them to change themselves from the inside.

That is the real medicine. That was always the real medicine. The transformation that ancient cultures named with their various words for renewal, for purification, for being made new — what they were describing was this. The biological work was happening alongside the psychological work all along. They had not separated them, because they did not need to. They knew, from long observation, that the body and the mind work together when given the chance, and that the chance must be of sufficient duration to let them.

You have given them that chance. The work that follows is the work of allowing what has been started to complete itself, and of receiving what comes through with the awareness it deserves.

Chapter 27

Preparing Your Body Before the Fast

* * *

For a long time I had been a teacher of this work. I had been a practitioner once, in a forest, at twenty-eight, and a great deal of what the forest had shown me about what I had not done well I spent the years afterward teaching to other people. Person after person after person came through my life. They learned some part of this from me, and they went back into their own lives carrying it.

And then a woman came into my life, some years ago, who came to live underneath my home. There was a room downstairs with its own bathroom, prepared for someone who would need to be under the same roof for a long time, and she had been on fifty separate medications when we met, which is not the kind of taper a person does in three months. She had skated at the highest level her sport allowed, and her body, by the time I met her, had been carrying more than a body is built to carry. The list had grown long. The seizures had begun. We worked together for two years to take the medications down, one at a time, and to ready her for the fast she was preparing to do. And before her fast began, she asked me to do it with her.

I told her I would. When her fast began it ran forty days on water and another eight on liquid afterward. Across those forty-eight days I did beside her everything she did, except the one thing. The one thing I had told her I would do with her, I kept not doing. I kept telling her. I kept not doing it. After a while she stopped asking.

Her fast ended. She did not leave. The room downstairs that had been the room of her preparation became the room of her recovery, and then, simply, the room she lived in, and a year and a half passed in which I kept teaching what I was no longer practicing while she was every day in the house. The teaching had grown, by then, into a kind of habit, and the habit into a kind of life. After long enough I no longer noticed that the habit had taken the place of the practice. The mask was good. It looked, from the outside, very much like the face. After long enough wearing it the face beneath it grew strange to me.

The gurgling had been there for some time. The body has a way of waiting that is not patient, exactly, but is steady. One morning, late in the third year of postponing, I sat with the question of whether I was still living what I was setting down, and the answer that came back was no longer the answer that had come back the year before. The decision was made in that hour. Day one was still months away.

I had done this work once before, in a forest, at twenty-eight, and a great many of the things I had not done well the first time had been things of preparation. The year and a half of postponing had given me long enough to be honest with myself about which of those errors had been errors of the body and which had been errors of preparation. Most of them had been errors of preparation. What was beginning, in the months that followed that morning, was the work I had not done the first time.

The flushes that followed were nights the liver worked differently than it had worked in years, and each next day arrived knowing something it had not known before. The daughter I had been teaching at the kitchen table to pay attention to her own small living world watched her father, without my naming it for her, do the same. The body, which is more honest than the mind, started showing up each morning a little more recognizable to itself.

By the time day one arrived, what was underway was not new. The body that began the fast had been turning toward it, by small degrees, for more than a year.

The first flush came in the first month. Five days of apple cider and water, a gallon of each across each day, the body opening slowly the way a long-locked house opens when the windows are taken down one at a time. The malic acid in the cider going through the bile ducts, softening what had been sitting there for years. By the fifth evening the body was a body that had not eaten solid food for a day, and the kitchen, in the late hour after the daughter had gone to bed and the woman downstairs had gone to her own quiet, was the kitchen of the work.

The Epsom salt at six. The grapefruit and the olive oil at ten. Then lying down on the right side, knees drawn up, the way the bile ducts open most easily, and waiting. The waiting, that first night, was the waiting of a man who had taught other people to wait through this and was now, alone in his own kitchen, doing what he had taught. The lying down on the right side was a small return. There were eleven hours between the oil and the morning and the body, in those hours, did something it had not done in a long time.

There is a thing in this work the body comes to know and to refuse. The Epsom salt is bitter in a way the body recognizes as wrong even before the tongue has decided. By the third dose of any flush — the morning dose, the one that pushes everything along to the gateway — the body understands what is coming and would, if allowed, turn its head. A man who has done many of these has learned that this is the moment the work asks something the protocol cannot, and he gets the third salt down because if the third salt does not go down, the night before becomes a night that did not finish.

What came out the morning after the first flush is the kind of thing a person who has not done this work cannot easily believe is possible. Small green stones, dark and rounded, of the kind the gallbladder makes when bile sits too long. There was a knock at the door of the bathroom — the daughter, who was homeschooled and so was up in the morning the way a person who knows the household is the school is up — asking, the way she always asked, can I see, papa. She had been asking this since she was four. She had grown up in a house where the body was not a hidden thing, and what came out of bodies, when something good was happening, was something to be seen and named. We named the stones.

The flushes ran one a month for six months. The first was the loudest. The second produced fewer stones than the first but lighter ones, the kind that have been sitting nearer the surface and were dislodged earliest. The third was quieter still, and the fourth quieter again. By the fifth there was almost nothing — a few small things, of the size and color the body releases when there is little left in the immediate reservoirs. The sixth produced more than the fifth, which surprised me until I understood: deeper rooms had finally opened, and what had been sitting in them for a longer time had begun to surface. The body was not running out of work to do. It was reaching down further.

After the sixth flush I stopped. There was a time — six months, in the end — when the body did the part of the work that has no protocol. The bile ducts, which had been worked monthly for half a year, were given the half-year that follows to find their own rhythm. The liver was given the long quiet to integrate what the flushes had reached. I did not do another flush in those six months. I ate carefully and I slept carefully and I let the body hold the work without being asked to do another piece of it, and the body, which is more honest than the mind, used the half-year well. By the end of those six months the morning gut was different than it had been in many years. The decision that had been made in an hour, eighteen months earlier, had reached the body by the long route.

The food on the counter had been changing in the household for a long time before the decision in the morning hour. When the woman moved into the room downstairs, two years earlier, she had brought a body that could not eat most of what the kitchen had been making. The reactions she had to ordinary food were many and severe, and the work of cooking for her — which fell, in those first months, partly to me — was the work of a kitchen that could not rely on the things kitchens of that decade ordinarily relied on. There were no sealed packets, no quick assembled dinners, no convenience that depended on someone else having decided what was in the food. There was the food itself, made from its parts, in the kitchen, by hand. She had not asked the household to change. Her body had asked, and the household had answered.

Before her arrival the kitchen had been a kitchen that bought carefully but did not, in the deeper sense, cook. The pizza in the freezer was organic. The pasta in the pantry was organic. The sauces were organic. A man and his daughter had been eating for years out of bags and boxes that had the right labels on them and that had been assembled by other hands in other places. None of it was wrong, exactly. None of it was right either. There is a kind of distance between a body and its food that a label cannot close, and the household, by the time the woman arrived, had been living inside that distance for a long time.

I had not eaten before the early afternoon for many years. That part of the daily shape was already in place when the prep year began. What changed, across the months that followed the morning of the decision, was the rest of the day. The two meals and the small grazings between them became two meals and nothing between. Then the lunch, which had never quite been a lunch, fell away, and there was an evening meal and a few small things across the afternoon. Then the few small things fell away, and there was an evening meal. By the last weeks of the prep year, the daily shape was one meal at the table at the end of the day, and the rest of the hours were hours that the body had once filled with food and now did not.

On many of those mornings the first thing the kitchen made was a smoothie. The daughter, who had grown up watching the work of the household but had not yet been inside it as a maker, asked early in the prep year if she could help. So we made the smoothies together — fruit and greens and a small amount of seed, the blender at seven, the two glasses on the counter, hers and mine. She loved the smoothies. She had been told a fast was coming and that the kitchen was changing because of it, and rather than receiving this as a deprivation she received it as a kind of arrival. Wait, we get to do flushes and fasting and we get to have smoothies? she said, when the new pattern was first explained to her. The smoothie hour became, across the months, a small ritual neither of us had asked for and both of us looked forward to.

What changed in the kitchen across those months was not, mostly, what the kitchen made. The kitchen had already been making what the woman downstairs needed, and the daughter had been eating the same food the kitchen made for her father and the woman, with small adjustments for a child's palate. What changed was the shape of the day around the food. The hours grew quieter between meals. The pantry held fewer things, because there were fewer reasons for the things to be there. The grocery list, which had been running long for as long as a man with a daughter and a household guest had been making it, began running shorter — not because anyone had decided to buy less, but because there was less the body was being asked to find a use for.

There is a principle in this kind of preparation that a person comes to understand only by living through it. The stomach made smaller across months while it is still being fed is a stomach that meets day one of the fast without finding day one a cliff. The body that has been eating one meal a day for a month enters the fast having already been doing, in a small way, what the fast asks. The descent across the prep year is its own kind of teacher, and the body that has been listening to that teacher arrives at the threshold knowing some things the body that arrives without the descent does not yet know. The work the household had been doing for two years, and the work the man had begun to do across the prep year, met at the threshold and were the same work.

By the time the month came near in which the fast would begin, the body had been doing the descent for so long that the descent itself had become the daily life. The juices that the existing protocol describes as a three-day bridge across the threshold had been the morning practice in the household for some time. The supplements that some preparations bring in across a final two weeks had come in earlier, when the woman downstairs had located the inventory and set the kitchen up for what was coming. The body was, by then, more ready than the mind was. The mind was the part that had not arrived.

There is a kind of waiting that the existing protocols do not describe and that a person who has done this work in their own kitchen comes to know. It is the waiting between the moment a body is ready to begin and the moment the mind agrees to begin. The body had been turning toward the fast for over a year. The household had been turning with it. What remained, in the final weeks, was the choosing of the day, and the choosing of the day was the part that had no protocol. I knew it was the month. I did not know which morning. The not-knowing began to make its own weather. There is a way the mind can use the absence of a chosen day to keep the day from arriving, and the longer the day was not chosen the more the mind found ways to make the choosing harder. I almost did not start. I came close enough to not starting that I want to say so plainly here, because a person preparing for this work should know that the last obstacle is not in the body. The last obstacle is the moment of saying now.

What the body had been bringing to the threshold was what the body had. I had slept four hours a night for most of my adult life, since the years in the military when sleeping longer was not the thing the work allowed.

The waking had often carried tension. Those facts were not facts the prep year was going to undo. The prep year was going to deliver the body it had to the threshold, and the body it had was a body that had been working hard for a long time and had not been resting the way bodies rest in lives that have not been working hard for a long time. The fast itself was going to address what the prep year could not. Knowing this, in the last weeks, was a quieter knowing than the knowing earlier in the year had been. The body was not perfect. The body was the body that was going to do this.

The thing about the prep year that had become true, across all of it, was that the household was a pair. My daughter and I had been a household of two for as long as I had been her father in the present-day sense, and the prep year had not been work I could do without her or beside her. It had been work the two of us did together. The flushes, the smoothies, the food on the counter, the shape of the day — none of it had been arranged by a man preparing alone. It had been arranged by a man and his daughter, both of them learning what the household was becoming. I knew, by the end of the prep year, that I would not finish the fast itself without her. I knew it the way a person knows what they have already been receiving. A great deal of the time had become easier because of her presence.

The juices in the morning had begun, in the way new patterns begin in households with children, to fail. She would drink some of hers and not the rest. The kitchen would tip the rest into the sink, and the next morning the same. So we changed the form. We took the juices and froze them. We added cashew powder and almond milk, a little vanilla, a heaping spoon of peanut butter, strawberries and mango and a half-dozen kinds of nuts and seeds. We poured the mix into a small machine and turned it into ice cream. I told her she could have her morning ice cream whenever she wanted, and she could. The juice had become something neither of us had to convince the other to take, and the work had become something we were inventing as we went, the way a kitchen invents what it needs in order to keep working.

When the day finally came it was not announced to me by the body. The body had been ready for weeks. The mind, which had been trying to find the day from outside the day, simply, on a morning, agreed. There was no ceremony in the agreeing. I asked my daughter, before the morning the agreement happened, whether she thought I was crazy for fasting for a month and not eating anything. She said she would let me know. She said she still loved me. The agreement that arrived the next morning was the kind of agreement a person makes with themselves after enough months of not making it. I am starting now, the mind said, and that was when it began.

The protocols that describe a final two weeks of supplements and a three-day juice bridge are honest descriptions of what a person who has not had a year of preparation must compress into the time available. They are at the back of this chapter for the reader who needs the structured version. What this chapter has tried to give before the protocols arrive is the longer view: a year of months turning into one another, a household learning what its kitchen could become, a body listening earlier than the mind, and a daughter who, at the end of all of it, was the one who said yes when there was no one else in the room to say yes. The fast began on the morning the mind finally arrived. The body had been there the whole time.

Chapter 28

How Do You Know You Are Done

* * *

This chapter answers what is, perhaps, the most important question of the entire process. When is enough, enough? When has the work been done? When is the right moment to exit the fast? Get this right, and the transformation completes itself with grace. Get it wrong in either direction — too early or too late — and the results are compromised.

The skill of recognizing completion is, in some ways, the most subtle skill the prolonged faster needs to develop. Everything that came before — the preparation, the protocol, the daily discipline — was relatively concrete. There were instructions. There were measurements. There were clear right and wrong choices. Knowing when to exit is different. It cannot be reduced to a single number on a calendar or a single reading on a meter. It requires reading the body, reading the signals, reading the convergence of many small indicators that together announce, when they align, that the work has been completed.

This chapter teaches you how to read those signals.

The Two Failure Modes

There are two ways to get the exit wrong, and they are roughly equally consequential.

The first is stopping too early. The deepest work has not yet been completed. Egg destruction cycles have not finished. Liver flukes are still active in the bile ducts. Within weeks of breaking the fast, symptoms can return as remaining eggs hatch and remaining adults reproduce. The result feels, to the practitioner, like reinfection — but it is not. It is incomplete clearing of an infection that was never fully addressed. The investment of weeks of fasting yields a fraction of the result that one or two more weeks would have produced.

The second is stopping too late. The body begins genuine catabolism beyond the therapeutic benefit zone. Muscle loss exceeds what is appropriate for the work being done. Mineral depletion becomes serious despite supplementation. Diminishing returns set in — the autophagy that was clearing damaged cells in week three is now beginning to break down healthy tissue in week six. Recovery from the fast becomes more difficult than it needs to be. The transformation that should have been gentle becomes a more taxing experience than the body can comfortably sustain.

The skill is recognizing when the work has been done — and exiting at that moment, neither earlier nor later. This is not, in the end, a calculation. It is a reading. Like any reading, it improves with practice.

The Convergence of Signals

No single signal indicates completion. The practitioner who tries to read any one indicator alone — even a strong one — will be misled. What matters is the convergence of signals across multiple categories, sustained consistently over several days. When the body is finishing the work, it announces this in many voices at once, and the harmony of those voices is what the practitioner is learning to hear.

There are seven categories of signals worth attending to. Each speaks in its own language. Together they tell a coherent story.

The Enema Returns

The most direct visual feedback during the fast is what comes out of the body during the morning and evening enemas. The returns tell, with little ambiguity, what work the body is currently doing.

While active work is continuing, the returns show what active work looks like. There is significant volume of debris. Mucoid material is releasing. Biofilm material is visible. Green sludge appears in the morning coffee enemas, sometimes in striking quantity. Stringy material comes through. Worm-like organisms or fragments of them appear, sometimes recognizable enough that the practitioner can identify what species they came from. The fluid going in looks substantially different from the fluid coming out.

As completion approaches, the picture changes. The returns become predominantly clear fluid. Debris becomes minimal. No mucoid material releases. The green sludge of the coffee enemas disappears, or appears only in occasional traces. No visible parasitic material is seen. The fluid going in begins to resemble the fluid coming out.

The critical pattern is consistency. A single clean return on a single day does not indicate completion — the body has rhythms, and one quiet day can be followed by another active day. What matters is three to five consecutive days of consistently clean returns, in both the morning and the evening enemas, with no new categories of debris appearing. When this consistency holds across several days, the work in the gut is approaching its end.

The Tongue and the Breath

The tongue is, by traditional accounts and by modern observation, one of the most reliable mirrors of internal state during fasting. The progression of the tongue's appearance through a prolonged fast follows a recognizable arc.

In the early weeks, the tongue develops a heavy thick coating. The coating represents the toxins being released through the tongue's surface — the body using every available elimination route, including the mucous membranes of the mouth. As die-off accelerates in the second and third weeks, the coating thickens further. It may shift in color from white to yellow, to grayish, to greenish, depending on what is currently being released. The shifts are not random. They reflect the categories of material the body is currently processing.

As the work approaches completion, the coating thins. The tongue begins to show pink underneath. By the time the practitioner is approaching the exit, the tongue is predominantly pink and clean, with only the lightest of coatings, sustained over five or more consecutive days.

The breath follows a similar arc. Strong fasting breath dominates the early weeks. The acetone smell of deep ketosis appears as the metabolic shift completes — a sweet, slightly chemical odor that confirms the body has fully entered the fasting metabolism. As the weeks pass, the breath neutralizes. By the time the work is approaching completion, the breath is clean, without odor or unusual taste, sustained.

A pink clean tongue with neutral breath, both maintained for many consecutive days, is one of the most reliable indicators that the deeper work has finished.

The Body Odor

The skin is the body's largest detoxification organ, and it speaks during fasting with a clarity that the practitioner sometimes finds surprising. In the first week or two, body odor often becomes strong and unusual. The smell may not be familiar. It may seem to come from places it never came from before. This is the body using the skin to release compounds that the gut and liver cannot process fast enough alone.

Through the middle weeks, the odor goes through phases as different toxin categories release in succession. The practitioner who is paying attention can sometimes notice these phases — a different quality of smell in week two than in week three, in week three than in week four.

As the work nears completion, the odor neutralizes. The skin returns to producing its natural light scent — the scent of a healthy human body, without the loud announcements of detoxification. When neutral or light natural body odor is sustained for many days, this is one of the converging signs that the deeper cleansing has finished.

Energy and Mental Clarity

The energy of the early fast is uncertain. It rises and falls in waves. Days of clarity alternate with days of fatigue. By the time the work is approaching completion, this fluctuation begins to settle. Energy becomes stable throughout the day. Significant afternoon crashes stop occurring. The baseline level of energy is sustained higher than it was before the fast began. Energy is available for activity, not just for survival. Sleep produces genuine restoration rather than the strange tired-but-not-rested quality that characterized some of the harder weeks.

Mental clarity follows the same arc. The clarity that came in flashes during the third week becomes sustained by the time the work is finishing. Calm focus is available consistently rather than appearing in unpredictable windows. Decision-making is clear and unhurried. Emotional stability returns with appropriate range — not the flatness of suppression, but the steadiness of a system no longer struggling against itself.

When the energy and the clarity are stable rather than fluctuating, when the mental quietness has become a baseline rather than an occasional visit, this is a signal worth listening to.

Internal Sensations

The body, throughout the fast, has been speaking through sensation. The gas and gurgling of accumulated material breaking down. The fullness and pressure of layers releasing. The occasional nausea of toxins mobilizing. The tenderness in the right side as bile work proceeds. The general internal busyness of a body engaged in significant clearing.

As completion approaches, these sensations quiet. The gas becomes minimal. The pressure releases. The nausea, if it had been present, departs. The right-sided abdominal area becomes quiet. There is a general sense of internal cleanness — a felt absence of the busyness that had been present for weeks.

This is sometimes the most subtle of the signals, and yet for many practitioners it becomes the most reliable. The body, at the moment of completion, sends a kind of internal message. A subtle but unmistakable signal. The deep work is done. The message is difficult to describe to someone who has not received it, but it is clear when it arrives. People who have completed multiple prolonged fasts describe it consistently. There is a moment, after weeks of work, when the body simply communicates that the work is finished. The signal is not loud. It is unmistakable.

Sleep and Dreams

Sleep through the middle weeks of a prolonged fast can be intense. Dreams are vivid, sometimes disturbing, sometimes ecstatic. The practitioner wakes with strong impressions that linger through the day. Sleep itself may be lighter than usual, more easily disturbed, sometimes punctuated by waking periods of unusual clarity.

As completion approaches, sleep settles. Falling asleep becomes easy. Sleeping through the night becomes the norm. Waking is refreshed rather than weary. Dreams calm. They become less vivid, less laden with material that needs processing. The dreaming mind, like the waking body, has finished much of its work.

When sleep is clean, restorative, and untroubled, sustained over several nights, this is part of the convergence pointing toward completion.

The Emotional State

Throughout the fast, emotional content has been surfacing. The negotiating mind of week three. The longing of week two. The grief of unexpected losses. The clarity of week four. The vulnerability of the final days. The emotional arc has been part of the work.

By the time the body is finishing the deeper work, the emotional state quiets. Major emotional releases have passed. A general sense of peace or contentment establishes itself. No major unresolved emotional content is still surfacing. The internal weather settles. The practitioner who has been navigating emotional storms for weeks finds themselves, somewhat suddenly, in calm.

This emotional quietness is not the same as emotional flatness. The capacity to feel remains. The depth of emotion remains. What has departed is the active processing of unresolved material. The room has been cleaned. The cleaning, for now, is finished.

When the Signals Align

When most or all of these categories show completion signals, sustained consistently for several days, the work is done. The body is announcing, in many voices at once, that the protocol has accomplished what it can accomplish in this particular fast.

For first-time fasters following the full protocol, this typically occurs between days twenty-eight and forty. For experienced fasters following the full protocol, it can occur between days twenty-one and thirty-five. For experienced fasters with a long history of clean eating — vegetarians, people who have been doing the work for years — completion can come between days eighteen and thirty.

The specific timeline within these ranges depends on individual factors. The history of accumulated burden. The current parasitic load. The state of the bile ducts. The microbiome composition. The genetic factors that influence how each body does this work. There is no single right number. There is the right number for this body, on this fast, at this moment.

Testing as Confirmation

For practitioners who want objective confirmation of completion, certain tests can supplement the body's own signals. The GI Map stool test uses DNA-based detection to identify parasites and pathogens, and it provides definitive confirmation of what has been cleared. It is best done four to six weeks after completing the protocol, when the body has stabilized and the test can establish a baseline for future monitoring. A comprehensive stool analysis examines microbiome composition, identifies remaining pathogens, and measures markers of gut health. It is useful for guiding the microbiome rebuilding work that follows the fast.

Blood work post-fast can confirm that the body is in good condition for refeeding. Inflammatory markers — C-reactive protein, ESR — can be checked. Nutritional status can be assessed. Liver and kidney function can be confirmed. The numbers, where they support the body's own signals, build confidence in the decision to exit. Where they conflict with the body's signals, they prompt the kind of careful reconsideration that the moment of exit deserves.

When to Trust the Body Over the Calendar

Sometimes the calendar says continue, but the body says enough. The practitioner has planned a forty-day fast. They are at day twenty-six. They had not expected to finish before day thirty-five at the earliest. And yet the signals are aligning. The returns have been clean for a week. The tongue is pink. The energy is stable. The mind is clear. The internal message has arrived.

Trust the body. The forty-day mark is a common framework, not a magic number. Some people need more days. Some need fewer. The body knows what it is finishing, and the practitioner who insists on continuing past the moment of completion is no longer doing the work the fast was designed to do. They are doing something else — sometimes proving something to themselves, sometimes proving something to others, sometimes simply unable to recognize that the work is finished. None of these is a reason to continue past the body's signal.

On the other hand, do not trust the body when its message is different. If hunger has returned strongly and persistently — different in character from the hunger of fasting itself, more like the body's request for nourishment than the mind's negotiation — pay attention. If energy is dropping significantly. If mental fog is returning. If extremities are cold and the body cannot warm itself. If genuine fatigue has set in beyond the baseline of a normal fasting day. These signals indicate the body is asking to break the fast not because the work is complete, but because reserves are depleted. This requires immediate but careful refeeding regardless of where the practitioner is in the planned protocol. The fast that should have ended at this moment, in this body, is not the same fast that ends in another body at another moment. Listening, in either direction, is the practice.

A Personal Note

The exit from the fast is one of the most important moments in the entire process. Approached with awareness, it transitions seamlessly into refeeding and the rebuilding phase. Approached carelessly, it can compromise everything that came before.

Take this moment seriously. Read the signals — all of them, across all the categories, sustained over several days. Trust the body when it announces completion. Honor what it has done. Exit when the work is complete, not before, not later.

The next chapter prepares you for what comes after. The breaking of a fast is its own art, with its own protocols, and the work of these final hours of fasting flows directly into the work of the first hours of eating again. The transition is delicate. It deserves the attention it requires. We will turn to it next.

Chapter 29

Breaking Your Fast

* * *

The body that has just completed a prolonged fast is in a particular condition. The lining of the small intestine is new tissue. The microbial communities that inhabited it for years have been swept down to bare ground. Insulin is low. Phosphate sits at the lower edge of normal, where the body has held it through weeks of using fat for fuel rather than glucose. The pancreas has been quiet. The liver has been processing at a slow, deliberate rhythm.

To meet that body with the eating habits of the body that began the fast is to ask something of it that it is not, in this moment, built to do.

What follows in this chapter is the protocol of the next two weeks. It is detailed, and the detail is necessary. Most fasters who run into trouble do not run into it during the fast. They run into it on the way out. The cleanse takes weeks to accomplish. Damage from incorrect refeeding can occur in hours.

Read this chapter carefully. Read it more than once. The chapter that follows turns to the longer arc — the months and years in which the work of the fast either consolidates into a different kind of life or quietly unravels. But the longer arc cannot be reached without these first two weeks. They are the bridge.

Refeeding Syndrome — The Real Risk

This is the medical concern that makes proper refeeding non-negotiable. After prolonged fasting, the body has adapted to using fat as primary fuel. Insulin levels are low. Cells have shifted their metabolic machinery for ketone use. Phosphate levels in the blood are lower than baseline.

When carbohydrates are reintroduced too quickly:

• Insulin surges in response.

• Cells suddenly demand phosphate to process glucose.

• Phosphate is pulled from blood into cells rapidly.

• Blood phosphate drops to dangerously low levels.

• This is **hypophosphatemia** — the central feature of refeeding syndrome.

Consequences can include:

• Cardiac arrhythmias, potentially fatal.

• Respiratory failure.

• Seizures.

• Muscle weakness.

• Confusion.

• Coma in severe cases.

Refeeding syndrome can be fatal. It is also entirely preventable through proper refeeding protocol. The protocol that follows in this chapter is what prevents it.

The Cardinal Rules of Refeeding

Five rules govern the refeeding process. Each is non-negotiable.

• **Start small.** The first food after a prolonged fast should be 4 ounces or less. Not a meal. Not a snack. A taste.

• **Start liquid.** Solid food on day one of refeeding is too much for the digestive system. Liquid forms first — broths, fresh juices, blended preparations.

• **Avoid concentrated carbohydrates.** Sugars, refined grains, sweet fruits in quantity — these trigger the insulin response that causes refeeding syndrome.

• **Phosphate awareness.** Begin with foods naturally containing minerals, including phosphate. Vegetable broths, leafy green juices, mineral water with electrolytes.

• **Rebuild slowly.** Each phase of refeeding takes the time it takes. Rushing to normal eating is the most common mistake. The first two weeks of refeeding deserve as much care as the fast itself.

A Sacred Transition

Treat the breaking of the fast with reverence. Set up the moment intentionally. Bless the food in whatever way is meaningful to you. Eat the first taste slowly, fully present to the experience. Notice everything — taste, texture, response.

This is a threshold moment, the bridge between the intensive cleansing phase and the rest of your life. The body remembers this moment. The relationship with food can be renewed in this moment. The intentions carried through the fast can be embodied in this moment.

Honor it accordingly. The first taste of food after weeks of fasting is, in its small way, one of the most memorable meals you will ever have. Make it worth remembering.

Day 1 — The First Taste

The day a fast ends is rarely a day of meals. It is a day of one cup of broth, often taken late, and a quiet evening that follows it. The body is not yet ready for more. The stomach has been at rest. The digestive secretions have slowed almost to a stop. To meet that condition with food in any quantity is to ask the system to wake up too quickly and to do work it is not yet built to do.

The first intake is small. Four ounces or less, taken slowly. Vegetable broth — homemade, well-strained, no salt added — is the most forgiving choice. A light bone broth, simmered for hours and skimmed of fat, is a good alternative for those who include animal foods. The temperature should be warm rather than hot. The volume should be measured rather than poured.

What enters with that first cup is mineral support and a gentle signal to the digestive tract. Trace minerals continue, as they have throughout the fast. A teaspoon of MCT oil, taken in or alongside the broth, begins the reintroduction of fat — and starts the ongoing daily practice of MCT or coconut oil that will continue indefinitely from this day forward.

Nothing else. Not a second cup. Not a piece of fruit. Not the reasoning that says "if a little is good, a little more cannot hurt." The body has had nothing for weeks. A little is enough.

The shape of Day 1

For grounding, a typical Day 1 takes a shape something like this:

- Late afternoon or early evening: 4 ounces of warm vegetable broth, taken slowly over fifteen or twenty minutes
- A teaspoon of MCT oil, in the broth or alongside it
- Trace minerals, as throughout the fast
- A second 4 ounces of broth, two to three hours later, if signals permit and the first cup was well-tolerated
- Water through the rest of the evening

What is not on the list is as important as what is. No solid food. No fruit juice. No herbal tea sweetened with anything. No second meal of a different kind. Day 1 is a single quiet reentry, not the first day of normal eating.

A note on the herbal protocol. The herbal stack that supported the fast does not stop at the breaking of the fast. It continues, modified, for several more weeks. The full schedule appears in the reference charts at the back of this chapter. The short version: clove continues at full dose; wormwood, black walnut, and the others step down on a schedule each tied to the specific work each one is still doing.

Days 2 to 3 — Building Liquids

From Day 2 forward, the eating window opens at midday. First intake at 1 PM. The window closes between 7 and 8 PM. Inside the window, intake comes every two to three hours, in small amounts. Outside the window

— through the morning, through the late evening, through the night — the body returns to the same rest it has had for weeks.

This rhythm is not a temporary refeeding rule. It is the long-term shape of how the practitioner now eats. The intermittent fasting window is the daily inheritance of the fast. A maximum of two meals per day, spaced inside that window, is the default rhythm from this day forward and through the coming months.

The morning beverages of Week 1 are simple. Water. Trace minerals. Nothing else. The post-fast body is sensitive in ways it has not been before, and caffeine — even decaf — runs harder through that sensitivity than the practitioner expects. Coffee and herbal tea wait until Week 2.

Within the window, what enters is liquid still. Warm vegetable broth. Light bone broth. Fresh vegetable juice — celery, cucumber, leafy greens — diluted with water. A half teaspoon of ghee may enter the broth on Day 2 or Day 3, joining the MCT oil that began on Day 1. Coconut milk in small amounts is permitted, particularly for those wanting to support continued ketone production. Aloe vera juice, taken in modest portions, soothes the lining as it continues to settle.

What stays out is concentrated sugar in any form, including sweet fruit juices. The pancreas is still quiet. To wake it sharply with a glass of orange juice is to invite the cascade — insulin surge, phosphate pulled hard from blood into cells — that the cardinal rules are written to prevent.

Volume builds slowly. Four to six ounces per intake on Day 2. Slightly more by Day 3 if signals are clear. The two-meals-maximum rule still holds: even broken into the small intakes the window calls for, the day's structure is two principal feedings, not five small meals scattered across the afternoon.

Days 4 to 7 — Soft Liquid Foundations

The fourth and fifth days bring ghee fully into the daily intake. A half teaspoon, then a full teaspoon, warmed into broth or stirred into the first blended foods. Ghee does work that MCT alone cannot do — it carries fat-soluble compounds, supports the lining as it integrates, and signals the gallbladder back into a gentle rhythm of activity.

The blended foods of this stretch are themselves a kind of liquid. Avocado, mashed thoroughly into broth, is the most forgiving of them. Steamed and pureed zucchini, summer squash, leafy greens — these enter in small portions, blended fine, taken inside the eating window. Soaked chia or flax in modest amounts adds gentle fiber and the omega-3 fats the rebuilding lining will draw on. The IF window remains in force: 1 PM to 7-8 PM, two meals as the default, intake every two to three hours inside the window.

The microbiome thread begins on Day 5. A small amount of sauerkraut juice — a tablespoon, taken with one of the day's intakes — is the first deliberate offering to the cleared microbial field. The volume is small on purpose. The point is to introduce, not to flood. A tablespoon of sauerkraut juice carries a startling density of organisms, and on a gut that has been swept down to bare ground, even a tablespoon registers.

By Day 7, two further additions enter. The first is a single-strain probiotic, low dose — Lactobacillus rhamnosus GG, or Bifidobacterium longum, in the range of one to five billion CFU, taken with a meal. The second is small amounts of kimchi or another fermented vegetable, joining the sauerkraut juice that began two days earlier. Both are introductions, not staples yet. Both will build over the coming weeks.

What does not enter, still, is solid food in any meaningful sense. The blended preparations of these days carry chewable substance, but they are taken as foods that have been broken down before they reach the gut. The first natural bowel movement has not yet occurred. Until it does, the gate to solid food remains closed.

Days 8 to 14 — The First Bowel Movement, and What Follows

The first natural bowel movement after a prolonged fast is the gate. Not Day 8. Not Day 10. Not whatever date the calendar offers. The gate is a body signal, and the protocol holds liquid until the body itself announces that the colon has resumed its work.

For most practitioners, this signal arrives somewhere between Day 8 and Day 10. For some it comes earlier; for others later. None of the variation is cause for concern. The colon has been emptied by the fast and has been receiving only small amounts of liquid for the better part of a week. What it has needed in order to begin moving again is something it has not yet had — a meaningful volume of plant fiber that its musculature can engage with, and a microbial community beginning to populate the lumen. Those things are entering now, in small amounts. The first bowel movement comes when they have entered in enough quantity that the colon has work to do.

When the gate opens, the first solid foods enter in modest portions, well within the eating window. Deeply steamed soft vegetables are the right place to begin — zucchini, summer squash, well-cooked carrots, well-wilted leafy greens, all cooked until they yield easily under a fork. Portions are small. The first plate of solid food is half what it would have been before the fast. The two-meals-per-day default holds. The intermittent fasting window holds.

What does not enter at the gate, regardless of what other writing about refeeding may suggest, is concentrated protein. No scrambled eggs as the first solid food. No meat. No dense legume preparations. The lining is still settling, the digestive enzymes are still recalibrating, and a heavy protein load on the first day of solid eating is the most common entry mistake practitioners make. Heavier foods come, but later, and gradually.

The shape of a first solid-food day

For grounding, a typical first solid-food day — whether it falls on Day 8 or Day 10 or Day 12 — takes a shape something like this:

- Morning: water, trace minerals, nothing else

- 1 PM: small bowl of warm broth with mashed avocado, a tablespoon of sauerkraut juice on the side, a few bites of deeply steamed zucchini

• Mid-afternoon: a small handful of soaked chia in coconut milk, or a second small bowl of broth with pureed vegetables

• 6 PM: a slightly larger plate — steamed vegetables, perhaps a small portion of avocado, a small spoonful of kimchi, the daily probiotic, MCT or ghee folded in for fat support

• Evening: water, herbal tea (now permitted, decaf only), nothing else

After the gate opens, the days that follow continue the same gradual expansion. Cooked fruits in small amounts — applesauce, baked apples, stewed pears — can enter on subsequent days, as the body shows it is handling the steamed vegetables well. Small portions of well-cooked whole grains are a careful addition late in Week 2, for those who include them: a few tablespoons of well-rinsed quinoa, or short-grain rice cooked soft. Soaked and cooked legumes follow a similar schedule, in small amounts only. Soft-cooked eggs can enter for those who eat them, but late in the week rather than at the gate.

The morning beverages widen at the start of Week 2. Water and trace minerals are joined by herbal tea and decaf coffee, taken in modest amounts. Caffeinated coffee waits longer; the post-fast nervous system is still sensitive, and the practitioner who pushes that sensitivity by Week 2 often regrets it.

The microbiome thread continues. The single-strain probiotic that began on Day 7 stays in place; kefir — goat or coconut, never cow — can enter for those who tolerate it; the variety of fermented vegetables widens.

The two-meals-maximum rule holds across this stretch. Even as solid food enters and portions begin to grow, the structure of two principal feedings within the eating window is the rhythm being established. To slip into three or four small meals across the day, however reasonable each one feels in isolation, is to begin recreating the eating pattern the fast has just dissolved.

The Long Arc Begins

By the end of the second week, the acute work of refeeding has finished its dramatic phase. You are eating again. The lining of the gut has integrated solid food. The microbial reseeding is underway. The first jar of kimchi has been finished and replaced; a glass of kefir water sits beside it on the door of the refrigerator. The morning herb dose, taken with breakfast, has begun to feel automatic — something the body now expects rather than something you are remembering to do. You are not, today, the body that began the fast. You are not, yet, the body the long practice will eventually produce. You are somewhere between.

What follows is longer than the two weeks behind it, and quieter, and in most lives more consequential. The work of the fast either takes root in the months and years that follow, or it slowly returns to whatever it was before. Almost no one tells you this. The book that brought you to the fast probably did not tell you. The friend who walked you through your first liver-gallbladder flush probably did not tell you. The dramatic phase is the part that gets written about. The long arc is the part that decides whether anything that was accomplished in the dramatic phase actually stays.

The next sections of this chapter set out what the long arc looks like, in the form it actually takes for a person living it.

The eating window

The intermittent fasting window you began at Day 2 is not a transitional measure. It is the long-term shape of how you now eat.

Most days, the first meal arrives a little after one in the afternoon. The last meal closes before the light leaves the sky — somewhere between seven and eight in the evening, depending on the season. Inside that window, two principal meals. Not three. Not five. Not the small steady grazing through the day that the modern food industry has trained most adults into.

The reasons converge from several directions. The morning, given to the body without food in it, is given to the slow inner work the digestive system can only do when nothing is arriving. The evening, closed early, lets sleep arrive on a body that is not still processing what was eaten an hour before. The two-meal default lowers the total insulin response of the day and gives the lining of the gut the long stretches of rest in which it does its quiet maintenance work — work that, in a body eating six small meals across twelve hours, never quite has space to happen.

None of this is restriction. The body that has come through the fast does not, on most days, want to eat at six in the morning. It wants to eat at one. The hunger that arrives in the early afternoon is a clean hunger — specific, undramatic, easily satisfied — rather than the noisy demand the body once produced from the moment it woke. What you are being asked to do, in this stretch of months, is to let the rhythm settle. The pressure to eat earlier and longer will come from outside — the social schedules, the workplace conventions, the family dinner that runs late, the weekend brunch — and joining those rhythms is, on any given day, the path that opens by default. The rhythm the body now wants takes a small ongoing act of attention to keep, against that current.

The herbal taper

The herbs that carried you through the fast continue into the months that follow, on a schedule that thins gradually toward an end.

The full schedule is in the chart at the back of the book, where you will return to it when you need to check what should be running this week and what should have stopped. What is worth saying in the prose is that the schedule has a shape: most of what you are taking thins toward absence across the first two months, and a small handful of things — clove, milk thistle — run longer because the work they are doing runs longer. By the end of Week 7, the herbal stack has substantially completed its work, and the small daily ritual of the morning dose ends without ceremony, the way most practices that have done their work end.

Clove is the one that matters most to keep through to the end. The reason has its own section in this chapter, a few pages further on, and it is worth reading carefully. The single most common cause of cleanse failure is stopping clove too early. The body that has been carrying parasites for years has eggs in tissue layers that the first weeks of clove cannot reach, and those eggs need the full seven weeks to be fully resolved.

The other herbs are doing more specific work, and they retire on the schedule that fits the work each is doing. The chart at the back has the dates. Most days, you will not need to look at it; the rhythm of taking what is on the kitchen counter that morning will become, after a few weeks, what you are doing without thinking about it.

The coffee enema

The coffee enema is also thinning.

In the early refeeding, it was happening every other day, or twice in the week. By Week 3 it has stepped down to twice weekly. By Week 4 to once weekly. By the end of Week 8, monthly maintenance only — the once-a-month return that keeps the bile flowing and gives the liver a small periodic helping hand. Beyond that, for most people, as the energy stabilizes and the signs settle, the enema goes to as-needed.

The schedule sits in the chart at the back. What matters in the prose is that the coffee enema is not a permanent feature of your life. It was the support the body needed while the larger work of repair was happening; once that work has substantially completed, the enema retires alongside the rest of the active interventions of the protocol. There are people who find it useful as an occasional return, in years when the body is being asked for more — a hard winter, a stretch of stress, a period after travel — and using it that way is fine. But the daily or weekly relationship you had with it in the early weeks ends, and the ending is itself a sign that the body has reached somewhere new.

What is happening underneath, without your noticing

While the eating window settles and the herbs thin and the enema retires, a different kind of work is happening, continuously, without your needing to do anything for it.

The microbial community of the gut — the small living world that the fast cleared down to bare ground, and that the first two weeks of refeeding began to reseed — continues to find its long-term shape across the months that follow. Each meal you eat is feeding it, or failing to. Each fermented food you keep on the counter is helping it, or its absence is letting it thin. Each new vegetable you bring home from the market gives a particular small population something it needed; each week without variety is a week in which some part of the community goes quiet for lack of what it eats.

You are not having to think about any of this. The community responds, on its own, to the conditions you put around it. Good conditions, kept steadily, produce a community that holds. Inattention, kept steadily, produces a community that thins. What that community is, what it does, and how it shapes nearly everything you experience as your own mood, your own clarity, your own steadiness — that is the subject of the chapter that follows this one. What is worth knowing here is only that it is happening, every day, mostly without your awareness, in the quiet of the gut.

What an ordinary day looks like

Three months past the fast, an ordinary day in your life now looks something like this.

You wake before the light, in a body that does not want food yet. The first thing that arrives, in the long minutes before you get out of bed, is the body's report — the breath, the mind's quiet, the small held places, the readiness or unreadiness for the day. You drink a glass of water. You take whichever herb is still active in the morning rotation. You move into the morning's work — the writing, the run, the children, the email, whichever life you are inside of — in a body that has begun to feel different from the one that started the fast. Lighter. Less reactive. Steadier in the chest.

A little after one, you eat. The meal is most days similar in shape: vegetables, dominant on the plate, with adequate protein folded in, with one of the fermented things included almost without thinking, with cooking oils your great-grandmother would have recognized. You sit at the table to eat it. You let the meal take the time it asks for. You do not eat again for some hours afterward, and the not-eating is not effortful; it is what the body has begun to ask for.

You eat once more in the early evening, before the light goes. The second meal is sometimes similar to the first and sometimes the simpler version of it — what is in the refrigerator, what comes together quickly, what the family wants tonight. You close the eating window before eight. The long hours of evening and night happen in a body that is no longer processing, and sleep, when it arrives, arrives onto a body that has been ready for it for some time.

You repeat this, day after day, across weeks and months.

The shift

What changes, across that repetition, is not the protocol. The protocol stays roughly what it has been since the second week of refeeding. What changes is your relationship to it.

In the first weeks, you are following something. By the second month, you are doing something. By the third month, what you are doing has stopped being a protocol. It is how you eat. The window is no longer something you remember; it is when meals happen. The fermented foods are no longer a deliberate addition; they are in the refrigerator, because the refrigerator is now the kind of refrigerator they live in. The herbal taper has finished, and the small daily attention it required ended without ceremony, sometime in the eighth week, and you noticed it had ended only when your hand reached, for the first time in months, for nothing.

This is the shift this chapter has been moving toward. Most of the gains of the fast are kept or lost in it. Reaching it, in your daily life, is something most modern adults never get the chance to accomplish — a rhythm of eating that is not arranged around the conveniences of a food industry but around the conditions the body itself, given the chance, has asked for.

The sections that follow set out the specific details of this longer arc: the reason clove continues, the specific shape the coffee enema takes in the months that follow, the considerations for those who are vegetarian, the reinfection precautions of the early months, and the signs that tell you whether the work is consolidating as it should be.

Why Clove Especially Must Continue

This deserves emphasis. The single most common cause of cleanse failure is stopping clove too early. A 28-day fast at full clove protocol has destroyed all pinworm eggs, all roundworm eggs, all tapeworm eggs, most intestinal fluke eggs, and most bile duct fluke eggs.

But likely still developing are eggs in liver tissue (the deepest reservoir), some Chinese liver fluke eggs from the oldest infections, and any eggs in mucus that was just released near the end of the fast.

If clove stops at day 28, these continue developing. If clove continues for one to three more weeks, they are destroyed. The difference between a complete cleanse and an incomplete one often comes down to those final weeks of continued clove.

Adapting the Coffee Enema for the Months That Follow

The coffee enema is not finished when the fast is finished. Its role simply changes from active intervention to maintenance.

Why continue at all:

- Liver continues processing released toxins.
- Bile flow benefits from periodic stimulation.
- Helps integrate the cleansed state.

The arc of the months that follow

The coffee enema does not end with the first two weeks. Its role thins. From a protocol practiced every other day or twice in the week, it steps down — first to a few times each week, then weekly, then monthly, then to as-needed only. The schedule below is the arc.

Modified protocol

- Week 3: twice weekly.
- Weeks 4 to 8: once weekly.
- Beyond Week 8: monthly maintenance.
- Standard solution — the additions like clove oil and black walnut tincture continue.

When to discontinue

- Once the practitioner has been eating normally for several weeks.

• Energy is sustained at high baseline.

• No signals indicating continued need.

• The body is integrated into post-fast equilibrium.

The full schedule sits in the Quick Reference Charts at the back of the book for return reference.

Avoiding Reinfection

The clean gut is also a vulnerable gut. Without established microbial communities, opportunistic organisms can establish more easily, and the practitioner who is most careful in the early refeeding window is the one who avoids the disappointment of an unnecessary recolonization.

Protective practices in early refeeding:

• Filter all drinking water.

• Wash all produce thoroughly.

• Avoid raw seafood and undercooked meat for first month.

• Be cautious with restaurant food in first few weeks.

• Continue herbal antiparasitic protocol at reduced level.

• Pay particular attention to food handling hygiene.

Specific Notes for Vegetarians

Most of what this chapter has set out applies to the vegetarian practitioner without adjustment. A few elements deserve specific attention, because the vegetarian protocol handles them deliberately where the omnivorous one handles them automatically.

• **Protein adequacy.** Lentils, beans, hemp seeds, pumpkin seeds, eggs (if included). Combine grains and legumes for complete proteins. Pumpkin seed protein powder is a useful supplement for those who want a concentrated source — though like most plant proteins it works best paired with legumes for the full amino acid profile. Adequate protein supports tissue rebuilding.

• **B12 attention.** Vegetarians often need B12 supplementation. Particularly important after a thorough cleanse. Methylated B12 forms preferred.

• **Iron consideration.** Pair iron-rich plant foods with vitamin C. Soaked legumes are more bioavailable. Cast-iron cookware adds dietary iron.

• **Zinc and minerals.** Continue trace mineral supplementation. Soaked nuts and seeds. Variety of legumes.

• **Omega-3 from plants.** Flax, chia, hemp seeds. Walnuts. Algae-based supplements if needed.

Signs the Continuation Is Working

The body sends clear signals when the post-fast continuation protocol is doing its work, and equally clear signals when something has gone off course.

During the first weeks of refeeding, signs that the work is consolidating:

• Energy continuing to improve rather than dropping.

• Mental clarity sustained.

• Digestion working well with reintroduced foods.

• No return of pre-fast symptoms.

• Continued sense of internal cleanness.

• Sleep deep and restorative.

Signs that suggest concerns:

• Return of fatigue or brain fog.

• Digestive symptoms reemerging.

• Skin issues returning.

• Symptoms suggesting parasitic activity returning.

• Energy crashes after meals.

If concerning signs appear, extend the continuation protocol and consider testing.

In the months that follow

The signs that tell the practitioner the work is consolidating change character as the months pass. The early signs are about absence — the absence of returning symptoms, the absence of energy crashes, the absence of the brain fog that drove the fast in the first place. The longer-arc signs are about something different: the gradual recognition that the patterns the chapter has set out are no longer being followed but lived. The eating window is the practitioner's ordinary rhythm, no longer something held against a current. The fermented foods are part of how the kitchen works. The herbal taper, once finished, has finished without ceremony, and the practitioner has not needed to think about herbs in weeks. When the protocol has stopped feeling like a protocol, the work has consolidated.

Reference Charts

The three charts that follow gather the protocol details for the first two weeks in one place, for use as a quick reference. The day-by-day prose above tells the story; these charts hold the schedule.

The Critical Two-Week Continuation

The two weeks immediately after breaking the fast deserve specific attention. The protocol during this window is what determines whether the work of the previous month consolidates or unravels.

Element	Week 1 of Refeeding	Week 2 of Refeeding
Clove tincture	3× daily — non-negotiable	Continuing 3× daily
Black walnut hull	Once daily at half dose	Continuing once daily at half dose
Wormwood	Once daily	Continuing once daily; discontinue at end of Week 2
Mimosa pudica †	Once daily	Continuing once daily
Berberine †	Once daily	Continuing once daily
L-glutamine	Daily	Continuing daily
Milk thistle †	Daily	Continuing daily
Coffee enema	Every other day	Twice in the week
Probiotics	Begin Day 7 (single strain, low dose)	Increase gradually
Fermented foods	Day 5 onward (small amounts)	Wider variety; kefir if tolerated

† **On capsule preparation during refeeding.** For the substances marked with † in the chart above, the same guidance from Chapter 19 applies during the first 1-2 weeks of refeeding: open the capsule and mix the powder into a small amount of water rather than swallow whole. Digestion is still re-establishing, capsule shells may not dissolve reliably, and the liquid diet of early refeeding doesn't provide the digestive activation that capsules need. Once you're eating solid foods well (typically by week 2-3), capsules can be swallowed normally.

Microbiome Reintroduction Timeline

Day / Week	Probiotics	Fermented Foods
During the fast	Do not take — can cause significant gas and discomfort	Do not consume
Day 5 of refeeding	Wait	Small amount of sauerkraut juice
Day 7 of refeeding	Begin: single-strain, low dose	Small amounts of kimchi or other fermented vegetables
Days 7-14	Increase gradually	Expanding variety
Week 2	Continue gradual increase	Kefir, fermented dairy if tolerated
Week 3 onward	Multiple strain formulations; spore-based	Full integration into daily diet

Quality matters. Choose refrigerated potency-guaranteed probiotic products and avoid cheap shelf-stable products with questionable viability. Different ferments contain different organisms — rotation builds a more diverse microbiome. Homemade ferments are often more potent than commercial.

Chart M — Fermented Foods Introduction

Item	Notes
Starting points (begin day 5 to 10 of refeeding)	
Sauerkraut juice	Small amount, 1 tablespoon to start
Kimchi juice	Similar small amount
Coconut water kefir	For those who avoid dairy
Kombucha	Small amounts to begin
Building over weeks	
Whole sauerkraut and kimchi	Build portions gradually
Cultured vegetables	In variety
Kefir	Dairy or coconut
Yogurt	For those who include dairy
Fermented beverages	Kvass, water kefir

A Window of Choice

Forty days have passed, and the body that began them is not the body that finishes them. The architecture of hunger has been disassembled and quietly rebuilt. The reflexive reaches — the cupboard at mid-morning, the drawer at three, the second helping that was never about hunger — have lost their grip, week by week, until they were no longer reaching at all. What kept them alive was use, and they have not been used.

The work that was done in those forty days is more difficult to name than the work of a single fast. Hunger was the smaller part of it. The larger part was the slow undoing of a relationship — between the body and what it had been asked to receive, between the day and the meals that punctuated it, between the practitioner and the patterns that had been quietly choosing on their behalf for years. That relationship has been dissolved. Not perfectly. Not forever. But thoroughly enough that, for a brief season, it does not run the day.

The body that breaks the fast is in a particular condition. The lining of the gut is new tissue. The small intestine has rested as it has not rested in years. The microbial community has been cleared down to bare ground and is only now beginning to reseed. The liver is processing again at a rhythm it has nearly forgotten. None of this is metaphor. The cells are different cells. The tissue is different tissue. To meet that body with the eating habits of the body that came before it is to ask something of it that it is no longer built to do.

And yet the old patterns wait. They are quieter now, but they are not gone. The hours that used to call for food still arrive on schedule. The cupboard is still where it was. The cultural rhythm of three meals or five meals or grazing through the waking hours still surrounds the practitioner on every side, and the muscle memory of participating in that rhythm has not been erased — only paused. To slip back into it would require no effort at all. It is the path that opens by default.

What is being asked, instead, is something the practitioner has never quite been asked before: to let the new body teach them how to eat. A meal taken at midday rather than at the cold edges of dawn. Two meals where there used to be four or five or six, scattered across the waking hours and the working hours and the hours that should have been for rest. A window of eating that closes before the evening lengthens, leaving the body the long hours of darkness for its quiet inner work, undisturbed by digestion. None of this is restriction. The body is no longer being denied. It is being offered, instead, the rhythm it would have asked for if it had been able to ask.

The window in which this choice is genuinely available will not stay open. Habits reform with surprising speed in the absence of others. Within months, whatever rhythm settles in will have become the new familiar — not because it was chosen, but because it was repeated. The cravings that once chose are quiet now, and the patterns that once decided are paused, but neither will remain so. What fills the space is what gets repeated in these particular weeks. Nothing else has the same chance to take root.

Forty days were spent dissolving a life. The question now is what gets built in the room that has been cleared.

Chapter 30

Rebuilding the Partnership

* * *

The Trace

There is a kind of morning that arrives, sometimes, in the weeks after a long fast. The light comes through the window early, and the sleep that preceded it was deep, and the body feels — there is no better word — quiet. A quiet that is not absence but presence. The mind is clear in a way that does not require effort. The breath comes easily. Hunger, when it arrives later in the morning, arrives as a clean signal rather than as a demand. The skin in the bathroom mirror looks like the skin of someone several years younger than the person who began the fast. There is a steadiness across the whole interior that the reader, in the years before, may have forgotten was even possible.

Most people, at this point, attribute the change to the fast. And the fast did, of course, do real work. The lining of the gut is new tissue. The liver is processing at a different rhythm. Insulin is low. Inflammation, at least for the moment, is quieter than it has been in years.

But almost none of what the reader is experiencing this morning is, strictly speaking, the work of the body that the reader thinks of as themselves. Most of it is the work of a partner. A partner the reader has never seen, has never thought about, has spent their entire life carrying without ever once being introduced.

A few grams of microorganisms, living in the dark of the colon, are the larger part of why this morning feels the way it feels. And the way they accomplish their work is not the way the reader, if they had to guess, would have guessed.

Consider only one thread. Begin with the steadiness of the mood — the calm that holds the morning. Trace it backward.

The mood is held, in part, by a population of cells living in the brain itself, called microglia. These are not neurons — they do not fire signals or carry thoughts. They are the brain's resident immune cells, its janitors and its guards, and they are present in vast numbers, perhaps one for every neuron in the entire central nervous system. When all is well they move through the brain tissue cleaning up debris, repairing small damage, and watching for threats, and they do this work quietly. When something disturbs them — an infection, a head injury, a chronic inflammatory signal arriving from elsewhere in the body — they shift state. They become reactive. They release chemical alarms that disturb every neuron near them. The mind, in that moment, becomes harder to live in. Concentration thins. Mood darkens. The internal weather changes.

This morning, the microglia in the reader's brain are calm. Why?

Because the level of certain inflammatory signals in the bloodstream is low this morning. Microglia, despite living behind the blood-brain barrier, are deeply responsive to what the rest of the body is doing — they read the chemistry of the blood that flows past them, and when that chemistry is calm, they are calm. This morning, the body's general inflammation is quiet, and the microglia have settled with it. Why is the body's inflammation quiet?

Because of the steady arrival, in the bloodstream, of a small fatty-acid molecule called butyrate. Butyrate is one of the most consequential molecules the human body deals with, and almost nobody who is not a microbiologist or a gastroenterologist has ever heard of it. It is the single most important food source for the cells of the colon wall — those cells will, given the choice, burn butyrate before they burn anything the bloodstream can deliver to them. But butyrate does much more than feed the colon. The portion of it that enters general circulation suppresses inflammation throughout the body. It acts on the immune system to calibrate response. It crosses, eventually, into the brain, where it influences the very microglia we have just been discussing. The skin is calmer this morning because of butyrate. The joints are quieter for the same reason. The sense of general internal ease the reader is experiencing is, in part, the work of a single small molecule, made elsewhere, traveling far. Why has there been adequate butyrate?

Because in the colon, an organism called *Faecalibacterium prausnitzii* has been doing the only thing it knows how to do. *Faecalibacterium* is, in the world of human gut bacteria, something close to a hero. It is one of the most abundant organisms in a healthy gut, sometimes accounting for as much as five percent of all bacteria present, and it is among the most reliably absent in nearly every disease of the gut yet studied — Crohn's disease, ulcerative colitis, inflammatory bowel disease, certain cancers. Researchers now use its presence as one of the basic markers of gut health, and its disappearance as one of the early warning signs that something has gone wrong. It does not move on its own; it does not pursue food; it has no nervous system and nothing resembling intent. What it does, all day every day, is eat certain kinds of plant fiber that arrive in the colon undigested by the body itself, and ferment them. The byproduct of that fermentation is butyrate. *Faecalibacterium* is, in plain terms, the body's most important butyrate factory.

Why has *Faecalibacterium* been thriving?

Because the meals of the previous days have included a variety of cooked vegetables and small amounts of fermented foods, and because the antibiotic load on the gut has been zero, and because the inflammatory environment that this organism cannot tolerate has, after the work of the fast, lifted. The bacterium is doing its work because it has been given the conditions to do its work.

A single bacterium, in the dark, eating a strand of fiber. A small molecule, made as a byproduct, crossing a wall. A signal, traveling a vein. A calming, two body systems away. The way the morning feels.

This is one chain. There are hundreds of others, running every minute, in every direction. The bacterium that ferments a different fiber and produces a different molecule that signals through a different pathway and ends up affecting the way an entirely different system behaves — repeated, in parallel, across the whole microbial community of the gut. The reader's interior is not, as the reader has likely been led to believe, a private space inhabited by a single self. It is something closer to a forest. The trees and the fungi and the soil organisms have been, for as long as there have been forests, in conversation. The forest is not the trees. The forest is the conversation.

There is a phrase for the kind of cause-and-effect at work here. A butterfly flaps its wings on one side of the world and a storm pattern shifts on the other, six weeks later, through a chain of consequences too long for any one observer to trace. The metaphor was originally used in mathematics, to describe systems where small changes at one scale produce large changes at another, through chains of intermediate steps. It applies, almost literally, to what is happening inside the body of the person reading this.

The bacterium does not "produce mood." The bacterium ferments fiber. The fermentation produces butyrate. The butyrate travels. The travel produces an effect on inflammation. The effect on inflammation reaches the brain. The brain, freed of inflammation, runs cleanly. The mood is steady. Six steps from a single anaerobe in the dark, eating something the body itself could not have eaten, six steps to the way the morning feels.

This is what is meant when scientists, sometimes too breathlessly, say that the gut influences mood. The reality is at once less direct than the breathless version and more astonishing. Less direct, because the bacteria do not make mood; they make a molecule, which makes another molecule, which influences a system, which influences another system. More astonishing, because the chain is genuinely that long, and the chain runs reliably, every day, in every healthy person who has ever lived.

The reader's morning is a chain. Most of the links are invisible. Most of them happen in the dark. Most of them are accomplished by organisms that have no nervous system, no awareness, no plan — only the metabolism they evolved with, and the food they happen to find in front of them.

The next chapters of the protocol — the practical work of probiotic introduction, fermented foods, prebiotic fibers, foods that feed the right organisms and avoid feeding the wrong ones — are not, in the end, about eating bacteria. They are about tending the chains. Each chain runs from a specific organism, through a specific food, through a specific molecule, to a specific effect in the body. The work of rebuilding the microbiome is the work of restoring the conditions under which the chains run reliably.

What the previous chapters did, quietly, was something rare. The fast cleared the gut of a great deal of what should not have been there. The first two weeks of refeeding began the work of putting back what should be there. What follows from here — the months in which the microbial community settles into its long-term shape — is when most of the chains either re-form, link by link, or quietly fail to.

The reader has, at this moment, an opportunity that most modern adults will never have. The opportunity to rebuild a partnership that has been quietly degrading, for most people, since childhood. The opportunity to plant a forest in cleared ground.

What follows is the work of that planting.

The Partnership in Outline

It is worth pausing, before going further, to say what the partner actually is.

The microbial community living in a healthy human colon is, by sheer count, larger than the body itself. Estimates have moved around in the research over the last fifteen years, but the rough proportion has held: there are roughly as many microbial cells in a healthy adult gut as there are human cells in the entire body, possibly more. By weight, the community runs to one and a half to two kilograms — a small dog's worth of organisms, carried inside a person, mostly without notice. The species count in a single healthy gut is usually somewhere between five hundred and a thousand distinct kinds of bacteria, with smaller populations of archaea, fungi, and viruses living alongside them. No two people's communities are identical. The fingerprint of microbes a person carries is more individual than a fingerprint, and it changes over a lifetime in ways that track that life — what was eaten, what illnesses passed through, which antibiotics were taken, which countries were lived in.

These organisms are not, as the cultural reflex has it, contamination. They are not invaders the body has somehow failed to expel. They are co-evolved. The lineage of bacteria living in the human colon today descends, without break, from organisms that lived in the colons of the early mammals, and before that in the guts of the reptiles those mammals descended from, and before that in the digestive tracts of the first multicellular animals to crawl out of the ocean. The relationship is older than backbones. It is older than lungs. There has never been an animal of any size or complexity that did not carry a microbial community inside it. The body has been a *we*, in the most literal biological sense, for as long as there have been bodies of this kind.

What has changed over evolutionary time is the depth of the partnership. The species of bacteria that thrive in a healthy human colon are species that depend on humans for their habitat — they cannot live for long outside the conditions of a particular kind of warm, wet, oxygen-poor, fiber-rich environment that only exists inside an animal of roughly this design. And the human body, in turn, has evolved to depend on what those bacteria produce. The colon wall feeds, as we have already seen, on a molecule it does not make for itself. The immune system depends on microbial signaling to develop properly in childhood; children raised in artificially sterile environments develop dysregulated immune responses that follow them through life. The brain forms, in part, in response to chemicals the gut microbes produce during early development. The skin's microbial layer, the mouth's microbial layer, the upper airway's microbial layer — these are not auxiliary; they are constitutive. Remove them, and what remains is not the human body. What remains is a system that has lost a working part and is failing.

The reader is not, in any meaningful biological sense, a single organism. The reader is a small ecosystem walking around in a particular shape. Most of what makes that ecosystem function is invisible to the reader and was, until quite recently, invisible to science as well. We are barely a generation into knowing this clearly.

What follows is what the partner does.

The Chains

The chain in the opening section traced one thread: from a meal of cooked vegetables, through a strand of fiber arriving in the colon, through *Faecalibacterium*, through butyrate, through the bloodstream, through inflammation, into the calm of microglia, into the steadiness of mood. One chain, six steps. There are a great many others.

What follows is not an exhaustive catalog. It is a small collection of chains, each one chosen because it ends somewhere the reader will recognize from their own body — the immune system, the skin, the hormones, sleep — and because each one shows a different shape of how the partnership works.

The chain through the immune system

About seventy percent of the body's immune tissue lies in or near the gut wall, most of it in the small intestine. This is not a small fact. It means that the largest single organ of the immune system is the lining of a tube, and the surface of that tube is in constant, intimate contact with the trillions of microorganisms living on the other side of it. The immune system, in the gut, is not a sentinel watching from a distance. It is a participant in a conversation that never stops.

The conversation, when it goes well, is one of the most sophisticated processes in all of biology. The immune cells in the gut wall must somehow recognize the bacterial species that have always belonged there and tolerate them, while simultaneously recognizing pathogens — bacteria, viruses, parasites — that do not belong, and mounting a swift, decisive response against them. The discrimination is enormously fine. A given strain of *Lactobacillus* may differ from a pathogenic strain by a small handful of surface proteins. The immune system is somehow able, in healthy gut tissue, to read those proteins and decide correctly, thousands of times per second, friend or foe.

How does it learn to do this? Through the conversation itself. From the moment a baby is born, the immune system in the gut is being trained by the bacterial community arriving there. Each microbial signal it receives — each surface protein it encounters, each metabolite it tastes — calibrates its sensitivity. By the time the immune system reaches adulthood, it has been shaped, profoundly, by the particular community it grew up next to. A child raised in a household with a healthy diverse microbiome and limited antibiotic exposure develops an immune system that is, on average, less reactive to harmless triggers and more decisive against real ones. A child raised in a more disrupted microbial environment — frequent antibiotics, processed food, low microbial diversity — develops an immune system that is, on average, more prone to overreacting to harmless things (allergies, autoimmune disease, asthma) and less effective at responding to real threats.

This training relationship does not end at childhood. The adult immune system in the gut continues to be tuned, every day, by the microbial signals it receives. A gut whose bacterial community has been disrupted — by a course of antibiotics, by a stretch of poor diet, by chronic stress — produces an immune system that drifts in measurable ways within weeks. A gut whose community has been restored — through fasting, through rebuilding, through the work of the next several months — produces an immune system that recovers its regulation within a similar window.

The reader, walking through a winter and not catching the cold that everyone around them is catching, is feeling, in a small way, a chain that runs from a fermented vegetable eaten three weeks earlier to an immune cell making a correct decision in the lining of the throat. A small molecule, made by a microbe, calibrating a cell, holding a wall.

The chain to the skin

The skin and the gut are, on a map of the body, far apart. Functionally they are neighbors.

What unites them is inflammation. The bloodstream connects every tissue to every other tissue, and inflammation traveling in the bloodstream — the same inflammatory signals that disturb the microglia in the brain — disturbs the cells of the skin in just the same way. A gut whose bacterial community is producing too little butyrate, too few other anti-inflammatory metabolites, too few signals of microbial calm, sends an inflamed bloodstream throughout the body. The skin reads that bloodstream. The skin responds.

Most chronic skin conditions of unclear cause — adult acne that refuses to resolve, eczema that flares without obvious trigger, psoriasis, rosacea — have, in recent research, been linked to gut inflammation more reliably than to any cause local to the skin itself. Treating the skin from the outside, with creams and washes, addresses the symptom. Treating the gut, in many cases, addresses the source. Practitioners who do prolonged fasts often report, in the weeks of refeeding, a quieting of skin conditions they had been treating topically for years. The chain runs through the bloodstream. The skin clears because the bloodstream cleared. The bloodstream cleared because the bacteria, finally, are doing their work again.

The cells of the skin live, on average, about a month. The skin the reader will see in the bathroom mirror two months from now is skin that does not yet exist. What that skin will look like is being decided, in part, by the microbial community currently establishing in the colon. The chain is that long, and that direct.

The chain through hormones

The body's hormonal systems — the thyroid, the adrenal axis, the reproductive hormones, insulin and the metabolic hormones — are deeply linked to the gut, in ways most of their carriers have never been told.

The clearest of these links runs through estrogen. The liver, after using estrogen for its various purposes in the body, packages it for excretion and sends it into the gut. There it meets a particular community of microbes — researchers have given the community its own name, the *estrobolome* — which produces an enzyme that can either keep estrogen on its way out of the body or unpack it and send it back into circulation. A healthy estrobolome, with its full range of organisms, regulates this process within a narrow band. A disrupted estrobolome — too little diversity, the wrong organisms in the wrong proportions — sends either too much estrogen back into the body or too little. The downstream consequences are felt across the entire endocrine system. Heavy or irregular cycles, mood changes around the cycle, certain breast and uterine cancers, the difficult years of perimenopause and menopause — all of these are influenced, sometimes profoundly, by a community of bacteria living in the colon, eating the body's discarded estrogen and deciding what to do with it.

The thyroid runs through a different chain but a similar logic. Thyroid hormone is converted into its active form, in part, by enzymes produced by gut bacteria. A disrupted gut produces a body that is hypothyroid in subtle ways even when the thyroid itself is fine — the conversion is not happening because the converters are not present in adequate numbers. The cortisol axis, the body's stress response, runs through the gut as well; chronic gut inflammation produces a chronic low-grade stress signal that the adrenal glands respond to as if real stress were occurring, and the consequences — sleep disruption, anxiety, the slow exhaustion of long-term elevated cortisol — follow from there.

The reader who has spent years tracking hormone numbers, watching them drift in inexplicable directions, may be feeling a chain that runs not from the glands themselves but from the microbial community that supports them.

The chain through sleep

The bacteria in the gut keep their own clock.

The microbial community as a whole runs on a daily rhythm that mirrors the body's own circadian cycle. Different species are more active at different hours; the chemistry of the colon shifts measurably between day and night; the metabolites produced by the community follow a daily curve. This rhythm is set, in part, by when the body eats and when it stops eating. The intermittent fasting window the reader has now established — eating closing in the evening, opening at midday — gives the microbial clock the long uninterrupted overnight stretch it evolved to expect.

When that clock is preserved, sleep deepens. Not because the bacteria are causing sleep directly — they are not — but because the body's sleep is tied to a great many systems that are themselves tied to the microbial rhythm. Inflammation drops at night in a healthy body, and that drop is partly microbial. Cortisol falls in the evening and rises before waking, and the curve of that fall and rise is partly microbial. Even the timing of certain neurotransmitters — serotonin's daily curve, for instance, which peaks in the gut during the day and feeds into the conversion to melatonin in the evening — runs through pathways the microbes are participating in.

The reader who has, in the weeks after the fast, begun to sleep the way they used to sleep as a child — falling asleep easily, waking rested without an alarm — is feeling a chain that runs from the dinner that closed before dark, to the long quiet hours during which the microbial community runs its overnight cycle uninterrupted, to the cortisol curve that rises gently into a clean morning, to the mind that wakes ready.

The cumulative architecture

There are more chains. The mood chain we traced first, the immune chain, the skin chain, the hormone chains, the sleep chain — these are five among many. The cardiovascular system, the urinary tract, the joints, the absorption of vitamins, the maintenance of bone density, the regulation of body weight, the body's resilience to physical and emotional stress — every one of these has microbial threads running through it that researchers are only now beginning to map clearly.

What matters is not the catalog. What matters is the shape of the catalog. The reader is not a body that happens to contain a microbial community on the side. The reader is a body whose every major system is, to some extent, a downstream effect of microbial work. The interior is not a self plus an addition. The interior is a partnership, all the way down.

When the partnership is healthy, the chains run reliably and most of the body's systems do their work quietly. When the partnership is disrupted — even partially, even temporarily — chains break, systems drift, and the reader feels a thousand small failures whose source is impossible to trace from the outside.

Most modern adults are, in microbial terms, partially disrupted. Have been for years. Often since childhood.

The next section is about how that happened.

Soil, Plants, and the Same Chemistry

Before turning to what has been broken, it is worth stepping briefly outside the body — onto the ground itself.

A handful of healthy soil contains, by recent estimates, more individual microorganisms than there are humans on Earth. Tens of thousands of distinct species, organized into communities as complex as any tropical forest, running an economy of nutrient exchange that the plants growing out of that soil depend on absolutely. The chemistry of the partnership in the soil is, in many cases, the same chemistry as the partnership in the gut — and not by coincidence. Both communities descended from common ancestors. Both run on similar metabolic logic. The bacteria that ferment plant fiber in the colon are first cousins, in evolutionary terms, to the bacteria that decompose plant matter in the forest floor.

A nitrogen-fixing bacterium living in a small nodule on the root of a clover plant takes nitrogen from the air — which the plant cannot use — and converts it into ammonia, which the plant can use. In exchange, the plant feeds the bacterium sugars from its roots. Neither one could do its work alone. The clover grows because the bacterium fixes nitrogen. The bacterium lives because the clover supplies sugars. The chain extends outward: the clover, having grown, is eaten by an insect, or dies and decomposes, or fixes nitrogen into the soil that the next plant relies on. The nitrogen that ends up in a leaf of grass was, six steps earlier, in the air; it traveled into the plant via the patient work of an organism the plant itself could not see.

This is the same architecture that runs in the colon. The reader cannot break down the cellulose in a stalk of celery. *Faecalibacterium* and its colleagues can. They do the breaking down. The byproducts — butyrate among them — feed the cells of the reader's colon wall, and travel onward through the body, and end up in the brain and the skin and the joints and the immune system. The reader provides shelter, warmth, and a steady arrival of plant material. The bacteria provide chemistry the body cannot do for itself.

The parallel goes deeper than analogy. A diverse plant community above ground produces a diverse microbial community below it; a monoculture of a single crop, repeated season after season, produces an impoverished soil that eventually cannot support even the crop it was planted to grow. The soil's diversity is a function of the plants' diversity. The plants' health is a function of the soil's diversity. Each one supports the other. Each one collapses when the other collapses.

The same is true inside the human body. A diverse plate produces a diverse gut community. A diet that runs on a small handful of foods, repeated every day for years, produces a gut community as impoverished as a field of corn grown for the fortieth season in a row. The species that depended on the foods no longer eaten go extinct in the gut, the way a species of bee goes extinct from a field that has been sprayed every spring for a generation. The community thins. The chemistry thins with it.

Carson saw this. *Silent Spring* was not, in the end, only a book about pesticides and birds. It was a book about the inseparability of the body's health from the soil's health, the soil's health from the plants', the plants' from the insects', the insects' from the birds'. *In nature nothing exists alone*, she wrote, and the line was the book's deepest claim. Sixty years later, the science has caught up with her in a particular direction she did not live to see — into the human gut, where the same logic of partnership and the same vulnerability to disruption are running, in the dark, every minute of every day.

The person who eats a diverse diet of plants is, in microbial terms, a person tending a diverse field. The person who eats narrowly is tending a monoculture. Both will, in time, have the soil they have built.

What Has Been Broken

The healthy microbial community described in the previous sections is increasingly rare.

Most modern adults in industrialized countries carry a microbial community that is a fraction of what their grandparents carried, and a smaller fraction still of what would have been present in any human gut from before the agricultural revolution. The diversity has dropped — the number of distinct species per gut has fallen, the populations of the most fragile species have collapsed entirely, and certain organisms that were nearly universal in pre-industrial humans are now nearly absent from the developed world. *Faecalibacterium* itself, the abundant butyrate-maker we met in the opening, is reduced in most modern guts to perhaps a third of what it would have been in a healthy ancestor, and absent altogether in many people. Other key species — the spirochete *Treponema* found in nearly every traditionally-living people studied, the methane-producing archaea, certain *Bacteroides* species — have disappeared from the developed-world gut so thoroughly that researchers have to travel to remote villages and Indigenous communities to study them in their natural state.

This loss did not happen all at once. It happened across generations, in small increments, mostly invisibly. A few of the contributing factors are worth naming.

Antibiotics in childhood. A course of antibiotics — even a single course — disrupts the gut microbiome severely. The most fragile species are killed outright; the more resilient species are reduced; the community as a whole undergoes a re-shuffling that takes months to settle. A healthy adult, given good food and some time, recovers most of what was lost. A child whose immune system is still being trained by the microbial conversation, however, may not. Each course of antibiotics in the first three years of life produces a measurable drop in microbial diversity that, on average, never fully recovers. The American child today receives, on average, roughly fifteen courses of antibiotics by age eighteen. The European child, somewhat fewer. The child raised in a traditional setting in a non-industrialized country, perhaps one or two. The cumulative effect, multiplied across the population over the last seventy years, is a generational thinning of the microbiome that compounds with each passing decade.

Antibiotics in the food chain. The animals raised for industrial meat and dairy in most of the developed world are routinely dosed with antibiotics for growth promotion and disease prevention. Residues of these antibiotics appear in the meat, the milk, and downstream in the water systems. The doses are small. They are also continuous. A person eating conventional meat and dairy and drinking municipal water in most modern countries receives a small but constant antibiotic exposure that, over years, performs its slow work on the gut community. The effect is less acute than a course of clinical antibiotics but more cumulative. By midlife, in many people, the damage rivals what a few rounds of clinical antibiotics would have done.

Glyphosate and other agricultural chemicals. Glyphosate, the active ingredient in the world's most widely-used herbicide, is toxic to certain kinds of bacteria — specifically the kind that include many of the most important species in the human gut. The chemical is now present, in trace amounts, in nearly all conventional grain products in the United States, in most conventional produce, in rainwater, and in the bodies of the great majority of tested humans. The amounts in any one meal are small. The exposure across years is constant. Whether the cumulative effect on the human microbiome is severe or modest is still being argued in the research literature; what is no longer in serious dispute is that the effect is real, and that it works in the same direction as everything else on this list.

The processed-food shift. A diet built mostly of refined grains, refined sugars, industrial seed oils, and concentrated additives — the diet that now constitutes the majority of caloric intake for most people in the developed world — is, microbially speaking, a starvation diet for the species that depend on plant fiber and plant polyphenols. *Faecalibacterium* cannot live without fiber. *Akkermansia*, the next character in this chapter, cannot live without polyphenols. A gut fed mostly on processed food is a gut in which these organisms slowly disappear, regardless of whether their host is otherwise well. The species that thrive on simple sugars and refined carbohydrates, on the other hand — many of which are inflammation-promoting and metabolically disruptive — flourish in the absence of competition from the species that have been starved out.

Chronic stress. The gut is exquisitely responsive to the body's stress response. A nervous system held in chronic low-grade alarm — through years of insufficient sleep, financial stress, relational stress, the diffuse stress of modern attention-fragmenting environments — produces a gut environment in which certain bacteria thrive and others die, and the direction of the shift is consistent. Stress narrows the microbiome. Calm broadens it. The reader who has spent years in chronic mild alarm has, during all of those years, also been hosting a slowly impoverishing community of bacteria.

The hygiene reflex. The cultural turn against microbial exposure — antibacterial soaps, sanitized environments, the avoidance of dirt, the discomfort with fermented and unpasteurized foods, the fear of any contact with microbes that has not been industrially controlled — has, over the last several decades, removed from most people's daily lives the steady microbial input that the body and its community evolved to expect. The skin community, the oral community, the respiratory community, and the gut community are all, in modern people, diminished partly by this. The body that meets very few microbes ends up with very few microbes living on it.

The cumulative effect of these factors, across a single lifetime, is a measurable disruption of the microbial community that most modern people carry without knowing. Across generations — a grandparent born in the 1930s, a parent born in the 1960s, a child born in the 1990s — the effect compounds. The grandchild inherits, at birth, a less diverse community than the grandparent did, and then proceeds to lose more of it across childhood than the grandparent ever did. The thinning is severe enough that some researchers now speak of a coming "microbial impoverishment" of the human species — a loss of the inherited partnership at a scale and speed without precedent in evolutionary history.

This is the stake. The reader, before the fast, was almost certainly carrying a partially disrupted community. Most of the symptoms that drove the reader to consider a fast in the first place — the digestive issues, the energy issues, the skin issues, the mood issues, the sleep issues, the slow and unaccountable thinning of vitality across the years — were, to a substantial degree, the symptoms of that disruption. Not all. But a substantial degree.

What the fast did, among other things, was clear the field. What follows is the rare opportunity to plant something different in the cleared ground.

The Window the Fast Just Opened

What happened in the colon during the fast is worth pausing on for a moment, because it is unusual and the reader should know exactly what was just done.

A prolonged fast empties the gut. Not just of food — that happens within the first day or two — but of the microbial communities that depend on a steady arrival of food to maintain their populations. The species that thrive on simple sugars and refined carbohydrates, including many of the inflammation-promoters and the species that should not be there in such abundance, collapse first. They have nothing to eat. The species that were already in lower numbers and that were already struggling — *Faecalibacterium* among them — also reduce. The biofilms that certain bacterial communities had built on the gut wall, layered structures that protect the inhabitants but also lock the disruption in place, are weakened and in many cases dissolved. The herbal protocol of the fast has, in parallel, killed the parasitic organisms that had been crowding the gut and competing with the bacteria for space. The result, by the end of a thirty- or forty-day fast, is a colon that has been, in microbial terms, returned to something close to bare ground.

This is rare. Most modern adults will go their entire lives without ever experiencing a microbial state like this one. The disrupted community they were born with, or developed in childhood, persists with them into the grave — adjusted at the margins by diet and stress, but never fundamentally re-set. Even the few interventions that approach this kind of clearance, like the prolonged courses of broad-spectrum antibiotics required for certain infections, do not produce the same condition; antibiotics kill organisms but leave their structural damage and their inflammatory signaling in place, and the community that re-establishes after them is often a worse one than the community that was there before.

The fast does something the antibiotics cannot do. It clears without leaving behind the chemical residue and the inflammatory signaling. It dissolves the biofilms and the parasitic load and the inflammatory environment together. It leaves a colon that is not damaged but emptied, and that is ready, biochemically, to receive whatever community is established next.

This is the window. It does not stay open. Within a few weeks of refeeding, whatever community has been seeded — by the first foods, by the first probiotics, by the first fermented vegetables, by the first prebiotic fibers — will have begun to establish. Within a few months, that community will be reasonably stable. Within a year or two, it will be the long-term resident community of the gut, and changing it after that will be much harder than seeding it now is. The bacteria that establish in the next three months are, in most cases, the bacteria the reader will be carrying for years.

This is why the work of this chapter matters. Not because the practical instructions are complicated — they are not — but because the moment in which they are applied is a moment of unusual leverage. What is planted now grows.

What follows is how to plant.

The Three Phases of Rebuilding

The work of rebuilding the microbial community happens in three phases. Each one has its own timing, its own focus, and its own characteristic mistakes. The chart below sets out the shape of all three at a glance.

Chart K — The Three Phases of Rebuilding

Phase	Window	What Happens
Seeding	Days 1 to 14	Introducing beneficial bacteria into the cleared gut. Establishing initial colonies. Setting up the conditions for diverse community establishment.
Establishing	Days 15 to 60	Bacterial colonies growing and stabilizing. Diversifying the species present. Strengthening the community structure.
Diversifying	Day 60 onward	Continuing to add diversity. Cultivating long-term resilience. Maintaining through ongoing practices.

The three phases are sequential but they are not separable. The work of seeding does not stop on Day 14; the practices of the seeding phase continue, modified, throughout the establishing and diversifying phases. The work of establishing does not stop on Day 60; the practices continue, in turn, into the long-term diversifying phase. Each phase builds on the one before it. None of them ends.

What changes between phases is not what the reader is doing but what the gut is doing in response. In the seeding phase, the gut is mostly empty, and what enters takes hold. In the establishing phase, the early colonies are competing for territory, and what enters joins or fails to join the existing community. In the diversifying phase, the community is settling into long-term shape, and the work shifts from establishing presence to encouraging variety.

The next sections walk through each phase in turn.

Phase One — Seeding (a brief recap)

The seeding phase covered the first two weeks of refeeding. Most of it has, by the time the reader is reading this chapter, already happened. The protocol of the previous chapter walked through the work day by day — the first broth, the first ghee, the sauerkraut juice on Day 5, the single-strain probiotic on Day 7, the kimchi and the kefir if it was tolerated, the first solid foods after the bowel-movement gate.

A single paragraph is worth saying here, in honor of what the reader has already done. Each of those introductions was a seeding event in its own right. A tablespoon of sauerkraut juice carries something on the order of a hundred million live organisms, most of them species the colon wants to receive. A capsule of single-strain probiotic delivers another billion. A small portion of kimchi adds another hundred million, of different species, with different work. The reader, whether they knew it at the time or not, was performing acts of microbial planting at every meal of the first two weeks. The colonies that have established by Day 14 are the foundation of everything that follows. They are small. They are precious. And they are, at this moment, beginning the work of growing into the long-term residents of the gut.

What follows is the establishing phase, which lasts roughly six weeks and does most of the work of building the community out from those small initial colonies.

Phase Two — Establishing

The second phase runs from Day 15 to roughly Day 60. The seeding work of the first two weeks gives way to something slower and steadier — colonies that were introduced settling into the gut, finding the conditions that suit them, beginning to outgrow or outlast the organisms that may have come along for the ride. The probiotic and fermented food practices that began in the first weeks continue through this phase, with their variety widening. What enters newly here is the food that the established colonies eat — the prebiotic fibers that feed bacterial diversity rather than the bacteria themselves.

The probiotic protocol, in particular, broadens during this phase. The single-strain probiotic that began on Day 7 — most often *Lactobacillus rhamnosus* GG, or *Bifidobacterium longum*, both of which are species that have been studied extensively in human guts and known to establish well — gives way, after seven to ten days, to a multi-strain formulation. The reasoning is simple: the gut wants variety, and a multi-strain formula introduces several species at once rather than one at a time. The dose climbs from the low billions of CFU of the early days to the ten-to-fifty billion range that is the standard maintenance dose for adult use. Refrigerated products, with strain counts that have been protected by cold storage, are reliably more potent than shelf-stable products of the same nominal CFU count.

A second class of probiotic enters during Phase Two as well: spore-based probiotics, particularly *Bacillus* species. These are different from the *Lactobacillus* and *Bifidobacterium* species in the multi-strain formula. The *Bacillus* organisms form spores — protective shells that allow them to survive stomach acid more reliably than other probiotic organisms — and they reach the colon in a higher proportion of viable cells than most other probiotic preparations. They also do different work. *Bacillus* species are particularly good at modulating the immune response in the gut and at producing metabolites that suppress harmful organisms. They join the multi-strain formula rather than replacing it. By the middle of Phase Two, a typical practitioner is taking both, alongside the daily fermented food intake.

Chart L — Probiotic Introduction Sequence

Type	Timing	Notes
Single strain	Begin around Day 7 of refeeding	Start with one well-studied strain — *Lactobacillus rhamnosus* GG or *Bifidobacterium longum*. Low dose initially, 1 to 5 billion CFU. Take with food. Build up over a week.
Multi-strain	After 7 to 10 days of single strain	Transition to multi-strain formula, 10 to 50 billion CFU. Look for diversity of strains. Refrigerated products preferred.
Spore-based	Add alongside traditional probiotics	Particularly valuable as a supplement to traditional probiotics. Survive stomach acid more reliably. *Bacillus* species are especially well-studied. Continue alongside traditional probiotics.
Soil-based	Optional addition	For those willing to use them. Approximate the bacterial diversity of natural environments. Build robust community structure. Take with caution if immunocompromised.

The fermented foods during Phase Two move from the small daily portions of the first two weeks to a more substantial place at the table. By the middle of this phase, a typical practitioner is having something fermented at most meals — sauerkraut at lunch, kimchi at dinner, a small bowl of kefir or yogurt as a snack. The variety widens. Different ferments contain different organisms; rotating through them builds a more diverse community than any single ferment can. Homemade ferments, where they are practical, are often more potent than commercial preparations because they have not been pasteurized for shelf stability.

What enters newly in Phase Two — and this is the conceptual shift of the phase — is the food the colonies themselves eat. The probiotics are bacteria that the reader is delivering to the gut. The prebiotics are foods that the bacteria, once they have arrived, can live on. The two are different kinds of work and they reinforce each other.

Chart N — Prebiotic Fibers

Fiber Type	Food Sources
Inulin	Onions, garlic, leeks, asparagus, Jerusalem artichokes
Resistant starch	Cooked and cooled potatoes, green bananas, properly prepared rice
Beta-glucans	Oats, mushrooms, barley
Pectin	Apples, citrus fruits
Acacia fiber	Supplemental form

Beyond the specific fiber sources above, leafy greens and seasonal berries belong in this rotation as well. They support microbial diversity through their varied phytonutrients rather than through a single named fiber, and the more colors on the plate across a week, the more diverse the community that grows from it.

The chart sets out the categories. What the chart cannot show is the way each category does its work. Inulin reaches the colon largely undigested by the body itself, and there it is fermented preferentially by *Bifidobacterium* — the genus that includes many of the gentlest and most beneficial gut species, and whose populations climb measurably within a week of inulin entering the diet. Resistant starch — the kind found in cooked-and-cooled potatoes, in green bananas, in properly prepared rice — reaches the colon similarly undigested, and there it is fermented into butyrate by the same *Faecalibacterium* and its colleagues that we met in the opening. Beta-glucans, found in oats and mushrooms and barley, are the food of yet another community of bacteria, ones that do work specifically on the immune system. Pectin, from apples and citrus fruits, supports a different group still.

A diet broad in prebiotic fibers feeds, by design, a broad community. A diet narrow in prebiotic fibers — the typical modern plate, heavy on refined grains and animal products and short on plants — starves whichever species depended on whichever fibers are missing. The bacteria do not move on. They die out. And the chemistry they were producing dies out with them.

The Thirty Plants Per Week

There is a number worth pausing on.

Researchers studying the microbial diversity of healthy human guts noticed, several years ago, that the people whose guts contained the most diverse and resilient communities had something in common in their diets. It was not a matter of total fiber, or total calories, or whether they ate animal products or did not. The common factor, oddly enough, was the count of distinct plant species they ate per week. People eating thirty or more different kinds of plants in a typical week had, on average, microbiomes substantially more diverse than people eating ten or fifteen.

The reason, in light of everything in this chapter so far, will be obvious. Each plant species carries a slightly different mix of fibers, polyphenols, and trace compounds. Each mix feeds a slightly different group of bacteria. A diet that includes thirty distinct plants per week feeds thirty distinct microbial neighborhoods; a diet that includes ten feeds ten. The bacteria that depend on the missing twenty have nothing to eat. They die out, or fail to establish, or persist only as marginal populations. The community thins.

Thirty plants in a week sounds like a lot. It is less than it sounds. A bowl of mixed greens at lunch — spinach, kale, arugula, romaine — is four plants. A vegetable stir-fry with onion, garlic, broccoli, mushroom, and ginger is five more. Berries on cereal in the morning — blueberries, raspberries, strawberries — is three more. A handful of nuts and seeds across a few days — walnuts, almonds, pumpkin seeds, sunflower seeds — is four more. By the second day, a moderately varied eater is already at fifteen or twenty.

But most people, when they actually count, are surprised to find that a typical week lands closer to ten. The same lunch every day. The same vegetables on rotation through the week. A fruit, a grain, a few staples. Variety, in modern eating, has narrowed without most people noticing. Tracking the count, even for a week, is often the single most useful exercise a practitioner can do for the long-term shape of their gut.

The number is not magic. Thirty is not a threshold above which everything works. But it is, in the research, a reliable rough marker of the level of plant variety that produces the kind of microbial diversity associated with long-term health. Most people, when they aim for it, end up eating thirty-five or forty in good weeks and twenty in lean ones, and the average across the year is what shapes the gut.

For the practitioner just past the fast, this is the time to begin tracking. Not anxiously. Just observantly. A list on the refrigerator, a column for each day of the week, a tick mark for each plant. Most people, in the first month of trying, double their plant variety without even particularly trying — simply by paying attention to what they have already been eating and noticing how narrow the rotation has become.

The gut grows as the plate grows. There is no faster way to widen the microbial community than to widen what it is fed.

Phase Three — Diversifying

From Day 60 onward, the community is settling. The seeding has happened. The establishing has happened. The major populations are in place. The work of Phase Three is different in character from the work of the previous phases — less about introduction, more about cultivation. Not what to add, but what to encourage; not new colonies, but the deepening of the colonies that are already there.

Three particular organisms deserve, at this point, proper introductions. They have appeared briefly in the chapter so far. They are worth meeting in full, because if the practitioner ends up cultivating any specific organisms in the long-term life that follows the fast, these are the three most worth the trouble.

Akkermansia muciniphila

The gut wall is lined, on its inner surface, with a layer of mucus. This mucus is not waste. It is a working component of the gut, secreted continuously by specialized cells in the gut wall, replaced every few hours, and serving as the buffer that separates the bulk of the gut contents — including the trillions of bacteria — from the gut wall itself. Without that mucus layer, the microbes would be in direct contact with the cells of the wall, and the immune system would respond to the contact with chronic inflammation. The mucus is the demilitarized zone that makes the partnership possible.

Akkermansia muciniphila lives in that mucus layer.

She is, by sheer name and appearance, an unlikely hero. She is a single-celled bacterium, found nowhere else in nature — only in the mucus layer of the gastrointestinal tract of mammals, where she has lived for tens of millions of years. What she eats is the mucus itself. Specifically, she eats the long sugar chains called mucins that the mucus is made of. As she eats them, she stimulates the gut wall to produce more — a feedback loop in which the act of consuming the mucus signals the body to make more mucus, which then becomes food for more *Akkermansia*, which produces more signal to make more mucus. The mucus layer of a gut with healthy *Akkermansia* populations is thicker, more protective, and more responsive than the mucus layer of a gut without her.

This work is, biologically, almost beyond praise. *Akkermansia* maintains the very wall that separates the partnership's inside from its outside. She is, in plain terms, the bacterium that keeps the boundary intact. Loss of *Akkermansia* — and she is one of the species most consistently lost in modern guts, in obesity, in type-2 diabetes, in inflammatory bowel disease, in metabolic syndrome — is loss of mucus layer integrity. And loss of mucus layer integrity is the first step on the road to what is sometimes called *leaky gut*: a gut wall that has begun to let pass into the bloodstream things that the body has spent its evolutionary history keeping out. Most of the chronic inflammation that drives modern disease begins, in some sense, with this failure.

What feeds *Akkermansia* directly — beyond the mucus she lives on — is a particular class of plant compounds called polyphenols. These are the molecules that give berries their dark color, that make pomegranate astringent, that flavor green tea, that color extra-virgin olive oil, that make dark chocolate dark. Most of them reach the colon largely undigested by the body itself, and there they feed *Akkermansia* preferentially. A diet rich in polyphenols produces a thicker, healthier mucus layer through the work of this single organism. A diet poor in them produces the opposite.

Akkermansia is, for these reasons, one of the most important targets of long-term cultivation. Polyphenols are her food. The work of the long-term diet is, in part, the work of feeding her well.

Faecalibacterium prausnitzii (returning)

The reader has already met *Faecalibacterium*, in the opening trace. There is more to say about her, and Phase Three is the place to say it.

Faecalibacterium is one of the most abundant bacteria in a healthy human gut — sometimes accounting for as much as five percent of the total population — and one of the most reliably absent in disease. The opening of this chapter mentioned her absence in inflammatory bowel disease and certain cancers. The list extends further: she is depleted in obesity, in type-2 diabetes, in metabolic syndrome, in major depression, in inflammatory bowel disease, in colorectal cancer, in chronic kidney disease, and in nearly every condition that involves chronic inflammation as part of its mechanism. The pattern is so consistent that researchers have proposed using her abundance as a single-organism marker of gut health — the *Faecalibacterium* count, on its own, predicting health and disease with striking accuracy.

What she does is what we have already seen: she ferments certain plant fibers — particularly the inulin and resistant starches discussed in the previous section — and produces butyrate as the byproduct. The butyrate feeds the colon wall, suppresses inflammation systemically, and reaches eventually into the brain. She is, more than any other single organism, the engine of the partnership's anti-inflammatory work.

What feeds her well is a diet rich in resistant starch and inulin. Cooked-and-cooled potatoes. Green bananas. Properly prepared rice. Onions, garlic, leeks, asparagus. A practitioner who eats these foods regularly is, in microbial terms, deliberately cultivating *Faecalibacterium*. A practitioner who does not is, by default, allowing the population to thin.

The butyrate producers as a family

Beyond *Faecalibacterium*, several other bacterial species produce butyrate as well — including organisms in the genera *Roseburia*, *Eubacterium*, and *Coprococcus*. They are quieter characters than *Faecalibacterium*, less abundant, less individually well-studied, but they are part of the same broader community of butyrate-makers, and their combined output is what the colon depends on for its baseline butyrate supply.

What feeds them, broadly, is the same plant fiber that feeds *Faecalibacterium*, with somewhat different specificities for different members of the family. A diet broad in plant fiber — many kinds, from many sources — feeds the whole family. A diet narrow in plant fiber feeds only the few members whose preferred fibers are still present.

The cultivation strategy, for the long term, is straightforward. Eat polyphenols for *Akkermansia*. Eat inulin and resistant starch for *Faecalibacterium*. Eat broad plant variety for the butyrate-makers as a group. The three strategies converge, in practice, on a single recommendation: eat lots of plants, of many kinds, with deep colors, prepared in various ways, every week.

The chapter has been building, one section at a time, toward exactly this conclusion. The next section names the foods.

Foods That Feed the Partnership Well

The foods that most reliably feed the partnership fall into three groups. None of them are exotic. Most of them are foods the practitioner already knows. What is new, after the chapter so far, is the reason behind each one.

Polyphenol-rich foods

These are the foods that feed *Akkermansia*, the keeper of the mucus layer. They are also food for a wider range of other beneficial organisms, but *Akkermansia* is the most consistent recipient.

• **Dark berries** — blueberries, blackberries, raspberries, the darker the better. The pigments that make them dark are the polyphenols in question.

• **Pomegranate.** Among the most polyphenol-dense foods that exist. The astringency on the tongue is the chemistry the colon will receive.

• **Dark chocolate,** 70 percent cacao or higher. The cacao itself is the source. Sugar in the chocolate works against the benefit, so darker is better.

• **Green tea.** A regular daily cup, unsweetened, is one of the cheapest and most reliable polyphenol deliveries available.

• **Olive oil,** extra virgin. The "extra virgin" matters; the polyphenols are concentrated in the unrefined oil and reduced or absent in the refined. The slight peppery bite at the back of the throat from a good olive oil is the polyphenols announcing themselves.

• **Red wine,** in moderation. The polyphenols are real, but the alcohol is its own complication, and the right amount of wine is no more than a glass, no more than a few times a week.

• **Coffee.** Yes, even after the cleanse. Coffee is among the densest polyphenol foods in the typical diet, and the practitioner who fully avoids it after refeeding is missing out on a substantial source.

Healthy fats supporting the microbiome

The microbial community responds to dietary fat differently depending on the kind. Industrial seed oils — soybean, corn, cottonseed, safflower, sunflower in its high-linoleic form — drive inflammation through pathways that the gut community is exquisitely sensitive to. The fats that support the partnership, by contrast, are the ones the body has co-evolved with.

• **Avocado.**

• **Coconut oil.** And MCT oil, the medium-chain fatty acid concentrate that has been part of the protocol since Day 1 of refeeding.

• **Olive oil,** the same extra-virgin oil noted above.

• **Ground flax, chia, and hemp seeds** for plant-based omega-3 fats.

• **Nuts and seeds,** particularly walnuts, soaked when possible to reduce the antinutrients that interfere with mineral absorption.

Specific microbiome foods

Some foods are not categorizable under either polyphenol or fat, but earn their place at the long-term table for what they do specifically for the gut community.

• **Fermented vegetables,** daily ideally. Sauerkraut, kimchi, fermented carrots, beet kvass. Each one contains a different microbial community.

• **Bone broth.** Supports the gut lining itself with the amino acids the lining draws on, and provides minerals that the lining uses in its repair work.

• **Mushroom variety.** Both as food and as a source of beta-glucans and other compounds that interact with the immune system through the gut.

• **Diverse colored vegetables.** The phytonutrients across the color spectrum — red, orange, yellow, green, purple — feed different bacterial communities. The colorful plate is, in microbial terms, the diversified plate.

These foods, taken together, are not a special diet. They are not unusual or expensive or hard to find. They are, in fact, mostly the foods that traditional cuisines around the world have arranged themselves around for centuries. The Mediterranean diet's olive oil and wine and produce. The Japanese diet's fermented soy and seaweed and green tea. The Korean diet's kimchi and fermented vegetables. The traditional Indian diet's variety of spices and legumes and fermented dairy. None of these traditions arose from microbiome research; the science is younger than any of them by centuries. But the people who developed and refined those traditions over generations were, without knowing it, building cuisines that fed the partnership well.

The partnership has been studied scientifically for perhaps thirty years. It has been fed correctly, by accident and by tradition, for thousands.

What Disrupts the Partnership

The chapter has, by this point, made the case for what to feed the community. There is a corresponding case for what not to feed it — what to keep out, or to reduce dramatically, particularly in the first sixty days when the new community is establishing.

The chart below sets out the items most worth restricting. Each one disrupts the partnership in a specific way, and the reasoning matters. A blanket restriction is easy to ignore; a restriction whose reason is understood is easier to honor.

Chart O — What to Avoid

Item	Why
At least for the first 60 days	
Processed foods	Stripped of minerals during processing; what remains feeds the wrong organisms
Refined sugar	Feeds the wrong organisms
Artificial sweeteners	Disrupt the microbiome
Industrial seed oils	Pro-inflammatory
Heavily processed grain products	Refining removes the bran, germ, and key minerals; what remains feeds the wrong organisms
Conventional dairy	Pesticide and antibiotic residues
Conventional meat	Antibiotic residues affect the microbiome
Long-term moderation	
Antibiotics	Only when truly necessary
Excessive alcohol	Disrupts the microbiome
Chronic stress	Directly affects microbial composition
Lack of sleep	Disrupts diurnal microbial rhythms
Sedentary lifestyle	Physical activity influences the microbiome

The pattern, looked at carefully, is the same pattern as the section on what has been broken. The disruptors are the same forces that produced the modern microbial impoverishment in the first place — antibiotics direct and indirect, processed food, chronic stress, sleep debt, the disrupted rhythms of modern life. A practitioner who has just spent thirty or forty days on a fast, and several months on a careful refeeding, is in a position to substantially reduce these disruptors going forward — not absolutely, but to the degree that real life allows.

Two notes on the long-term moderation list are worth adding.

On antibiotics specifically. Antibiotics, when genuinely needed, are needed. A serious bacterial infection is not the moment to refuse antibiotics in service of the microbiome; the cost-benefit shifts entirely when the alternative is a life-threatening illness. But many of the antibiotic prescriptions in the modern world are, by the consensus of careful prescribers, not strictly needed — given prophylactically, given for viral infections that antibiotics do not affect, given to satisfy a patient's expectation rather than to treat an underlying condition. The practitioner who has rebuilt a careful microbiome will, going forward, want to be a more selective consumer of antibiotics. Asking the prescribing physician whether the antibiotic is genuinely needed for the specific condition, and whether the more targeted narrow-spectrum option is available rather than the broad-spectrum option, is a reasonable conversation to have.

On sleep. The microbial community runs, as the earlier section discussed, on a daily rhythm that mirrors the body's. Chronic sleep debt is, in microbial terms, chronic interruption of that rhythm. The practitioner who works to establish a steady sleep pattern after the fast — going to bed near the same time, sleeping in the dark, allowing the long uninterrupted overnight period — is, without thinking about it as such, supporting the microbial community as much as supporting their own sleep. The two are the same support.

The disruptors above are not a list to be perfect about. Real life includes occasional restaurant meals, occasional disrupted sleep, occasional courses of antibiotics that genuinely help. What matters is the average. A community fed mostly well, disrupted occasionally, recovers between disruptions and remains intact. A community disrupted constantly, with brief windows of being fed well, never recovers and slowly impoverishes.

How to Know It Is Working

The signs that the partnership is reestablishing well are felt across the body, not just in the gut. By the time the reader has spent a few months in this work, the changes will be obvious — but they will be obvious in places the reader did not expect them.

Positive signs:

- **Energy stable and high.** Not the artificial spikes of caffeine or sugar, but the steady, low-grade aliveness that holds across a day.

- **Mental clarity sustained.** Concentration that does not require effort. Thinking that moves cleanly from one thing to the next.

- **Digestion working well across diverse foods.** The capacity to eat what is in front of one without anxiety about what it will do.

- **Stool quality good** — well-formed, regular, not requiring strain. The downstream signal of a functional colon.

- **No return of pre-fast symptoms.** The conditions that drove the fast — the digestive issues, the energy issues, the skin issues — staying quieted.

- **Skin clear and healthy.** The chain through the bloodstream we traced earlier, working as it should.

- **Sleep deep and restorative.** The body using the night for the work of repair.

- **Mood stable.** Not the absence of difficult feelings, but the presence of an inner ground that holds across them.

- **Immune function evident** — fewer minor illnesses, faster recovery from the ones that pass through.

• **General sense of vitality.** The animal aliveness that the reader, in the years before the fast, may have forgotten was the baseline.

Signs of concern:

• Return of digestive symptoms.

• Energy issues returning.

• Mood changes.

• Skin issues recurring.

• Frequent minor illness.

• Brain fog returning.

If concerning signs appear, the work is to assess and adjust. Sometimes specific testing helps identify what is happening — a comprehensive stool analysis can distinguish a return of parasitic load from a microbial imbalance from a gut-lining issue, and the appropriate response is different in each case. More often, though, the cause is identifiable from the practitioner's own experience: a stretch of disrupted sleep, a stretch of disrupted eating, a course of antibiotics taken for an unrelated reason. Returning to the practices that worked — the fermented foods, the prebiotic-rich diet, the steady sleep, the eating window — usually returns the partnership to its work within a few weeks.

The body is patient with this. The microbial community responds to good conditions quickly. What was lost in a course of antibiotics can be substantially recovered in a month of careful eating. What was lost across years of disrupted living takes longer, but the direction of recovery is, in most people, available.

Closing — The Trace, Returned

There is a kind of morning that arrives, sometimes, in the months after a long fast.

The light comes through the window early. The sleep that preceded it was deep. The body feels quiet — that particular quiet that is not absence but presence. The mind is clear in a way that does not require effort. The breath comes easily. Hunger arrives, when it arrives, as a clean signal. The skin in the bathroom mirror looks like the skin of someone several years younger than the person who began the fast. There is a steadiness across the whole interior.

The reader, this time, knows what is happening.

The morning is a chain. The steadiness of the mood is the calm of the microglia is the quiet of the inflammation is the steady arrival of butyrate is the work of *Faecalibacterium* on yesterday's serving of cooked vegetables. The clear skin is the same chain, branching through the bloodstream. The deep sleep is the long uninterrupted overnight stretch in which the microbial community ran its rhythm undisturbed. The immune function is the conversation between the gut wall and the bacteria on the other side of it, settling, day by day, into something closer to right calibration. The hormonal steadiness is the estrobolome, doing its work with diversity restored.

The morning is the chain. The chain is the partnership. The partnership is the work of every meal, every night of sleep, every day of the kind of living that allows the community to do its work.

Tend it, and the morning holds.

Neglect it — through stress that goes uncaught, sleep that thins, diet that narrows, antibiotics taken without thought — and the morning thins with it. The chain still runs. It just runs through a thinner forest, with fewer organisms, producing less of what the rest of the body depends on. The reader will, in that case, gradually notice the morning becoming less of what it was. Not dramatically. Not all at once. The way most modern people experience their bodies as the years pass.

The work is daily. It is also, mostly, simple. Eat plants of many kinds. Eat fermented foods. Eat the fats the body co-evolved with. Sleep in the dark, in long unbroken stretches, on a rhythm. Avoid antibiotics when they are not needed. Spend time with the kind of microbial input the body evolved to expect — outside, in dirt, with other living things, away from sterile surfaces and recirculated air. Allow the partnership to do what it has, in the lineage of organisms the reader descends from, been doing for a billion years.

The fast cleared the field. The first weeks of refeeding planted the seeds. The months that follow are when the forest grows.

There will be no single moment when the work is finished. It is not that kind of work. There will only be, gradually, the recognition that the morning the reader is now experiencing is the morning that, in the years before, they had stopped expecting. That the body they are walking around in is the body they were always supposed to have. That the partnership, which has been doing its work in the dark of the gut for as long as there have been bodies of this kind, is finally, and quietly, being allowed to.

The forest tends itself, when it is given the conditions.

The reader's part is the conditions.

Chapter 31

The 30-Day Refeeding Plan

* * *

The thirty days after the breaking of a fast ask for as much care as the fast itself. These are templates, not rigid prescriptions. Adapt to your specific situation, dietary preferences, and food availability. The principles are what matter — slow buildup, quality foods, diverse plants, adequate protein, continued microbiome support. The schedule below is the day-by-day version of those principles, translated into the food on your plate.

Days 1 to 3 — Liquid Foundation

Day 1:

• Morning: 4 oz fresh celery juice diluted with 4 oz water.

• Late morning: 4 oz vegetable broth.

• Midday: 4 oz bone broth (light, well-strained).

• Afternoon: 4 oz coconut water.

• Evening: 4 oz vegetable broth with 1/4 tsp ghee.

• Throughout: trace minerals, mineralized water.

Day 2:

• Slightly larger portions — 6 oz each.

• Add: pureed avocado in broth (1 tablespoon).

• Add: small amount of fresh leafy green juice.

• Continue mineral supplementation.

Day 3:

• 6 to 8 oz portions.

• Add: small amount of pureed steamed zucchini in broth.

• Add: 1 tsp ghee in evening broth.

• Begin: small amount of fermented vegetable juice.

Days 4 to 7 — Soft Foods Introduction

Day 4 sample:

• Breakfast: smoothie — coconut milk, half avocado, small handful spinach, 1 tsp coconut oil.

• Lunch: bone broth with pureed cauliflower, 1 tablespoon olive oil.

• Snack: coconut water with trace minerals.

• Dinner: vegetable broth with pureed sweet potato, 1 tsp ghee.

Days 5 to 6 progression:

• Adding well-cooked oatmeal with coconut milk.

• Adding pureed steamed vegetables in variety.

• Adding small amounts of soft cooked egg if applicable.

• Adding fermented vegetable juice — 1 tablespoon.

Day 7:

• Three small meals plus snacks.

• Soft cooked vegetables.

• Pureed soups.

• Beginning probiotic supplementation.

• Small portions of cooked legumes if tolerated.

Week 2 (Days 8 to 14) — Building Solid Foods

Sample Day 10:

• Breakfast: soft scrambled eggs with avocado and steamed spinach (or for vegetarians: a small bowl of well-cooked lentils with avocado and steamed spinach).

• Mid-morning: small piece of fruit, half banana.

• Lunch: vegetable soup with quinoa and well-cooked vegetables.

• Afternoon: coconut yogurt with berries.

• Dinner: well-cooked lentils or hemp-seed-crusted vegetables with steamed greens, small portion of rice.

• Throughout: continued hydration, herbs at reduced doses.

Day 14 broader options:

• Soft cooked grains in modest portions.

• Variety of well-cooked vegetables.

• Cooked legumes building up.

• Soft cooked eggs daily for those who eat them.

• Small portions of well-cooked lentils or hemp seeds in soft preparations.

• Fermented vegetables with meals.

Week 3 (Days 15 to 21) — Expanding the Diet

Sample Day 18:

• Breakfast: oatmeal with berries, walnuts, coconut milk, cinnamon.

• Mid-morning: apple with small amount of almond butter.

• Lunch: quinoa bowl with roasted vegetables, sauerkraut, tahini dressing, avocado.

• Afternoon: green smoothie with kefir.

• Dinner: lentil soup with cooked greens, sourdough bread (small portion).

• Continued mineralization.

Adding through this week:

• Raw foods, beginning gradually with small portions.

• Salads, starting with tender greens, well-chopped.

• Nuts and seeds, soaked when possible.

• Greater variety of fruits, including some raw.

• More substantial protein portions.

• Sourdough or sprouted bread in moderate amounts.

Week 4 (Days 22 to 30) — Approaching Normal Eating

Sample Day 25:

• Breakfast: smoothie bowl with kefir, berries, granola, hemp seeds, ghee.

• Mid-morning: hard-boiled egg with sauerkraut.

- Lunch: large salad with quinoa, roasted vegetables, chickpeas, avocado, fermented vegetables, olive oil.
- Afternoon: apple with cheese (if tolerated) or hummus.
- Dinner: roasted seasoned lentils with roasted vegetables, sweet potato, large green salad.
- Evening: herbal tea, small piece of dark chocolate.

Approaching normal eating:

- Three balanced meals plus snacks.
- Wide variety of foods.
- All food groups except processed foods.
- Fermented food at most meals.
- Continued attention to hydration and minerals.
- Continued modified herbal protocol if appropriate.

Beyond Day 30 — The New Normal

Day 31 and forward is integration into long-term healthy eating. The intensive phase is complete. What remains is the sustained, daily practice that maintains what the intensive phase accomplished.

Core principles continuing:

- **Plant diversity.** Aim for 30+ different plant species weekly. Rotate through colors, families, and varieties. Seasonal eating naturally provides diversity.
- **Fermented foods daily.** Include something fermented at most meals. Variety across the week.
- **Adequate protein.** For tissue maintenance and rebuilding. Variety of sources.
- **Quality fats.** Olive oil, avocado, coconut, nuts, and seeds. Continue MCT or coconut oil for some ketone capacity.
- **Whole foods focus.** Minimize processed foods. Cook from scratch primarily. Quality ingredients.
- **Continued mineralization.** Trace minerals daily. Mineralized water habit continued.
- **Continued microbiome support.** Probiotics ongoing or via fermented foods. Prebiotic-rich foods regularly. Avoid microbiome disruptors.

What to Watch For During Refeeding

Positive signs:

• Energy continuing to improve.

• Digestion working well.

• Mental clarity sustained.

• Sleep good.

• Mood stable.

• Continued sense of cleanness internally.

Signs that suggest going slower:

• Bloating after meals.

• Gas or digestive discomfort.

• Energy crashes.

• Brain fog returning.

• Sleep disruption.

• Skin breakouts.

If concerning signs appear, slow the progression, return to simpler foods, and identify potential triggers.

A Few Reminders

The refeeding period is not just about reintroducing food. It is about establishing new patterns, rebuilding the microbiome with intention, honoring what the cleanse accomplished, and setting up the long-term gains. Take it seriously. Move slowly. Pay attention. Adjust as needed. The 30 days of refeeding determine, in many ways, how well the gains of the fast persist into the months and years that follow.

Chapter 32

Long-Term Parasite Prevention

* * *

The cleanse cleared what was there. The continuation protocol consolidated the work. The refeeding rebuilt the microbiome. Now comes the question that determines everything: how do you protect what you have achieved?

The honest answer begins with a clarification. Total permanent prevention is unrealistic. You live in a world where parasitic exposure is part of biological reality. Even the most careful person will be exposed periodically. But — and this matters — exposure is not the same as infection. A strong immune system, healthy microbiome, and intact intestinal barrier handle most parasitic exposures naturally without establishing infection. What you have built through the cleanse and refeeding is a body capable of handling exposure without succumbing to establishment.

Prevention, therefore, is about two things. Reducing unnecessary exposure. Maintaining the strong defense that handles unavoidable exposure.

Practical Prevention Practices

Water — your first defense.

• *Drinking water:* Always filter — minimum carbon filter, reverse osmosis ideal. When traveling, bottled water from reputable sources. Avoid drinking from natural sources without proper treatment. Be especially cautious in foreign countries.

• *Cooking water:* Use filtered water for cooking too. Particularly important for foods that absorb water during cooking — rice, pasta.

• *Ice:* Often forgotten, but ice in restaurants can be a source of parasitic exposure. Particularly important when traveling — request drinks without ice. Even at home, use filtered water for ice.

• *Swimming:* Public pools — chlorine kills most pathogens but not all (Cryptosporidium is resistant). Lakes and rivers, variable risk depending on location. Hot tubs, higher microbial load. Be aware of swallowing water during swimming.

Food preparation.

• *Produce:* Wash all fresh produce thoroughly. For greater safety, soak in filtered water with apple cider vinegar for 10 minutes. Particularly important for produce eaten raw. Organic does not equal parasite-free — wash everything.

• *Meat and fish:* Cook meat to proper internal temperatures. Particularly important for pork (Trichinella), beef (tapeworm), fish (Anisakis). Be cautious with sushi — know the source and preparation standards. Frozen fish for sushi should be commercially frozen at proper temperature.

• *Restaurants:* Choose establishments with good hygiene reputation. Be cautious with raw foods at unknown places. When traveling, pay attention to reputation and reviews.

Personal hygiene.

• *Hand washing:* before eating, after using toilet, after contact with soil or animals, after contact with raw meat or fish.

• *Bathroom hygiene:* wipe thoroughly, wash hands after every bathroom use. Be aware that pinworm transmission especially happens through hand contact.

• *Clothing and bedding:* hot wash bedding regularly. Particularly important if anyone in household has parasitic infection. Pinworm eggs survive on surfaces for weeks.

Lifestyle awareness.

• *Footwear outdoors:* Wear shoes when walking on soil. Particularly important in warm climates where hookworm and Strongyloides are present. Beach walking — be aware of contaminated sand.

• *Pets:* Regular deworming for pets is essential. Wash hands after pet contact. Especially important if pets sleep with you. Indoor cats less risk than outdoor cats.

• *Travel:* Heightened awareness in countries with different sanitation standards. Bottled water exclusively. Avoid raw produce in higher-risk areas. Cooked and hot foods safer. Consider preventive herbal protocol during and after travel.

Maintenance Protocols

The maintenance work scales in three layers — quarterly light protocols, annual resets, and periodic major cleanses every several years.

Quarterly herbal protocol. Every 3 months, a brief preventive cleanse.

One-week protocol:

• Black walnut hull tincture — 1 teaspoon twice daily.

• Wormwood tincture — 4 drops twice daily.

• Clove tincture — 4 drops three times daily.

• Mimosa pudica — 1 capsule twice daily.

• All with piperine.

This catches any new exposures before they establish, maintains pressure on any small populations, supports continued microbiome health, and keeps the parasite garden weeded.

Annual reset. Once per year, a more thorough but shorter intensive period.

Two-week protocol:

• Full daily herbal protocol.

• Daily enemas.

• Coffee enema 2 to 3 times in the period.

• Strict dietary discipline during this period.

This serves as comprehensive maintenance, periodic intensive cleansing, a relationship with the protocol that sustains awareness, and significant ongoing prevention.

Periodic major cleanses. Every 3 to 5 years, consider another prolonged fast. Even with maintenance, some accumulation occurs. Major life events, illness, antibiotic use can disrupt the gains. Periodic deeper work maintains the optimal state long-term. Subsequent fasts build on previous ones — each is more effective than the last because the foundation is already in place.

Timing considerations: after significant antibiotic use, after major travel to higher-risk areas, when symptoms suggest accumulation, or as preventive maintenance even without specific signs.

Building Strong Defense

Beyond avoiding exposure, strengthening the body's response to exposure is the second pillar of prevention. A strong defense handles routine exposures without consequence.

Microbiome maintenance:

• Continued fermented foods daily.

• Continued prebiotic-rich foods.

• Continued plant diversity.

• Periodic probiotic supplementation.

• Avoiding microbiome disruptors when possible.

Immune system support:

- Adequate sleep.
- Stress management.
- Regular movement.
- Sun exposure for vitamin D.
- Adequate protein.
- Avoiding chronic inflammation triggers.

Intestinal lining maintenance:

- L-Glutamine periodically.
- Bone broth regularly.
- Healthy fats including coconut oil.
- Avoiding gut disruptors — gluten for sensitive individuals, processed foods, excessive alcohol.

Liver function:

- Periodic liver-supporting practices.
- Milk thistle periodically.
- Coffee enema occasionally.
- Adequate hydration always.
- Avoiding excessive toxic load.

Living With Awareness, Not Paranoia

All of this could create anxiety. That is not the goal. The healthy mindset is awareness of exposure routes, reasonable precautions where they make sense, trust in the body's defense capability, periodic maintenance practice — not obsession or anxiety.

You can travel. You can eat at restaurants. You can have pets. You can live a normal life. The point is to live normally with awareness, not to avoid life out of fear.

The mindset that serves you over the long term is one in which reasonable precautions become automatic, periodic maintenance is integrated into life, awareness of warning signs exists without hypervigilance, trust in the cleansed and supported body is the default, and you remain engaged with the world rather than withdrawn from it.

Warning Signs Worth Noting

If any of these appear over time, consider whether maintenance protocols need intensification:

• Return of pre-cleanse symptoms.

• New digestive issues.

• Energy declining without clear cause.

• Mental fog returning.

• Skin issues recurring.

• Sleep deteriorating.

• Mood changes.

These signs do not necessarily mean parasitic activity — many factors can cause them. But they are worth investigating, including consideration of whether parasitic activity is reestablishing.

Testing as Tool

For those who want objective confirmation:

• Annual GI Map test.

• Provides ongoing baseline.

• Catches new establishment early.

• Confirms maintenance is working.

• Guides any needed adjustments.

This is especially valuable for those at higher exposure risk — international travelers, agricultural workers, healthcare workers, and others whose lifestyle places them in regular contact with elevated parasite exposure.

A Long-Term Perspective

Your relationship with parasitic exposure is now lifelong. But it can be a relationship of informed awareness rather than ignorance. Of strong defense rather than vulnerability. Of periodic maintenance rather than chronic accumulation.

What you have built through this protocol is something you can maintain. With relatively modest ongoing effort, you can preserve the gains for decades. The major work is done. The maintenance is comparatively light. The benefits continue. This is what makes the intensive work worthwhile — not just the immediate transformation, but the decades of sustained health that follow when the work is properly maintained.

Chapter 33

The Long Partnership

* * *

There is a kitchen, in a small house at the edge of a town, where a man cooked for the first months after his fast the way the book had taught him to cook.

A wide blue ceramic bowl on the counter, filled with whatever vegetable the season offered. A jar of olive oil beside the stove. On the refrigerator door a tall jar of kimchi, and beside it a glass of water-kefir from the mother culture in the cupboard. He ate his first meal a little after one in the afternoon, at the small wooden table by the window, slowly, watching the light move across the floor of the room. He ate his last meal before the light left the sky. The body that had come back to him after the long fast was the body that the kitchen, in those months, was tuned to support.

The first season passed. The second season passed. By the eighth month the kitchen had begun, very gently, to change.

The blue bowl was still on the counter, but it held two oranges and a banana that was beginning to brown. The olive oil was still beside the stove, although a bottle of vegetable oil had appeared next to it some weeks ago. The kimchi jar that had lived on the refrigerator door for the first six months was gone — the last one had finished in May, and he had been meaning to buy another. The water-kefir mother had thinned in the warm weeks of July without anyone noticing, and the empty jar had been moved to the back of the cupboard. He still ate at the small wooden table when he was home. But he was home less. And the meals had started arriving earlier and ending later, until on most days the table was being used from ten in the morning until nine at night.

None of these changes had been decided. A visitor would not have seen them at all. Only the man, if he had stopped and looked carefully, would have seen them, and he had not been looking carefully.

If you had asked him whether he was still keeping the practice, he would not have said no. He would have said something like mostly, or for the most part, and he would have meant it. He had not abandoned anything. The fermented foods had simply gone quiet in his kitchen the way certain birds go quiet in a wood when the soil beneath the trees has changed. Nothing dramatic had happened. Nothing was missing in any way that called attention to itself. The kitchen was still a kitchen. It only failed, slowly and almost invisibly, to be the kitchen the body needed it to be.

By the end of the first year the body had begun to remember a little of how it had felt before the fast. Not all of it. The brain fog had not fully returned, and the joints were quieter than they had been, and the sleep was better than it had been. But the morning energy had thinned. The skin was a little less clear. The clean signal of hunger that had arrived, in the early months, near the middle of the day, had given way again to the older, noisier hunger of the body that ate from the moment it woke.

This is the first failure mode of the long practice. Not the dramatic abandonment, the falling-off-the-wagon, the conscious return to old patterns. The slow, almost invisible thinning of the practice into something that looks, from outside, like the same practice. The same kitchen. The same intentions. Less and less of the actual work.

It is also, structurally, the first failure mode of a long marriage.

A marriage does not usually end in a fight. It ends in a slow thinning of attention across years, in which the conversations that used to happen at bedtime stop happening one at a time and never with announcement, until one day one of the partners looks up and notices that the other person has become a presence in the room rather than a person being attended to. The marriage was still a marriage. It only failed, slowly and almost invisibly, to be the marriage the partners needed it to be.

This chapter is about what is required to prevent that thinning. In a body. In a kitchen. In a relationship that has to last decades.

What is required, it turns out, is the same thing in all three.

* * *

Most people who do a prolonged fast and a careful refeeding do not maintain the gains a year later. The statistics on this are not encouraging. Even among practitioners who came to the work seriously, who did the protocol carefully, who experienced the changes the work produces, the majority drift back, across the months and years that follow, toward the patterns that produced the problem in the first place.

This is not because the protocols were wrong. The protocols are sound. The book the man in the opening had read was a careful book, and the practice it described was a real practice, and the body it gave him back was a real body. The protocols held while he was paying attention. They thinned when he stopped.

The same is true of marriages. Most long marriages that end did not end because the partners had irreconcilable differences, or because something fundamental was wrong with the partnership. They ended because attention thinned. The conversations that used to happen at bedtime stopped happening, one at a time, never with announcement, always with reason. The work changed, the days got long, the children needed something, a parent got sick. None of these were the year the marriage ended. Each was an ordinary stretch of difficult life. The marriages that lasted through such years lasted because the partners kept paying attention to each other across them. The marriages that did not last did not lose the attention all at once. They lost it the way the kimchi jar disappeared from the refrigerator door — once, in May, and never quite replaced.

This is the failure mode the chapter is about. Not the dramatic one. The quiet one.

It is worth saying clearly that the dramatic failure modes — the practitioner who decides on a Tuesday to start eating processed food again, the spouse who walks out — are easier to defend against than the quiet ones, precisely because they announce themselves. The body and the partner both know what is happening when the dramatic failure occurs. There is a moment of decision; the decision can be reconsidered. The quiet failure has no moment of decision. It happens through cumulative inattention, in tens of thousands of small omissions, none of which look serious in the moment. By the time the cumulative effect is visible, years have passed and the work of recovery is much larger than the work of prevention would have been.

What goes missing, in both cases, is not knowledge of the protocol. The man in the opening still knew, in his eighth month, that the kimchi belonged on the refrigerator door. He knew the eating window was supposed to close before the light left the sky. The knowledge had not left him. What had left him was the daily, low-level attention to the practice that translated knowledge into action.

What goes missing in a long marriage is, in just the same way, not knowledge of the partner. The husband who has been married twenty years still knows, in the abstract, what kind of person his wife is. He could describe her to a stranger. He could list her preferences. What he has stopped doing, without noticing, is reading her — the small daily reading of what kind of mood has just walked into the room, what kind of cup of coffee would land well this morning, what kind of evening the day has been preparing her for. The reading was the practice. The reading was what kept the marriage actually a marriage rather than a shared address.

The same kind of reading is what keeps a body actually a partnership rather than a vehicle.

* * *

What ends a marriage, and what ends a long practice, and what ends the partnership a person has with their own body, is the same thing. It is the gradual loss of a particular kind of attention. The word attention needs to be pinned down here, because it does too much work in ordinary use, and the version this chapter is asking for is specific.

It is not vigilance. It is not the practitioner who scans the body each morning for warning signs and waits for one of them to appear. That version produces, in time, a body that responds to its owner's anxiety by becoming more anxious, less regulated, harder to read. The body, like a partner, withdraws when the looking is fearful.

It is not a checklist. It is not a daily journal of what was eaten and when, what was felt and how strongly, what was slept and how well. The checklist has its uses in the early months, when the practice is new and the body is still teaching the practitioner what its signals mean. But the practice that holds across decades is not a practice of recording. It is a practice of recognizing.

The version this chapter is asking for is the kind that runs below conscious thought. Consider what happens, on an ordinary morning, in the kitchen of a couple who have been married for thirty years.

He is at the counter, making coffee. The water heating, the grounds measured, the kettle small and loud. He is not thinking about his wife. He is not thinking about anything. He is making the coffee. She walks in. He looks up. The looking up takes less than half a second, and in that half-second his eyes register, without any of it requiring conscious thought, that she has not slept well, that she is wearing the soft grey cardigan she wears on the mornings she wants the house to be quiet, and that she is carrying the kind of mood that will lift if a cup of coffee arrives in front of her without her having to ask for it. He pours the coffee. He sets it on the table by the window. She sits down, wraps her hands around it, exhales. None of the exchange registers in either of them as anything. It happens almost every morning. It is the practice the marriage is built on.

The half-second of looking up is the practice. The cup of coffee is the visible tip of it. Below the surface lies an enormous accumulated reading, gathered across thousands of mornings, that the husband does not have to think about because the practice of reading has become the way he inhabits the room his wife is in.

The same kind of reading is possible with a body, and is what the long practice consists of.

It does not look like much, from outside. It looks like a person who, in the first moment of waking, before the eyes have fully opened, already knows what kind of morning the body has given them. It looks like a person who, halfway through a meal, registers without having to think about it that something at this particular dinner is sitting heavily and that the body would like the meal to end soon. It looks like a person who, walking through an ordinary week, notices that the energy is lower than it was last week and adjusts the week accordingly — earlier sleep, lighter food, a longer walk, a quieter weekend — without ever quite formulating the adjustment as a decision.

This kind of reading is not effortful. The body, like a long-married partner, is producing signals continuously. The signals arrive whether anyone is reading them or not. The question is whether anyone is reading them.

The reader who has been paying this kind of attention to their body for years arrives at a place that is, in its essential structure, identical to the place the long-married husband has arrived at by his thirtieth year of marriage. The reading happens automatically. The body becomes a presence whose current state is steadily available, the way a long-married partner's current state is steadily available, in the first half-second of looking up. Most days, the answer is fine. On the days when the answer is not fine, the response begins early, while the not-fine is still small.

What the chapter is calling attention is this: the steady, low, almost automatic reading of what is currently true about a partner — body or person — who has been read, daily, for years. It is the mechanism by which long marriages remain alive. It is the mechanism by which long practices hold. The seven pillars that come next are not seven things to do. They are seven different aspects of this reading, applied to the seven aspects of the body that most reward being read.

What that practice looks like, day to day, is what comes next.

* * *

The practice begins, on most days, before you are fully awake.

There is a moment, after sleep has lifted and before the eyes have opened, when the body's report arrives unsolicited. The breath is moving easily, or it is not. The mind is quiet, or it is not. The shoulders are soft, or there is the small held tightness that means the day before was harder than you registered. The jaw is unclenched, or it is held. Hunger has not arrived, or it is arriving early in a way that suggests something at last night's dinner is still being processed. Most mornings, the answer is fine. The body has done its slow inner work in the dark, and the morning that follows will be an ordinary morning.

You do not have to ask for this report. The body sends it. What the practice asks of you is that you receive it.

Most mornings the receiving takes less than a few seconds. The eyes open. The body's state has already been noted. The day proceeds. You get up, you drink water, you move into whatever the morning is.

On the days when the report comes back different, the receiving takes a little longer. The breath was tight in the lower ribs; the dinner sat heavily; the energy is low in a way that resembles other late winters. None of this produces alarm. The reading is not the kind of reading that turns small signals into large fears. It is the kind that produces small adjustments. A lighter breakfast. A walk before the work begins. Earlier sleep tonight. A quiet weekend, if the body has been asking for one for several days. The adjustments are not decisions, exactly. They are the body's request being honored without ceremony.

This is the daily form of the practice. It is not effortful. It does not involve a journal, or a morning checklist, or a sustained interior conversation with the body about what it needs. It is closer to the way a long-married partner reads the mood of the person who has just walked into the kitchen — already known, by the time the looking up has happened, in a half-second.

There is also a periodic form of the practice, which moves on a longer rhythm.

Once a week, there is a morning when you take a slightly longer measure. Sunday, perhaps, when the week ahead is being prepared for. The body across the past week — was it, on the whole, well? Where did it ask for something it did not get? What is the energy beneath the day's energy, the steadier reading that comes from looking at seven mornings rather than one? Once a season, there is a longer measure still. Has the body, across the past three months, been moving in the direction it was moving the season before? Is something thinning that should not be? Is something arriving that wants attention now while it is small?

The seasonal measure is the one that catches what the daily measure misses. Some changes in a body are slow enough that no single morning can see them; only the comparison of mornings, across months, reveals the slope. The practitioner who keeps the seasonal measure will catch, in early autumn, the small thinning that began in late spring, while it is still small, while it is still easy to address.

None of this should be confused with anxious self-monitoring.

There is a version of bodily attention that is not the practice. It is the version in which the body becomes a thing to be inspected for signs of failure — a project to be managed, a system to be monitored, a daily report card to be filled out. That version produces a particular kind of suffering. It produces the practitioner who lies awake at three in the morning interpreting a small twinge as the beginning of something serious. It produces the practitioner who cannot eat a meal in company without analyzing it. It produces the body that responds to its owner's vigilance by becoming, over time, more reactive, less regulated, harder to read.

The practice is not that. The practice is closer to the way you would read the mood of a child you have raised. Calm. Familiar. Already informed by years of looking. Quick to notice when something is off, but not searching for things to be off. The body is not a problem to be solved. It is a partner to be lived with. The discipline of noticing is the discipline of staying available, daily, to a partner who has been there all along.

What you are noticing, when you do this well across the years, is the subject of the next section. There turn out to be seven distinct things worth noticing, and each one is worth its own consideration.

* * *

There are seven of them. The number is not magical. The number is what falls out, in practice, when the work of keeping a body well across decades is broken into the distinct kinds of attention it actually asks for. The pillars overlap. They reinforce each other. They are not, in any strict sense, separate practices. But each one names a particular kind of looking, and naming them separately makes the looking easier to do.

The pillars below are walked through as forms of attention. The practical specifics are real and matter — they live in the chart at the end of the chapter, in their working-tool form. The prose names what each pillar is asking you to notice.

The first pillar is attention to the small living world inside you.

The body you are walking around in is not, strictly speaking, only yours. Inside it lives a community — billions of small organisms, distributed mostly along the lining of the gut, that participate in nearly everything you do. They digest your food. They make vitamins your body cannot make. They send signals to your brain. They are the invisible partner in nearly every meal you have ever eaten.

The first pillar is the practice of feeding this community well. Not as a rule. As a relationship. The kimchi on the side of the lunch plate is for them. The variety of vegetables across the week is for them — they are not one organism but thousands, and the thousands need different foods to thrive, the way a garden needs different plants to support its insects and birds. The occasional yogurt, the sauerkraut, the small fermented things that show up across the week: these are the ways you feed the community that has been feeding you. Attention here looks like a kitchen that makes room, daily, for one or two small fermented things, and that varies, across the week, what is on the plate.

The second pillar is attention to the wall that holds the community.

The lining of the gut is the boundary between the inside and the outside of you. It is a single layer of cells, in most places, which is a startling thing — a single layer of cells, deciding, all day, what is allowed to cross into your bloodstream and what is not. This wall is rebuilt continuously. It has to be. It is doing one of the most demanding jobs in the body, and it pays the price in turnover.

The second pillar is the practice of supporting the wall while it does its work. Bone broth, made well, with the long simmer that pulls collagen into the liquid, has been doing this since people first kept fires. L-glutamine, in periodic short cycles, gives the cells of the wall the specific amino acid they need most. Adequate fats, of the kind the body has co-evolved with — olive oil, butter from animals that ate grass, the occasional spoonful of coconut oil. Attention here looks like a kitchen that has bone broth in the freezer through the winter, and that does not run out of olive oil.

The third pillar is attention to the slowness of digestion.

The body did not evolve to eat in eight minutes between meetings. The digestive system runs on rhythms that take an hour at the table and several hours afterward to do their work properly. Eating fast, eating distracted, eating while the nervous system is still in the day's rush — these short-circuit the work the system was built to do, and the body pays for it.

The third pillar is the practice of making the meal a meal again. Sitting down. Putting the work away. Chewing. Letting the meal take the time it asks for. Not eating again for some hours afterward, so the digestive system can do the long work it does between meals — the slow sweeping motion of the gut clearing itself, which only happens when nothing new is arriving. Attention here looks like a person who, at midday, closes the laptop, sits at the table, and eats a meal that is not also a status update or a phone call. It is a small practice with disproportionate effects.

The fourth pillar is attention to the slow fire that runs beneath everything.

There is a low, quiet chemical fire that the modern diet keeps lit in most bodies. It is not a fever. It is not visible. It is the slow inflammation that runs from the foods the body did not co-evolve with — the industrial seed oils, the refined sugars, the processed substitutes for things that used to be grown — and it is the background condition for nearly every chronic illness of the modern world.

The fourth pillar is the practice of keeping that fire low. Daily fish, or another source of omega-3s. The polyphenol-rich foods that the body recognizes as medicine — the dark berries, the green tea, the turmeric, the olive oil. Avoiding the foods that keep the fire lit. Attention here looks like a kitchen where the cooking oil is olive or coconut, where there are berries in the freezer, and where the foods that smolder the fire — the fast food, the soda, the things in plastic bags — have, gradually, stopped appearing.

The fifth pillar is attention to the nervous system that talks to the gut all day.

The gut and the brain are connected by a thick bundle of nerve fibers called the vagus nerve, and the conversation across that bundle never stops. When the brain is calm, the gut works well. When the brain is in alarm — the alarm of a long week of work, the alarm of a difficult relationship, the alarm of a life that has not been resting properly — the gut responds. Digestion slows. The lining gets less of the resources it needs. The microbial community shifts. Stress is not a metaphor in the gut. It is a chemistry.

The fifth pillar is the practice of caring for the nervous system as a way of caring for the gut. Not as a separate self-improvement project. As part of the same practice. The walks. The sleep. The breathing practice, or the prayer, or the meditation, or the time in the garden, or whatever form of nervous-system care has actually worked, in your own life, to bring you back to yourself. Attention here looks like a person who, when a hard week is arriving, makes more room for sleep rather than less, who walks in the evening, who keeps the relationships in their life that are nourishing and lets thin out the ones that are not.

The sixth pillar is attention to what is in the water and on the food.

A modern body, even one being cared for well, is taking in a steady low load of substances the body did not evolve to process. Some of them come from the water supply. Some come from the residues on the produce. Some come from the household products that quietly off-gas into the air of the rooms a person sleeps in. The body has capable detoxification systems. Those systems are not unlimited.

The sixth pillar is the practice of reducing the load while supporting the systems. The water filter. The organic produce when it can be afforded. The cleaning products that are not industrial chemistry. The personal-care items that do not have unpronounceable substances at the top of the ingredient list. Periodic milk thistle, gentle, when the liver has been working hard. Sweating, regularly, through exercise or warmth, which is one of the body's primary ways of clearing what the liver releases. Attention here looks like a kitchen with a water filter, a pantry that has slowly emptied of foods that came in plastic, and a household that has gradually replaced its cleaning supplies with simpler things.

The seventh pillar is attention to the longer rhythm.

The first six pillars run on the rhythm of days and weeks. The seventh runs on the rhythm of seasons and years. There are practices that the body benefits from in periodic, intensified form — not as the daily practice, but as the larger waveform that sits beneath it.

Once a quarter, a one-week return to the herbal antiparasitic protocol — not because reinfection is likely, but because the pulses of those particular herbs, kept in the rotation, prevent any small thing that might be re-establishing from getting comfortable. Once a year, a two-week intensification — a longer fasting period, the herbal protocol at heightened intensity, the kind of week that returns the practitioner to the conditions of the original work. Every three to five years, the consideration of another prolonged fast, a comprehensive reassessment, the larger return that catches what the smaller returns missed. The seventh pillar is the practice of keeping these longer rhythms in the calendar, on purpose, as part of the year. Attention here looks like a calendar in which one week of each quarter is held for the maintenance protocol, one annual stretch is held for the deeper return, and the practitioner, at fifty, is considering the next fast at fifty-three with the same care they brought to the first one.

These are the seven. They overlap. They reinforce each other. The microbial community feeds on the polyphenols that quiet the inflammation that supports the lining that the chewing helped digest in the calm nervous system the rested body produced. None of them is independent. None of them, alone, is the practice.

The practice is all seven, held together, daily and periodically, across the long stretch of years the practitioner has remaining.

The chart at the end of this chapter is the working-tool version of all seven. It belongs by the kitchen, or in the back of a notebook, or wherever the practitioner keeps the small references they actually return to. The chart is what to do. The prose above is why.

* * *

There is a thing that has to be said clearly, before this chapter becomes a chapter about discipline.

The practice you are being invited to keep across the years is a human practice, not a perfectionist one. Your daughter will turn nine on a Saturday in October. There will be cake. You will eat the cake, and you will eat it without measuring, and you will eat it in the company of a child who is trying to read your face for whether the cake is being received as the gift she means it to be. You will receive it. You will eat the slice she cut for you, and possibly a second one. The practice is not asking you to refuse this.

A friend will call on a Thursday in summer and ask you to come have a beer at the place by the water where you used to go in your twenties, and you will go, and you will have a beer, and the conversation will be the kind of conversation that two old friends have when they are sitting outside at the end of a long day. The practice is not asking you to refuse this either.

There will be a wedding. There will be a reunion. There will be a Tuesday when your wife is tired and the only thing in the house that wants to be made is pasta with cream and you do not feel like asking the body what it wants tonight; you want pasta with cream. The practice is not asking you to refuse the pasta.

What the practice is asking is that the next morning you come back.

The discipline is not the absence of the cake or the beer or the pasta. The discipline is the return. Most mornings of your life are in the practice. A few mornings are not. You drift, and you come back. You drift, and you come back. The drift is not the failure. The failure to come back is the failure. The reader who has understood this will spend the rest of their life inside a practice that contains, comfortably, the cake and the beer and the pasta, because the practice is the bed they sleep in, and an evening out is not a different bed.

This is the human shape of the long practice. It is not a regime. It is not a moral test. It is a way of living, with built-in room for the things that make a life worth living. Without the cake on your daughter's birthday, the practice would be turning you into someone who refuses cake on his daughter's birthday, and that is not the person you set out to become.

What happens, when you keep coming back over a long enough stretch of years, is something you will not anticipate.

A friend who used to find a reason to drink most days of the week will mention, one evening, that he has cut back. He will not say why. He will not say it has anything to do with you. But he will have noticed, somewhere along the way, that you have a steadiness he does not have, and the noticing will have produced a question in him that he has begun, in his own time, to answer. Another friend will tell you, half-apologetically, that he is eating less meat. A third will mention, in passing, that his wife has been reading about the cleanse and has ordered the herbs. A fourth will appear at your door one Saturday and ask, with some embarrassment, whether you would talk him through what you actually do.

You will not have proselytized. You will not have lectured. You will, in most cases, not have brought any of this up at all. What people will have noticed is the way you carry yourself across a meal. The clarity of your skin, in the seventh year. The color of your hair, in the tenth. The way you are still, at sixty-five, the person you were planning to be at thirty. They will read these signs the way the long-married husband reads his wife across the kitchen — without conscious thought, in the half-second of looking up — and the reading will produce, in them, their own slow turning toward something.

A practice held steadily, for long enough, becomes a quiet invitation to the people around the practitioner. The invitation goes out without being sent. It is received without being addressed. Some of the people who receive it will turn toward their own version of the practice. Some will not. None of this is your work to do; the practice is your work, and the practice is enough.

But the community that grows up around a person who has held the practice for thirty years is, in the end, a different community than the one that would have grown up around the same person if they had not. There are healthier marriages in it. There are children growing up watching adults who pay attention. There are friends who, having seen something in you that produced their own question, are now living more carefully than they would otherwise have lived. None of this was promised, and none of it can be insisted upon, and the practitioner who undertakes the practice in order to produce these effects in others has misunderstood the practice from the start. But for the practitioner who undertakes the practice for its own sake — for the morning energy, for the clear mind, for the body that still feels like a partner at sixty-five — the radiating effect is real, and over the long arc of a life it is one of the finer things the practice produces.

You become, without intending to, a pivotal person in the lives around you. Not because you set out to be. Because you stayed.

* * *

There is something the chapter has not said yet, and the chapter would be incomplete without it.

The long version of this practice is more interesting than the short version. Not less. Not the same. More.

This is counterintuitive enough that it deserves to be set out carefully, because most people, when they look at a long discipline from the outside, see only its repetitions. The same kitchen, year after year. The same fermented vegetables on the plate. The same hour, more or less, when the eating window opens and closes. The same Sunday morning of slightly longer review. From outside, the practice looks like a smaller and smaller life — a person doing the same things over and over, while everyone else is having more variety, more spontaneity, more of whatever the spontaneous-looking life seems to offer.

This view of the practice is wrong, and it is wrong in a way that is worth understanding.

Consider, again, the long marriage. A couple who have been together for thirty years and who have not lost each other are not, at year thirty, doing different things from what they were doing at year three. They are still eating dinners together. They are still going on walks. They are still talking about the same kinds of things — work, family, the future, the small specific complaints of being alive. From outside, the marriage looks repetitive. But from inside, the marriage at year thirty is not the marriage at year three. The conversations are deeper, because each one is happening on top of three decades of accumulated reading. The dinners are richer, because each one carries the weight of every other dinner the couple has shared. The partner at year thirty is more interesting than the partner at year three, not less, because the partner is a person who has continued to change, and who has been continuously read, and the reading has produced a knowing that did not exist at year three.

The same is true of a body.

The body at year three of careful attention is not the body at year one. The body at year ten is something else again. The body, like the long-married partner, is alive. It changes. It surprises. It develops, across the years, particular signals and rhythms that did not exist when the practice began. The reader who pays attention across years comes to know things about their body that no first-year practitioner could know.

In the third year, you notice that your energy has a rhythm across the seasons that you did not see at first. There is a particular kind of low-grade tiredness in late February that is not winter and is not depression — it is the body asking for a quieter week before the spring asks more of it. In the fifth year, you notice that certain foods you used to eat happily now produce a particular small heaviness in the next morning that the body did not used to produce, and the body is teaching you, slowly, where its current limits are. In the seventh year, you notice that your relationship to hunger has become something that earlier practitioners describe but that you had not yet experienced — a clean, predictable arrival of hunger near the middle of the day, and an equally clean disappearance of it a few hours after the eating window closes, with no noise in between. In the tenth year, you notice that your body has begun teaching you things about your own emotional life — that anxiety, when it arrives, has a specific texture in the lower ribs, and that the texture means something is unprocessed, not that something is wrong. In the fifteenth year, you notice — and here the chapter has to step carefully, because what is being noticed is not exactly nameable — that you have a relationship with your body that you did not know was available when you started. You inhabit it differently. You read it differently. The body, in turn, is offering itself to be read in ways it could not offer itself to be read at year one.

This is the romance. Not heightened sensation. Not the pursuit of perfect health. The slow accumulation of mutual reading between a person and their body that produces, over the decades, a relationship of unusual depth.

The practice, from outside, looks like repetition. From inside, it is the opposite of repetition. It is the long unfolding of a partner — the body — who has been continuously alive, continuously changing, continuously revealing things that earlier years had not yet made available. The reader at year fifteen is not bored by the practice. The reader at year fifteen finds the practice more interesting than they did at year three, because the body that is being read has continued to be a presence whose interior keeps surfacing in new ways.

This is the gift the long version of the practice offers. The short version offers a clean body and a return to function, which is not nothing, but which is not the gift the long version offers. The long version offers an actual partnership across the decades a person has remaining — a partnership in which the practitioner becomes, slowly, a person who knows the body they live in, and the body becomes, slowly, a body that knows it is being known.

Most of the people you have ever met do not have this kind of relationship with their bodies. Most of them never will. The practice is the small daily price of being one of the few who do.

* * *

The chart that follows is the seven pillars in working form. It is meant to be photographed, printed, taped to the inside of a cupboard door, kept in the back of a notebook, or otherwise placed where the practitioner will actually see it across the years. The chart is not the chapter. The chapter is the prose above. The chart is the chapter's working tool, and is best used by a reader who has already understood what the seven pillars are forms of attention to. Read the prose for the why. Use the chart for the what.

Pillar	Practical specifics
1. Microbial community	Daily fermented food (kimchi, sauerkraut, yogurt, kefir). Plant variety across the week.
2. Gut wall	Bone broth weekly. L-glutamine in periodic short cycles. Olive oil, butter from grass-fed animals, occasional coconut oil.
3. Slowness of digestion	Sit-down meals. Adequate chewing. Several hours between meals.
4. Inflammation	Daily omega-3s. Polyphenol-rich foods (dark berries, green tea, turmeric, olive oil). Avoid industrial seed oils, refined sugars, processed foods.
5. Vagus nerve / nervous system	Adequate sleep. Daily walks. Breathing practice or meditation. Nourishing relationships kept; depleting ones thinned.
6. Toxin load	Water filter. Organic produce when feasible. Simple cleaning products. Periodic milk thistle. Regular sweating.
7. Longer rhythm	Quarterly: one-week antiparasitic maintenance. Annually: two-week intensification. Every 3-5 years: consideration of another prolonged fast.

* * *

There is a particular look that sometimes crosses the face of a person who has been paying close attention to their own body for many years. It is not the look of vitality, though vitality is often part of it. It is something quieter. A small ease at the eyes. A way of sitting in the kitchen on an ordinary morning that suggests the person sitting there is not trying to be anywhere else, in any sense of the word.

The look is rare in modern adult life. Most adults, by the third or fourth decade, have stopped paying close attention to their bodies, and the bodies have responded the way any partner responds to being unattended — by going quiet, by withdrawing, by becoming a vehicle the person rides around in rather than a presence the person lives with. There is no particular tragedy in this; it is the ordinary outcome of an ordinary life. But it is what the look of long attention is rare against.

The few who keep paying attention produce, across the decades, a different face. The face is not glowing. It is not radiant in the way self-help advertising would have the reader believe. It is something less dramatic and more lasting — the calm of a person who knows the body they are sitting in, and who has been knowing it for years, and whose mornings have become, by accumulation, a small steady pleasure rather than a small obligation.

The people in this person's life see the look without naming it. The friend who has been finding reasons to drink less mentions, casually, that the practitioner has a steadiness about them. The grown daughter notices, on a visit, that her father seems younger than the fathers of her friends, and does not understand quite why. The wife of thirty years, across the kitchen, sees the look every morning and reads it the way she has been reading it for decades, without conscious thought, in the half-second of looking up. The look is part of how the household is. It has become part of how the community is.

This is what the long partnership produces. Not a perfected body. Not a guarantee against time. The long partnership produces a person who, across an ordinary morning, in an ordinary kitchen, is more in the body they were given than they would otherwise have been, and who is, through that fact alone, more in the lives of the people around them than they would otherwise have been.

The kitchen is still the kitchen the chapter began in. The body is still the body the fast and the careful refeeding gave back, eight months ago, more or less. The decades that follow are still the decades that follow. What changes is what the practitioner brings to them.

They keep paying attention.

That is the long partnership.

Chapter 34

The Numbers: A Practitioner's Guide to the Blood Work of a 28-Day Fast

Companion chapter to The Long Quiet

Why This Chapter Exists

There is no other book in the prolonged-fasting literature that hands the reader the actual lab panel and explains, in practitioner's language, what each number means, why it shifts on a long fast, why it matters during refeeding, and why you retest it across the year that follows. This chapter is that document. If you read nothing else in this book, read this and the safety chapter.

Every number below is one your body is keeping for you whether you ask for it or not. The fast does not change whether the numbers exist. The fast changes whether you know what they are. A practitioner who watches the numbers gives himself the gift of a second pair of eyes on a body that is doing something extreme. A practitioner who refuses to watch the numbers is choosing to trust the body's signals exclusively, and the body's signals on Day 25 are sometimes the loudest liars in the room.

This is not medical advice. This is the teaching of one practitioner to another. Take what serves you. Test what you can. Read your own results. Bring the strange ones to a clinician who knows what fasted blood is supposed to look like.

The Frame: What Blood Work Is Actually Doing

Blood is a courier. Every cell in your body either makes a deposit into the bloodstream or takes a withdrawal from it, hundreds of times a second. A blood draw is one frame of a film that has been playing for as long as you have been alive. What you see in the frame is not the cells themselves — it is the residue of what those cells have been doing, the inventory in transit between organs, the regulatory signals the body uses to coordinate work across distances larger than any single cell can see.

When you fast for 28 days, the cells do not stop working. They start working differently. They stop expecting glucose from food and start manufacturing ketones from fat. They stop building tissue and start carefully cannibalizing the tissue they have built. They downshift the thyroid because they no longer need to spend energy at the rate the daily-fed body spends it. They release stored minerals from bone, fat-soluble vitamins from liver, and toxins from anywhere those toxins have been hiding. All of this shows up in the blood as numbers that look strange compared to the normal-fed reference ranges that the lab will print on your results.

This is the central confusion of fasting lab work: the reference ranges on your printout are calibrated to people who ate lunch. You did not eat lunch. You did not eat lunch for 28 days. Some of your numbers will be flagged as abnormal by the lab software, and the lab software will be wrong, because the software does not know you are on Day 28 of a planned protocol. Other numbers will look normal and actually be hiding something serious. The only way to read fasted blood work is to know, for each test, what the fast does to it and what to expect. That is what this chapter is for.

Tier 1 — The Refeeding-Safety Floor

These tests exist for one reason: refeeding syndrome. After an extended fast, the body's electrolyte handling is not the same as it was before the fast. The first food — even broth, even a few sips — triggers a cascade. Insulin rises (it has been near zero for weeks). Rising insulin tells cells to pull electrolytes out of the blood and into the cells, especially phosphorus, magnesium, and potassium. If the blood levels were already low from the fast itself, the post-meal drop can be catastrophic. Cardiac arrhythmia. Seizures. Respiratory failure. Heart stoppage. In hospitals that treat anorexia patients and concentration-camp survivors, refeeding syndrome is the number one cause of death in the first 72 hours of food reintroduction. This is not a hypothetical risk. This is the most common way long-fast practitioners die — not during the fast, but in the first 72 hours after they break it.

The Tier 1 panel is the cheap insurance policy. Roughly $100 cash-pay. Every one of these numbers needs to be known before the first solid food, ideally before the first broth.

Comprehensive Metabolic Panel (CMP)

What it measures:

A bundle of 14 individual tests in one draw: glucose, BUN (blood urea nitrogen), creatinine, sodium, potassium, chloride, CO2 (bicarbonate), calcium, total protein, albumin, alkaline phosphatase, ALT, AST, and bilirubin. This is the workhorse of every medical panel — kidney function, liver function, electrolytes, and basic metabolic state, all in one tube of blood.

Normal range:

Each component has its own range. Glucose 70-99 mg/dL fasting. Sodium 135-145 mEq/L. Potassium 3.5-5.0 mEq/L. The lab prints all ranges on the report.

What extended fasting does to this number:

Glucose will be very low — often 50-70 mg/dL, sometimes lower. This is expected and not dangerous as long as you are in deep ketosis (BHB elevated), because your brain is running on ketones, not glucose. BUN will be elevated because the body is breaking down some protein for gluconeogenesis and the urea is the waste product. Creatinine may be unreliable because muscle mass has changed. Albumin holds reasonably steady on a clean fast — if it drops significantly, the fast has gone too long. Liver enzymes (ALT, AST) often rise modestly because the liver is working hard processing fat for ketone production.

Why it matters at refeed:

Sodium and potassium handling can shift fast in the first 24-72 hours after food. Low potassium plus rising insulin is the classic refeeding-arrhythmia setup. Albumin tells you whether your blood can hold fluid properly when you start eating — low albumin means edema risk.

Why deficiency or imbalance is dangerous in a normal (non-fasting) person:

Sodium too low: confusion, seizures, brain swelling. Potassium too low or too high: cardiac arrhythmia, can be fatal. Calcium too low: muscle cramps, tetany, seizures. Albumin too low: fluid leaks out of vessels into tissues, causing edema in legs, lungs, abdomen. The body cannot hold itself together without these baseline numbers in range.

Why it goes off in a sick person who isn't fasting:

Diabetics show elevated glucose. Kidney disease shows elevated BUN and creatinine. Liver disease elevates ALT and AST. Dehydration concentrates everything. Diuretic medications drop potassium. Vomiting and diarrhea drop multiple electrolytes at once. People who 'feel sick' usually feel sick because one or more of these numbers has drifted.

Why we retest it on the follow-up schedule:

Day 3 (Draw 2) and Day 7 (Draw 3): the refeeding-syndrome danger window is 24-72 hours after first food and remains elevated through Day 7. Confirming electrolytes stay in range during this window is the single most important data point in the entire schedule. Day 30 (Draw 5) and beyond: tracks recovery of liver enzymes, kidney function, and protein synthesis as you rebuild.

Phosphorus

What it measures:

The level of inorganic phosphate dissolved in your blood. Phosphorus is the P in ATP — adenosine triphosphate — the energy currency of every cell in your body. It is also a structural mineral in bone, a buffer in blood pH, and a component of DNA.

Normal range:

2.5 to 4.5 mg/dL in serum.

What extended fasting does to this number:

Often drifts toward the lower end of normal during an extended fast. Stored phosphorus in bone and muscle continues to be available, but circulating levels can drop. The cells become hungry for phosphorus precisely because ATP production is shifted to ketones and the system is running on a thinner phosphate margin.

Why it matters at refeed:

This is the single most dangerous number in refeeding syndrome. The moment you eat carbohydrate, insulin rises. Insulin drives phosphorus from blood into cells to make ATP for processing the incoming glucose. If your starting phosphorus is already at the low end, the post-meal drop can crash it below 1.0 mg/dL within hours. Below 1.0 mg/dL: cardiac muscle cannot generate enough ATP to contract, respiratory muscles fail, red blood cells cannot deliver oxygen properly. People die. This is the number that has killed long-fast practitioners who broke their fast carelessly. Knowing your pre-refeed phosphorus is the difference between knowing whether you can have broth and oil tonight, or whether you need to take supplemental phosphate first.

Why deficiency or imbalance is dangerous in a normal (non-fasting) person:

Beyond refeeding: chronic low phosphorus causes muscle weakness, bone pain, fragility, confusion, and red blood cell dysfunction. Severe deficiency can be fatal. People with kidney disease often have the opposite problem — phosphorus too high — which calcifies arteries and damages organs.

Why it goes off in a sick person who isn't fasting:

Alcoholics, diabetics in ketoacidosis, people on certain antacids, people with severe burns, and refeeding patients of any kind. Chronic kidney disease pushes it the other direction.

Why we retest it on the follow-up schedule:

Days 3 and 7 are non-negotiable. If your baseline today is below 2.8 mg/dL, you supplement phosphate before the first solid food and recheck in 24 hours. If your Day 3 number drops by more than 30% from Day 1, you slow the refeed. After Day 7, the danger window closes, and you only retest if symptoms suggest a problem.

Magnesium (RBC, not serum)

What it measures:

Magnesium concentration inside the red blood cells, not just in the serum. RBC magnesium is a far more accurate picture of true body magnesium status than serum magnesium, because the body holds serum magnesium in a narrow range by pulling from cellular stores when serum drops. By the time serum magnesium looks low, intracellular magnesium has been depleted for months.

Normal range:

RBC magnesium: 4.2 to 6.8 mg/dL. Serum magnesium: 1.7 to 2.2 mg/dL (less useful).

What extended fasting does to this number:

Often low in modern practitioners even before the fast, because soil depletion and processed food have made magnesium deficiency endemic. A long fast can deplete it further if supplementation is inadequate. Symptoms of low magnesium during a fast: muscle cramping (especially calves at night), heart palpitations, insomnia, anxiety, headaches, twitching eyelids.

Why it matters at refeed:

Same mechanism as phosphorus. Insulin drives magnesium into cells when food returns. Low starting magnesium plus a meal can drop serum magnesium fast. Symptoms of acute low magnesium: muscle tetany, cardiac arrhythmia, seizures.

Why deficiency or imbalance is dangerous in a normal (non-fasting) person:

Magnesium is a cofactor in more than 300 enzymatic reactions in the human body. Severe deficiency: muscle spasms, arrhythmia, seizures, and a kind of free-floating anxiety that no amount of mental work will resolve. Moderate chronic deficiency is one of the most under-recognized contributors to chronic disease in the modern world — implicated in hypertension, type 2 diabetes, migraines, depression, and osteoporosis.

Why it goes off in a sick person who isn't fasting:

Diuretic use, alcoholism, chronic diarrhea, proton-pump inhibitor medications, type 2 diabetes, and the standard American diet, which provides perhaps half the magnesium humans need.

Why we retest it on the follow-up schedule:

Days 3 and 7 to confirm refeed stability. Day 14 and Day 30 to confirm repletion as supplementation continues. Magnesium deficiency takes months to fully correct, so the longer-term retests track whether the repletion is actually working.

Potassium

What it measures:

The level of potassium ion in your blood. Potassium is the dominant intracellular cation — most of your body's potassium is inside cells, not in blood. The blood level is a tightly regulated narrow band, because the heart will not tolerate much variation.

Normal range:

3.5 to 5.0 mEq/L.

What extended fasting does to this number:

Usually holds steady on a well-supplemented fast. Can drift low if you are losing it via enemas, sweat, or inadequate intake of mineral-rich water. Symptoms of low potassium during a fast: muscle weakness, fatigue, constipation, palpitations.

Why it matters at refeed:

Third pillar of the refeeding-syndrome triad with phosphorus and magnesium. Insulin pushes potassium into cells. Low starting potassium plus a meal can drop serum potassium into dangerous range. Below 2.5 mEq/L is medical emergency territory.

Why deficiency or imbalance is dangerous in a normal (non-fasting) person:

Cardiac arrhythmia. Muscle paralysis. Severe weakness. Potassium runs the electrical system of the heart, and the heart is unforgiving when potassium goes out of range — in either direction. Too high (hyperkalemia) is just as dangerous as too low, and is what kills people in kidney failure.

Why it goes off in a sick person who isn't fasting:

Diuretics, chronic diarrhea, vomiting, laxative abuse, and certain blood pressure medications. People on a standard American diet who do not eat vegetables are often modestly low.

Why we retest it on the follow-up schedule:

Same as phosphorus and magnesium — Days 3 and 7 are the critical reads. Beyond that, only if symptomatic.

CBC with Differential

What it measures:

Complete blood count. The numbers and types of cells in your blood: red blood cells (RBC), white blood cells (WBC) broken down by subtype, platelets, hemoglobin (the oxygen-carrying protein inside red cells), hematocrit (the percentage of your blood by volume that is red cells), and MCV (mean corpuscular volume — the average size of your red blood cells).

Normal range:

Many components, each with its own range. Hemoglobin: men 13.5-17.5 g/dL, women 12-15.5. Hematocrit: men 41-50%, women 36-44%. MCV: 80-100 fL. WBC: 4-11 K/µL.

What extended fasting does to this number:

Hemoglobin and hematocrit may rise slightly as plasma volume decreases (concentration effect) and may drop slightly as red cell turnover catches up. MCV is especially useful: elevated MCV (macrocytosis) is a flag for folate or B12 deficiency, both of which become more pressing on a long fast. White cells often drop modestly during fasting — this is part of the autophagy and immune-renewal effect of prolonged fasting, where old immune cells are recycled and new ones are generated when refeeding begins. Platelets usually hold steady.

Why it matters at refeed:

Not directly a refeeding-syndrome marker, but anemia (low hemoglobin) compounds the cardiovascular stress of refeeding. If you are anemic going into refeed, you tolerate the metabolic load less well.

Why deficiency or imbalance is dangerous in a normal (non-fasting) person:

Anemia: fatigue, breathlessness, lightheadedness on standing (orthostatic hypotension), decreased exercise tolerance, cognitive fog. Low white cells: increased infection risk. Low platelets: bleeding risk. The CBC is the most-ordered blood test in medicine because it catches a wide range of problems.

Why it goes off in a sick person who isn't fasting:

Anemia has many causes — iron deficiency, B12/folate deficiency, chronic disease, blood loss, hemolysis. Elevated white cells suggest infection or inflammation. Elevated platelets suggest inflammation. Low everything suggests bone marrow failure or severe nutritional deficiency.

Why we retest it on the follow-up schedule:

Days 7, 14, and 30. Tracks whether the bone marrow is responding to refeeding by producing new red cells. If MCV is elevated and folate/B12 supplementation is in place, MCV should normalize over 8-12 weeks as new red cells with proper folate replace the old macrocytic ones.

Thiamine (Vitamin B1, whole blood)

What it measures:

The level of thiamine inside red blood cells — the body's most accurate measure of thiamine status. Thiamine is a critical cofactor in glucose metabolism, especially in the brain.

Normal range:

70-180 nmol/L whole blood (lab variation).

What extended fasting does to this number:

Often low after extended fasting because thiamine has been used continuously and dietary intake has been zero. Many practitioners are mildly deficient even before the fast because thiamine is not stored in large quantities — the body holds only about a 2-3 week reserve.

Why it matters at refeed:

This is the second most dangerous part of refeeding after phosphorus. When you reintroduce carbohydrate, your body needs thiamine to metabolize the glucose. If thiamine is depleted, the brain cannot process the incoming glucose properly, and this can cause Wernicke's encephalopathy — a neurological emergency presenting with confusion, ataxia (loss of coordination), and ophthalmoplegia (eye movement problems). Untreated, it progresses to Korsakoff's syndrome, which is permanent brain damage. Some hospitals now give prophylactic thiamine to all refeeding patients before any carbohydrate exposure precisely to prevent this. A $10 thiamine supplement is cheap insurance.

Why deficiency or imbalance is dangerous in a normal (non-fasting) person:

Beriberi: a deficiency syndrome with two forms. Wet beriberi affects the heart (high-output heart failure). Dry beriberi affects the nerves (peripheral neuropathy, weakness, foot drop). Wernicke-Korsakoff syndrome in alcoholics is the same thiamine deficiency mechanism, made worse by alcohol blocking thiamine absorption. Severe deficiency is fatal.

Why it goes off in a sick person who isn't fasting:

Alcoholism, malabsorption syndromes, bariatric surgery, chronic vomiting, kidney dialysis, refeeding any starved patient, and certain genetic variants that impair thiamine transport.

Why we retest it on the follow-up schedule:

Day 7 retest catches whether supplementation has corrected the deficiency. Beyond that, only if symptoms suggest persistent issues.

Tier 2 — Nutrient Status

These tests answer the question: now that the fast is done, what does my body actually have in storage? Many of these nutrients were depleted to varying degrees during the fast itself. Some were already low going in, which is the case for most modern people. The Tier 2 panel tells you what to eat for the next year, which supplements actually matter, and which deficiencies will limit your recovery if left uncorrected.

Vitamin B12 (active B12 / holoTC preferred; otherwise serum B12)

What it measures:

Cobalamin level in blood. B12 is the largest and most chemically complex vitamin, used for DNA synthesis, red blood cell production, and myelin sheath maintenance on nerves. Active B12 (holotranscobalamin) measures only the B12 that is actually available to your cells. Total serum B12 includes inactive forms and is a less precise picture.

Normal range:

Serum B12: 200-900 pg/mL (but the lower part of this range is functionally deficient for many people). HoloTC: above 50 pmol/L is generally adequate.

What extended fasting does to this number:

B12 is stored in the liver in large quantities — a healthy person has 3-5 years of B12 reserve. A 28-day fast does not deplete it meaningfully. However: many people enter a fast with low B12 already (vegetarians, vegans, people on metformin, older adults with poor stomach acid). The fast can be the moment you discover the pre-existing deficiency, because subtle neurological symptoms get noticed when the body's other distractions go quiet.

Why it matters at refeed:

Not a direct refeeding-syndrome risk. But low B12 plus folate supplementation alone can mask a B12 deficiency: folate corrects the anemia (the visible sign) while B12 deficiency keeps progressing silently and damages nerves permanently. This is why folate and B12 are always tested and supplemented together.

Why deficiency or imbalance is dangerous in a normal (non-fasting) person:

Macrocytic anemia. Peripheral neuropathy (tingling, numbness in hands and feet). Cognitive decline, depression, even dementia-like symptoms. Damage to the spinal cord (subacute combined degeneration) can be permanent if deficiency is severe and prolonged. B12 deficiency is one of the great mimics in medicine — it can look like dementia, like depression, like multiple sclerosis.

Why it goes off in a sick person who isn't fasting:

Vegan/vegetarian diets without supplementation, atrophic gastritis (common in adults over 60), pernicious anemia (autoimmune destruction of intrinsic factor, the stomach protein that binds B12), bariatric surgery, metformin, proton-pump inhibitors, alcoholism.

Why we retest it on the follow-up schedule:

Day 7 and Day 30 — checks whether supplementation is working. Methylcobalamin is the bioactive form and corrects faster than cyanocobalamin. If B12 is severely low at baseline, intramuscular injections are more reliable than oral.

Folate (serum) — REPEAT TEST

What it measures:

Folate (vitamin B9) level in blood. Folate is essential for DNA synthesis, red blood cell production, and methylation — the chemical process that regulates gene expression, neurotransmitter production, and detoxification.

Normal range:

Serum folate: greater than 5.4 ng/mL is generally adequate. Below 3.1 ng/mL is clinical deficiency. Between 3.1 and 5.4 is borderline / insufficient.

What extended fasting does to this number:

Folate stores are smaller than B12 stores — only about 3-4 months' worth in the liver. A 28-day fast can meaningfully deplete folate, especially in someone who was already borderline or who has an MTHFR genetic variant (about 40% of the population has at least one MTHFR variant that impairs folate metabolism). The patient's baseline result of folate below 3.1 ng/mL — clinical deficiency — is exactly the picture expected at the end of a long fast without folate-rich supplementation. This is not a crisis, but it requires immediate correction during refeeding.

Why it matters at refeed:

Folate is critical for the rapid cell production that happens during refeeding — new red blood cells, new intestinal lining cells, new immune cells. Inadequate folate during refeeding slows recovery across the board.

Why deficiency or imbalance is dangerous in a normal (non-fasting) person:

Macrocytic anemia identical in appearance to B12-deficiency anemia. Birth defects (neural tube defects) in pregnancy — which is why prenatal vitamins contain folate. Elevated homocysteine, which is an independent risk factor for cardiovascular disease and dementia. Mood symptoms because folate is required for serotonin and dopamine production.

Why it goes off in a sick person who isn't fasting:

Inadequate dietary intake (leafy greens, legumes are the main sources), alcoholism, malabsorption (celiac, Crohn's), pregnancy and breastfeeding (increased demand), MTHFR genetic variants, certain medications (methotrexate, phenytoin, sulfasalazine).

Why we retest it on the follow-up schedule:

Day 7, Day 14, Day 30. Folate corrects relatively quickly with methylfolate supplementation (the bioactive form, which bypasses MTHFR issues) plus dietary folate from leafy greens, asparagus, lentils. Folic acid (the synthetic form in cheap supplements) is poorly converted in many people — always use methylfolate (5-MTHF).

Vitamin D, 25-hydroxy

What it measures:

The storage form of vitamin D in blood. Vitamin D is technically a hormone, not a vitamin, and regulates calcium absorption, immune function, mood, and over 1,000 genes' expression.

Normal range:

30-100 ng/mL (some experts argue optimal is 50-80).

What extended fasting does to this number:

Vitamin D is fat-soluble and stored in fat tissue and liver. A 28-day fast does not significantly deplete it. However, most modern people are deficient at baseline because of indoor living, sunscreen use, dark skin (which requires more sun exposure), and high latitudes. The fast often reveals a chronic deficiency that has been present for years.

Why it matters at refeed:

Not directly a refeeding risk, but adequate vitamin D supports the immune recovery and bone remineralization that should happen in the weeks after a fast.

Why deficiency or imbalance is dangerous in a normal (non-fasting) person:

Osteomalacia (soft bones in adults), osteoporosis, increased fracture risk, increased infection susceptibility, muscle weakness, depression, and probably increased risk of autoimmune disease, cardiovascular disease, and some cancers. The 'sunlight vitamin' is actually one of the most important regulators of the immune system.

Why it goes off in a sick person who isn't fasting:

Indoor lifestyle, sunscreen, high latitudes (north of 37° latitude, you cannot make adequate vitamin D from sun for half the year), dark skin without supplementation, obesity (vitamin D gets trapped in fat tissue), malabsorption.

Why we retest it on the follow-up schedule:

Day 30 and Day 90. Vitamin D takes weeks to months to correct. Supplementation should be paired with vitamin K2 to ensure the calcium absorbed goes into bones rather than soft tissues.

Ferritin + Iron + TIBC + Transferrin Saturation

What it measures:

The full iron picture. Ferritin is your iron storage protein — it tells you how much iron is in the bank. Serum iron is how much is in transit right now. TIBC (total iron binding capacity) is the total carrying capacity of transferrin (the iron-shuttle protein). Transferrin saturation is what percentage of your shuttles are currently loaded. Together these four numbers tell you whether you are iron deficient, iron overloaded, or fine.

Normal range:

Ferritin: 30-400 ng/mL (men), 13-150 ng/mL (women). Functional optimum is 50-150. Serum iron: 60-170 µg/dL. TIBC: 240-450 µg/dL. Transferrin saturation: 20-50%.

What extended fasting does to this number:

Iron metabolism is unusual on a fast. Ferritin may rise because of the inflammation and tissue breakdown of fasting (ferritin is also an acute-phase reactant — it rises with any inflammation). Serum iron may drop because no dietary iron is coming in. Hemoglobin holds reasonably steady because red cell lifespan is 120 days and the fast is only 28.

Why it matters at refeed:

Not a direct refeeding-syndrome risk. But iron status affects oxygen delivery during the recovery period.

Why deficiency or imbalance is dangerous in a normal (non-fasting) person:

Iron deficiency anemia: fatigue, weakness, pale skin, breathlessness, cold extremities, pica (craving non-food items like ice or dirt), restless leg syndrome, hair loss. Severe iron deficiency impairs cognitive function and immune function. Iron overload (hemochromatosis) is the opposite problem and damages liver, heart, joints, and pancreas — it is one of the most underdiagnosed genetic conditions and affects perhaps 1 in 200 people of Northern European descent.

Why it goes off in a sick person who isn't fasting:

Iron deficiency: blood loss (menstruation, GI bleeding from ulcers or colon cancer, donating blood), inadequate intake, malabsorption (celiac), pregnancy. Iron overload: hemochromatosis genetic mutation, excessive supplementation, multiple blood transfusions.

Why we retest it on the follow-up schedule:

Day 30 and Day 90. Iron repletion is slow and requires either dietary iron (red meat, organ meats, legumes) or supplementation. Iron supplements are often poorly tolerated (constipation, GI upset) and absorption is improved with vitamin C and impaired with calcium, coffee, and tea taken at the same time.

Zinc (RBC zinc)

What it measures:

Zinc level inside red blood cells. Zinc is a cofactor in over 300 enzymes and is especially important for immune function, wound healing, taste and smell, testosterone production, and DNA repair.

Normal range:

RBC zinc: 11-15 mg/L. Serum zinc: 60-130 μg/dL (less accurate).

What extended fasting does to this number:

Often depleted during long fasts. Zinc is not stored in large quantities (only about 2-3 grams total body zinc) and is continuously used. Symptoms of zinc deficiency that often appear late in a long fast: loss of taste and smell, slow wound healing, white spots on fingernails, hair thinning, increased frequency of cold sores or other immune issues.

Why it matters at refeed:

Not directly. But adequate zinc supports the rebuilding of intestinal lining, immune cells, and tissues during refeeding.

Why deficiency or imbalance is dangerous in a normal (non-fasting) person:

Impaired immune function, increased infection risk, slow wound healing, loss of taste and smell, hair loss, skin problems, low testosterone in men, infertility.

Why it goes off in a sick person who isn't fasting:

Vegan/vegetarian diets without careful planning, alcoholism, malabsorption, chronic diarrhea, age (absorption declines), certain medications.

Why we retest it on the follow-up schedule:

Day 30 and Day 90. Zinc and copper compete for absorption — supplementing one long-term can deplete the other, so they are tested together.

Copper

What it measures:

Serum copper level. Copper works in close partnership with zinc and is essential for iron metabolism, connective tissue formation, neurotransmitter synthesis, and antioxidant defense (via the enzyme superoxide dismutase).

Normal range:

70-140 µg/dL.

What extended fasting does to this number:

Usually holds reasonably steady. Modern people are more commonly copper-overloaded than deficient, because of copper water pipes and certain supplements.

Why it matters at refeed:

Not direct.

Why deficiency or imbalance is dangerous in a normal (non-fasting) person:

Anemia that does not respond to iron (copper is needed to mobilize iron from storage), neutropenia (low white cells), neurological symptoms similar to B12 deficiency, connective tissue weakness.

Why it goes off in a sick person who isn't fasting:

Zinc supplementation without copper, malabsorption, bariatric surgery, rare genetic disorders (Menkes disease — deficiency; Wilson's disease — overload).

Why we retest it on the follow-up schedule:

Day 90. Less urgent than other nutrients.

Selenium

What it measures:

Serum selenium level. Selenium is a critical cofactor in thyroid hormone activation (converting T4 to T3) and in the body's primary antioxidant enzyme system (glutathione peroxidase).

Normal range:

70-150 ng/mL.

What extended fasting does to this number:

May be depleted on a long fast, especially in regions where soil selenium is low (much of the U.S. midwest is selenium-poor).

Why it matters at refeed:

Adequate selenium supports thyroid recovery from the conservation mode the fast induces.

Why deficiency or imbalance is dangerous in a normal (non-fasting) person:

Impaired thyroid function, weakened immune function, increased oxidative stress. Severe deficiency is rare in developed countries but is implicated in Keshan disease (a heart muscle disorder) in selenium-deficient regions of China.

Why it goes off in a sick person who isn't fasting:

Geographic — soil selenium varies widely. Malabsorption. Strict vegan diets without Brazil nuts or supplementation.

Why we retest it on the follow-up schedule:

Day 90 if low at baseline. One or two Brazil nuts daily corrects most selenium deficiency.

Reticulocyte Count

What it measures:

The percentage of immature red blood cells in your bloodstream. Reticulocytes are the precursors of mature red blood cells, freshly released from the bone marrow.

Normal range:

0.5-2.5%.

What extended fasting does to this number:

Typically low during a long fast because bone marrow downregulates red cell production when nutrients are scarce.

Why it matters at refeed:

Not direct.

Why deficiency or imbalance is dangerous in a normal (non-fasting) person:

Low reticulocyte count plus anemia suggests the bone marrow is failing to produce red cells — could indicate severe nutrient deficiency (iron, B12, folate), bone marrow disease, or chronic disease. High reticulocyte count plus anemia suggests the body is trying hard to make red cells but they are being lost or destroyed faster than produced.

Why it goes off in a sick person who isn't fasting:

Bone marrow disorders, severe nutritional deficiency, kidney disease (low erythropoietin), recent blood loss (high), hemolysis (high).

Why we retest it on the follow-up schedule:

Day 14 to confirm bone marrow has responded to refeeding by ramping up red cell production. Should rise sharply in the first 2 weeks after refeeding begins if folate, B12, and iron are adequate.

Tier 3 — The Metabolic Snapshot

These values will change within hours of your first food. The Tier 3 panel captures the deep-fasted metabolic state for the historical record. You cannot get these numbers again from this fast. Whether they matter for the book or for your personal practice, they represent a state your body has been in that very few measured humans have been in. Capture them while you can.

Beta-hydroxybutyrate (BHB), serum

What it measures:

The level of beta-hydroxybutyrate, the dominant ketone body in extended fasting. BHB is the molecule your liver makes from fat that your brain, heart, and muscles burn as fuel in place of glucose.

Normal range:

Normal fed state: less than 0.5 mmol/L. Nutritional ketosis (low-carb diet): 0.5-3.0. Extended fasting day 7+: 4-6 typical, sometimes higher. Diabetic ketoacidosis (a dangerous condition, different from fasting ketosis): often 10+, but with simultaneously high blood sugar and low pH.

What extended fasting does to this number:

Day 28 of a clean water fast: BHB will likely be 4-7 mmol/L. This is deep nutritional ketosis. Your brain is running 70-80% on ketones. Your insulin is at the floor. This is the metabolic state hunter-gatherer ancestors entered during seasonal food scarcity and that monastic fasting traditions have engineered intentionally.

Why it matters at refeed:

Not a refeeding-syndrome marker. Will drop quickly with first food.

Why deficiency or imbalance is dangerous in a normal (non-fasting) person:

BHB is not something you can be 'deficient' in — it is a state, not a nutrient. The point of measuring it is to document the depth of the fasted state.

Why it goes off in a sick person who isn't fasting:

Ketogenic diet, prolonged exercise without carbs, diabetic ketoacidosis (in conjunction with high glucose and metabolic acidosis — this is medical emergency, very different from fasting ketosis).

Why we retest it on the follow-up schedule:

Once is enough for this fast. Future fasts can be tracked with finger-stick ketone meters for ongoing measurement.

Insulin, fasting

What it measures:

Insulin is the hormone your pancreas releases in response to rising blood sugar, telling cells to take up glucose. Fasting insulin tells you how much insulin is circulating when no food is in the system.

Normal range:

Normal fasted (well-fed person): 2-10 μIU/mL. Optimal is below 5. Pre-diabetic and insulin-resistant people: 10-25. Diabetics: variable.

What extended fasting does to this number:

Day 28 of fasting: insulin will be near the floor — often below 1 μIU/mL, sometimes undetectable. This is the lowest insulin the body produces. This number alone is worth the price of admission for the metabolic-health story — it documents what the body looks like in true nutritional rest.

Why it matters at refeed:

Will rise sharply with first food. The rate of rise is what drives the phosphorus/magnesium/potassium intracellular shift that causes refeeding syndrome.

Why deficiency or imbalance is dangerous in a normal (non-fasting) person:

Insulin is not something you want to be 'high' in chronically — high fasting insulin is the earliest sign of insulin resistance and metabolic dysfunction, often present 10+ years before type 2 diabetes is diagnosed. Low fasting insulin is actually a marker of metabolic health.

Why it goes off in a sick person who isn't fasting:

High: obesity, insulin resistance, prediabetes, type 2 diabetes, polycystic ovary syndrome, certain medications. Low: type 1 diabetes (autoimmune destruction of the insulin-producing cells), advanced type 2 diabetes (pancreatic burnout), Addison's disease.

Why we retest it on the follow-up schedule:

Day 30, Day 90 — compares fasting insulin pre-fast (if available) to post-fast to document metabolic improvement. A long fast often resets insulin sensitivity significantly.

Glucose, fasting

What it measures:

Blood glucose level after at least 8 hours without food. In your case, after 28 days without food.

Normal range:

Normal fasting: 70-99 mg/dL. Prediabetic: 100-125. Diabetic: 126 or higher.

What extended fasting does to this number:

Day 28 fasting glucose will be very low — often 50-70 mg/dL. This would be hypoglycemic and dangerous in a fed person, but is fine in someone in deep ketosis because the brain is running on ketones. The body maintains exactly the small amount of glucose required for red blood cells (which cannot use ketones) and for the small portion of brain function that still requires glucose.

Why it matters at refeed:

Will rise with first food. The first carbohydrate exposure after a long fast can spike glucose more dramatically than expected because the muscle's GLUT4 transporters have been downregulated.

Why deficiency or imbalance is dangerous in a normal (non-fasting) person:

Symptomatic hypoglycemia in a fed person (shakiness, sweating, confusion, anxiety, hunger) is medical emergency below 50-55. Asymptomatic low glucose in a deep-fasted person on ketones is normal. Chronic high glucose damages every blood vessel in the body and is the engine of diabetic complications.

Why it goes off in a sick person who isn't fasting:

High: diabetes, stress, certain medications, Cushing's syndrome. Low: insulin overdose in diabetics, rare insulin-secreting tumors, severe liver disease, sepsis.

Why we retest it on the follow-up schedule:

Day 30, Day 90 — tracks recovery of glucose regulation post-fast and confirms it returns to a healthy fasting range.

Hemoglobin A1c

What it measures:

The percentage of your hemoglobin that has glucose chemically attached. Because red blood cells live about 120 days, A1c is an average of your blood glucose over the prior 3 months.

Normal range:

Normal: below 5.7%. Prediabetic: 5.7-6.4%. Diabetic: 6.5% or higher.

What extended fasting does to this number:

Reflects the 3-month average that includes the fast and the time before. Will be lower than pre-fast A1c if the fast brought average glucose down.

Why it matters at refeed:

Not relevant immediately. Becomes meaningful again 3 months post-refeed.

Why deficiency or imbalance is dangerous in a normal (non-fasting) person:

Elevated A1c is the gold-standard marker of long-term glucose dysregulation. Every percentage point above 6 increases cardiovascular risk substantially.

Why it goes off in a sick person who isn't fasting:

Type 2 diabetes, prediabetes, insulin resistance, certain anemias can falsely lower it, certain genetic hemoglobin variants can falsely affect it.

Why we retest it on the follow-up schedule:

Day 90, Day 365 — A1c becomes meaningful again on those timescales because it represents 3 months of glucose averages.

Uric Acid

What it measures:

Uric acid is the waste product of purine metabolism. Purines are components of DNA and RNA, and during fasting or any rapid tissue turnover, purines are released and converted to uric acid for excretion.

Normal range:

Men: 3.4-7.0 mg/dL. Women: 2.4-6.0 mg/dL.

What extended fasting does to this number:

Often elevated during long fasts because of accelerated tissue turnover and reduced kidney excretion (the kidneys preferentially excrete ketones over uric acid). Some practitioners experience gout flares during long fasts because of this — sudden joint pain, especially in the big toe.

Why it matters at refeed:

Will normalize over days to weeks as refeeding restores kidney handling of uric acid.

Why deficiency or imbalance is dangerous in a normal (non-fasting) person:

Chronically elevated uric acid causes gout (uric acid crystals in joints), kidney stones, and is associated with metabolic syndrome and cardiovascular disease.

Why it goes off in a sick person who isn't fasting:

Genetics, high purine intake (organ meats, shellfish, beer), kidney disease, certain medications (diuretics), psoriasis, leukemia, fructose consumption.

Why we retest it on the follow-up schedule:

Day 30 confirms it has normalized post-fast.

Tier 4 — Thyroid Panel

The thyroid is the body's metabolic thermostat. On a long fast, the body deliberately downregulates thyroid activity to conserve energy. This is not pathology — it is intelligence. The body does not want to burn calories at the daily-fed rate when no calories are coming in. The thyroid downshift includes reduced T4-to-T3 conversion (T3 is the active hormone), often with elevated reverse T3 (an inactive form that competes with active T3 for receptor binding). This pattern would look hypothyroid in a non-fasting person and warrant treatment. In a fasting person, it is expected and reverses on refeeding.

TSH (Thyroid Stimulating Hormone)

What it measures:

The signal the pituitary gland sends to the thyroid telling it to make more thyroid hormone. Counterintuitively, high TSH means the thyroid is underactive (more shouting is needed to get hormone produced), and low TSH means the thyroid is overactive (no shouting needed).

Normal range:

0.4-4.5 mIU/L. Optimal is generally considered 0.5-2.5.

What extended fasting does to this number:

Often slightly suppressed during a long fast because the body is intentionally downshifting metabolic rate. May rise during refeeding as the body signals for thyroid hormone to restart normal metabolism.

Why we retest it on the follow-up schedule:

Day 30, Day 90 — confirms thyroid recovery from conservation mode.

Free T3

What it measures:

The active thyroid hormone, free and unbound, available to bind cellular receptors and regulate metabolism.

Normal range:

2.3-4.2 pg/mL.

What extended fasting does to this number:

Often significantly suppressed during prolonged fasting — this is the heart of the conservation response. Will rise over days to weeks of refeeding.

Why we retest it on the follow-up schedule:

Day 30 and Day 90 are the key checks. If T3 has not recovered by Day 60-90, the body may need additional support (selenium, zinc, tyrosine, adequate carbohydrate).

Free T4

What it measures:

The storage form of thyroid hormone, free and unbound. T4 is converted to T3 in peripheral tissues, primarily by enzymes that require selenium.

Normal range:

0.8-1.8 ng/dL.

What extended fasting does to this number:

Usually holds steady or modestly low during fasting. The shift during fasting is mostly in T4-to-T3 conversion, not in T4 production itself.

Why we retest it on the follow-up schedule:

Day 30, Day 90.

Reverse T3

What it measures:

An inactive form of T3 that the body produces when it wants to slow metabolism. Reverse T3 binds to T3 receptors without activating them, blocking active T3 from working.

Normal range:

9-24 ng/dL.

What extended fasting does to this number:

Often elevated during prolonged fasting — the body intentionally producing reverse T3 to slow metabolism further. The ratio of free T3 to reverse T3 is a more useful number than either alone. Should normalize within weeks of refeeding.

Why we retest it on the follow-up schedule:

Day 30, Day 90. Persistent elevation of reverse T3 with normal T4 is a sign of ongoing stress, illness, or inflammation.

Tier 5 — Inflammation, Methylation, Lipids

These tests look at the body's inflammatory state, the methylation cycle (which depends on folate, B12, and B6), and the lipid picture. Long fasting often dramatically reduces inflammation, sometimes improves the lipid panel, and reveals methylation problems that were hidden by the noise of daily eating.

hs-CRP (High-Sensitivity C-Reactive Protein)

What it measures:

The most sensitive blood marker for systemic inflammation. C-reactive protein is made by the liver in response to inflammatory signals from anywhere in the body.

Normal range:

Optimal: below 1 mg/L. Moderate cardiovascular risk: 1-3. High risk: above 3.

What extended fasting does to this number:

Often dramatically lower after a long fast than before. This is one of the most reliable benefits of prolonged fasting — systemic inflammation drops substantially.

Why deficiency or imbalance is dangerous in a normal (non-fasting) person:

Chronic inflammation is the engine of nearly every chronic disease — cardiovascular disease, diabetes, autoimmune disease, cancer, dementia. Elevated CRP independently predicts cardiovascular events and overall mortality.

Why it goes off in a sick person who isn't fasting:

Acute infection (very high), chronic disease, obesity, smoking, poor sleep, chronic stress, autoimmune disease, periodontal disease.

Why we retest it on the follow-up schedule:

Day 30 confirms the anti-inflammatory effect persists. Day 90 and beyond tracks whether daily life is keeping it down.

Homocysteine

What it measures:

An amino acid that accumulates when the methylation cycle is impaired. Homocysteine should be efficiently converted to either methionine (via folate, B12, B6) or cysteine (via B6). When those conversions fail, homocysteine builds up and damages blood vessels.

Normal range:

Optimal: below 7 µmol/L. Acceptable: 7-12. Elevated: above 12.

What extended fasting does to this number:

Variable. May be elevated if folate or B12 deficiency is present (which is your case, given the folate result).

Why deficiency or imbalance is dangerous in a normal (non-fasting) person:

Elevated homocysteine is an independent risk factor for cardiovascular disease, stroke, dementia, and Alzheimer's. Some research suggests it is more predictive of cardiovascular events than cholesterol.

Why it goes off in a sick person who isn't fasting:

Folate, B12, or B6 deficiency. MTHFR genetic variants. Kidney disease. Hypothyroidism.

Why we retest it on the follow-up schedule:

Day 30, Day 90. Should normalize with adequate methylfolate and B12 supplementation.

Lipid Panel

What it measures:

Total cholesterol, LDL (low-density lipoprotein), HDL (high-density lipoprotein), and triglycerides.

Normal range:

Total cholesterol: below 200 mg/dL desirable. LDL: below 100 optimal, below 70 for high-risk patients. HDL: above 40 men, above 50 women. Triglycerides: below 150.

What extended fasting does to this number:

Surprising patterns. Triglycerides often drop dramatically (this is one of the cleanest benefits of long fasting). Total cholesterol and LDL may rise transiently because fat is being mobilized from storage. HDL may rise. The pattern usually normalizes and improves over weeks to months.

Why deficiency or imbalance is dangerous in a normal (non-fasting) person:

Elevated LDL, particularly small dense LDL, is associated with cardiovascular disease. Low HDL is also a risk. High triglycerides are a marker of metabolic dysfunction. The lipid panel alone is a crude tool — advanced lipid testing (LDL particle number, apolipoprotein B) is more informative but more expensive.

Why it goes off in a sick person who isn't fasting:

Genetics (familial hypercholesterolemia), diet, exercise, metabolic syndrome, hypothyroidism, kidney disease, certain medications.

Why we retest it on the follow-up schedule:

Day 30, Day 90, Day 180. The lipid panel is dynamic and worth tracking over time.

GGT (Gamma-glutamyl Transferase)

What it measures:

A liver enzyme particularly sensitive to bile duct issues and oxidative stress. GGT is also induced by alcohol and certain medications.

Normal range:

Men: below 50 U/L. Women: below 30 U/L. Optimal is significantly lower (below 20 in both sexes is associated with the best outcomes).

What extended fasting does to this number:

May rise modestly during a fast as the liver works hard processing fat and as bile is mobilized aggressively (especially with coffee enemas).

Why deficiency or imbalance is dangerous in a normal (non-fasting) person:

Elevated GGT is one of the most underappreciated markers in medicine — it correlates strongly with all-cause mortality, cardiovascular disease, and diabetes. Even within the 'normal' range, lower is better.

Why it goes off in a sick person who isn't fasting:

Alcohol consumption (very sensitive), fatty liver, bile duct disease, certain medications, oxidative stress.

Why we retest it on the follow-up schedule:

Day 30 and Day 90 — tracks liver recovery and ongoing oxidative status.

Bilirubin (direct and indirect)

What it measures:

Bilirubin is the breakdown product of hemoglobin. Indirect (unconjugated) bilirubin is the form produced when red blood cells are broken down; direct (conjugated) is the form the liver has processed and is ready to excrete in bile.

Normal range:

Total bilirubin: 0.1-1.2 mg/dL. Direct: 0.0-0.3.

What extended fasting does to this number:

Often slightly elevated during fasting because of red blood cell turnover and reduced liver throughput. People with Gilbert's syndrome (a common benign genetic variant) often show notably elevated indirect bilirubin during fasting.

Why deficiency or imbalance is dangerous in a normal (non-fasting) person:

Elevated direct bilirubin suggests bile duct obstruction or liver disease. Elevated indirect bilirubin suggests hemolysis (red cell destruction) or Gilbert's syndrome.

Why it goes off in a sick person who isn't fasting:

Liver disease, bile duct obstruction (gallstones, tumors), hemolytic anemia, Gilbert's syndrome.

Why we retest it on the follow-up schedule:

Day 30 if elevated at baseline.

Tier 6 — Hormones (Recovery Baseline)

The hormonal system takes longer to recover from a long fast than the metabolic system. Testosterone often drops significantly during a fast (this is well-documented and not gender-specific — testosterone in women drops too). Cortisol may rise modestly. DHEA can drop. These changes usually reverse within weeks to months of refeeding, but they are worth measuring as a baseline.

Cortisol, AM

What it measures:

The level of cortisol, the body's primary stress hormone, measured in morning blood (when cortisol naturally peaks).

Normal range:

AM cortisol: 6-23 μg/dL. Should be highest in the morning and decline through the day.

What extended fasting does to this number:

Often slightly elevated during fasting because fasting is a controlled stressor. Should normalize with refeeding and adequate sleep.

Why deficiency or imbalance is dangerous in a normal (non-fasting) person:

Too high (chronic): metabolic syndrome, hypertension, immune suppression, sleep disruption, abdominal weight gain. Too low: adrenal insufficiency, fatigue, hypotension. Cortisol dysregulation (high at the wrong times, low at the wrong times) is more common than absolute high or low.

Why we retest it on the follow-up schedule:

Day 30, Day 90.

Testosterone (total and free)

What it measures:

Total testosterone is the total amount in blood. Free testosterone is the unbound fraction, which is biologically active. Both are needed for the full picture.

Normal range:

Men: total 300-1000 ng/dL, free 5-25 ng/dL. Women: total 15-70 ng/dL, free 0.3-1.9 ng/dL.

What extended fasting does to this number:

Often drops significantly during long fasts in both sexes. Usually recovers within weeks of refeeding, but in some cases requires 2-3 months of full nutrition for full recovery.

Why deficiency or imbalance is dangerous in a normal (non-fasting) person:

Low testosterone in men: fatigue, low libido, depression, muscle loss, slow recovery from exercise, decreased erectile function, mood changes. Low testosterone in women: low libido, fatigue, mood changes, reduced muscle mass.

Why we retest it on the follow-up schedule:

Day 60 is the typical recovery checkpoint. Day 90 confirms full recovery or identifies persistent low T that may need other intervention.

DHEA-S

What it measures:

Dehydroepiandrosterone sulfate, an adrenal steroid hormone that is a precursor to testosterone and estrogen.

Normal range:

Highly age-dependent. Adult men: 100-400 µg/dL. Adult women: 60-300.

What extended fasting does to this number:

May drop during prolonged fasting as adrenal reserves are taxed.

Why deficiency or imbalance is dangerous in a normal (non-fasting) person:

Low DHEA-S is associated with fatigue, low libido, and possibly accelerated aging.

Why we retest it on the follow-up schedule:

Day 90.

Tier 7 — Kidney Function

Kidney function tests are tricky in someone who has lost muscle mass, because the standard marker (creatinine) is a breakdown product of muscle. Less muscle means lower creatinine, which makes kidney function look better than it actually is. Cystatin C is a more accurate marker in this context.

Cystatin C

What it measures:

A small protein produced by all cells in the body at a steady rate, filtered by the kidneys. Cystatin C is independent of muscle mass and is the most accurate marker of kidney function in someone whose muscle mass has changed.

Normal range:

0.5-1.0 mg/L.

What extended fasting does to this number:

Should remain in the normal range during fasting. If elevated, suggests true kidney impairment (not just muscle loss).

Why deficiency or imbalance is dangerous in a normal (non-fasting) person:

Elevated cystatin C indicates reduced kidney filtration. Chronic kidney disease is asymptomatic until severe.

Why we retest it on the follow-up schedule:

Day 30 if baseline is abnormal.

Urinalysis

What it measures:

Examines urine for protein, glucose, ketones, blood, specific gravity, pH, and microscopic elements.

Normal range:

Negative for protein, glucose, blood. Ketones will be strongly positive in a fasted person. Specific gravity usually 1.005-1.030.

What extended fasting does to this number:

Strongly positive ketones (expected). Possible mild proteinuria from the fast itself, should resolve. Specific gravity may be high (concentrated urine) if hydration is borderline.

Why deficiency or imbalance is dangerous in a normal (non-fasting) person:

Protein in urine suggests kidney damage. Blood suggests infection, stones, or other pathology. Glucose suggests diabetes.

Why we retest it on the follow-up schedule:

Repeat if any abnormality at baseline.

Follow-Up Schedule — The Reasoning

The schedule of follow-up draws is not arbitrary. Each draw catches a specific physiological window. Here is the reasoning for each.

Draw 1 — Today, before first food

Captures the only chance to document the deep-fasted metabolic state for this fast. Beta-hydroxybutyrate, fasting insulin, fasted thyroid, baseline electrolytes, baseline nutrient status. The Tier 1 results determine whether you can safely begin refeeding immediately or whether supplementation is needed first.

Draw 2 — Day 3

The refeeding-syndrome danger window is 24-72 hours after the first food. This draw is short and cheap (Tier 1 only) but absolutely non-negotiable. Phosphorus is the critical number. If phosphorus, magnesium, or potassium have crashed since Day 1, the refeed is escalated too fast and needs to be slowed or supplemented urgently.

Draw 3 — Day 7

End of the immediate refeeding window. Confirms electrolytes have stabilized. Adds folate and B12 retests because supplementation should be showing effect by now. Thiamine retest if baseline was low. This is the decision point for moving from liquids to soft foods.

Draw 4 — Day 14

Two weeks post-refeed. Full nutrient panel to confirm repletion is happening across the board. hs-CRP to confirm gut inflammation is calming as foods are reintroduced. Reticulocyte count to confirm bone marrow has ramped up red cell production.

Draw 5 — Day 30

First major checkpoint. The 'after' snapshot that compares to the pre-fast 'before.' Metabolic markers (insulin, glucose), thyroid (recovery from conservation mode), lipid panel, inflammation, nutrient status. The single most valuable post-fast draw for documenting outcomes.

Draw 6 — Day 60

Hormone recovery checkpoint. Testosterone typically rebounds by Day 60 if it is going to. Final confirmation of nutrient repletion. Thyroid recheck if Day 30 showed incomplete recovery.

Draw 7 — Day 90

Quarterly comprehensive. Hemoglobin A1c is now meaningful again (3-month average). This draw is the comparison point against Draw 1 for the book — what does this man look like 90 days after a 28-day fast?

Draw 8 — Day 180

Six-month checkpoint. Includes a stool analysis (separate test, not blood) to document the gut microbiome and any residual parasites. Final confirmation that repletion has held.

Draw 9 — Day 365

One year out. The full-circle data point. Annual labs become normal health baseline from here forward.

When You Can Stop

After Draw 9, the intensive cadence ends. Annual comprehensive labs are appropriate for anyone, fasted or not. If everything is stable at Year 1 and no symptoms suggest a problem, you can shift to once-yearly going forward.

The non-negotiable draws — the ones that exist for safety, not for documentation — are Draws 1, 2, and 3. Refeeding syndrome is the primary cause of death after prolonged fasting, and these three draws are designed to catch it. If budget forces a choice, these are the ones to keep.

Everything beyond Draw 3 is recovery documentation and book material. Valuable. Worth the money if you can. But not safety-critical.

A Final Note for the Practitioner Reading This

If you are reading this chapter as a practitioner considering your own long fast, hear this: the labs in this chapter are not optional. They are the equivalent of checking your parachute before a jump. You do not have to test every single number. You do have to test the Tier 1 panel before breaking your fast. If you cannot afford a hundred dollars for the refeeding-safety floor, you cannot afford the fast. Reschedule for when you can.

This is not because the body cannot survive a careless refeed. Many people refeed carelessly and survive. It is because the people who do not survive a careless refeed do not get to tell you about it. The history of long fasting is told by the survivors. The casualty list is shorter than the survivor list, but the casualty list is real.

Take the labs. Read the numbers. Then break your fast with broth and walk into the next chapter of the life you came here to live.

— Mark W. Boutwell II

Post-Fast Lab Follow-Up Schedule

A reference schedule for the first year after a prolonged fast.

9 draws over 12 months. Tapers from weekly (refeed window) to monthly (recovery) to quarterly (long-term). Refer to the Lab Requisition document for the full test list referenced by tier.

WHEN YOU CAN STOP

After Draw 9 (one year post-fast), annual labs become your normal health baseline — same cadence most people should follow. The intensive 6-month cadence ends. If everything is stable at Draw 9, you can shift to once-yearly comprehensive plus once-yearly basic.

Stop sooner if: budget forces it. The non-negotiable draws are 1, 2, and 3 — the refeed-safety window. After Draw 3, every subsequent draw is valuable but not safety-critical.

BARE MINIMUM SCHEDULE (if budget is tight)

Draw 1 (today, full panel) — done.

Draw 2 (Day 3, refeeding safety, ~$100) — non-negotiable.

Draw 3 (Day 7, refeed + nutrients, ~$175) — non-negotiable.

Draw 5 (Day 30, full picture, ~$450) — single best 'after' snapshot for the book.

Skip the rest if needed. Total minimum: ~$725 on top of today's draw.

TOTAL COST RANGE

Bare minimum (4 draws): ~$1,750–$2,400 over the year

Full schedule (9 draws): ~$4,750–$6,400 over the year

All prices assume cash-pay through Ulta Lab Tests or similar direct-to-consumer service. Hospital prices would be 3–5x.

Chapter 35

Special Considerations

* * *

Some readers come to this work carrying something that changes how it should be approached. Those who have done extended fasting before. Those undertaking subsequent fasts after their first. Vegetarians with specific considerations. Those who have done previous parasite cleanses.

The protocol is the same. But the experience and the timeline can be quite different depending on what you bring to it. The body that arrives at this work having done it before is a different body from the one that arrives entirely new, and the protocol that worked the first time will work differently — usually faster, often deeper — the second and third times.

For Those With Previous Fasting Experience

Each subsequent fast builds on the last. The body has metabolic memory of the fasted state. The mind has psychological familiarity with the rhythm. The work that was done previously has not been undone, and the new work begins from a foundation that the first fast had to build from scratch.

What changes from first to subsequent fasts:

Ketosis transition:

• First fast: 3 to 5 days for full transition.

• Second fast: 1 to 2 days typically.

• Subsequent fasts: sometimes within 24 hours.

• Body has metabolic memory of the fasted state.

Initial difficulty:

• First fast: first three days are typically the hardest.

• Subsequent fasts: often surprisingly easier from the start.

• The mental component is largely already known.

• The physical transition is more efficient.

Cleansing depth:

• First fast: surface and middle layers primarily.

• Second fast: deeper layers and remaining accumulation.

• Third and subsequent fasts: increasingly deep work.

• Each fast addresses what the previous left behind.

Egg elimination:

• First fast: may not fully eliminate all egg deposits.

• Subsequent fasts: work through what remained.

• Multiple fasts often required for complete fluke elimination.

Timeline Adjustments for Returning Fasters

The compressed timeline of subsequent fasts is one of the most striking features of returning to the practice. The body that has already done this work needs less time to do it again.

Process

First Fast

Subsequent Fasts

Ketosis establishment

3-5 days

1-2 days

Surface clearing

7-10 days

3-5 days

Mucoid plaque release

10-21 days

5-14 days

Adult worm clearing

7-14 days

5-10 days

Egg elimination

Full timeline

Reduced timeline

Liver fluke clearing

14-21 days

10-14 days

Total fast duration commonly

28-40 days

21-30 days

Why the timeline compresses: less initial accumulation to clear; the body knows the process; the immune system is primed from previous experience; the mental preparation is already done; the refeeding protocols are already understood.

What Subsequent Fasts Often Reveal

Each fast reveals what the previous one missed. The pattern is consistent enough to be predictable.

Second fast often clears:

- Liver flukes that survived the first fast.
- Deeper biofilm communities.
- Older accumulation from earliest decades.
- Emotional content that did not surface previously.

Third fast often addresses:

- The deepest tissue level work.
- Patterns the body was not ready to release earlier.
- Heavy metal accumulation.

• Stored emotional content from very early life.

Each subsequent fast reaches what was previously inaccessible, builds on the foundation of the previous work, achieves greater depth in less time, and often produces different emotional and spiritual experiences than its predecessors.

Considerations for Those With Previous Cleanse Attempts

Many readers will have tried other cleansing protocols before this one. The experience of having done partial cleanses changes how the protocol unfolds the next time.

If previous protocols were incomplete:

• This protocol can complete what others started.

• The clove protocol especially addresses what is commonly missed.

• The integrated approach typically achieves what fragmented approaches do not.

If previous protocols caused issues:

• May need extended preparation phase.

• Slower entry into the full protocol.

• Particular attention to electrolytes.

• Possibly shorter initial duration with subsequent fasts.

What previous protocols often missed:

• Egg destruction (no clove or insufficient clove).

• Liver fluke specifically (most protocols do not address).

• Bile duct work (no coffee enemas).

• Mineral support adequacy.

Physical Adaptations Across Multiple Fasts

The body learns. Each fast trains the body, and subsequent fasts inherit that training.

• **Metabolic adaptation.** Each fast trains metabolic flexibility. Ketosis becomes a more accessible state. Fat utilization more efficient. Less metabolic stress with each subsequent fast.

• **Detoxification capacity.** Liver function improves with each cycle. Detoxification pathways more efficient. Less Herxheimer reaction with subsequent fasts. Better tolerance of die-off processes.

• **Microbiome resilience.** Beneficial bacterial populations more established. Stronger response to herbal interventions. More robust rebuilding capacity. Greater resistance to dysbiosis.

Psychological Adaptations

The mental component changes as well as the physical.

• **Less fear.** The process is no longer unknown. Difficult phases are familiar. Confidence is based on previous successful completion.

• **More acceptance.** Of difficult days. Of emotional surfacing. Of body signals. Of the time required.

• **Deeper engagement.** More attention to subtle signals. Greater appreciation for the process. More sophisticated relationship with the practice. Often deeper spiritual or psychological dimensions.

When Multiple Fasts Become Beneficial

This is worth considering carefully. The decision to undertake another prolonged fast deserves the same kind of intentionality as the decision to undertake the first one.

Reasons to consider multiple fasts:

• First fast clearly incomplete based on signs.

• Specific parasites confirmed not fully cleared.

• Major life events disrupted between fasts.

• Periodic deep maintenance for ongoing health.

• Continued personal development through the practice.

Reasons not to multiply fasts:

• The current results are good and sustained.

• Maintenance protocols are working well.

• Compulsion or anxiety driving the impulse.

• Disordered eating patterns emerging.

Healthy frequency for prolonged fasts:

• After full integration of the previous fast.

• With at least 12 to 18 months between intensive fasts in most cases.

• When clear specific reasons indicate value.

• Not as routine practice but as intentional intervention.

A Note on This Book's Author

The context here is relevant. The author of this book — having guided approximately 500 people through prolonged fasting and being currently in a second 40-day fast — represents a profile worth noting:

• Substantial direct experience.

• Significant time integrating previous fasts.

• Vegetarian for 12 years.

• Medical professional context.

• Returning to the practice with full preparation.

This is the appropriate context for prolonged fasting: genuine experience, integration time between intensive practices, lifestyle supporting maintenance, professional knowledge base, returning by choice rather than compulsion. This book is written from that context. Readers approaching prolonged fasting should consider what context they bring to the practice.

Final Thoughts on the Returning Faster

If you are reading this section because you are returning to prolonged fasting, you bring more than first-time fasters bring. The protocol can do more for you because of what you have already done. The work is potentially deeper — not just because of what you remove, but because of what you can access.

Use that experience. Trust what your body has learned. Allow the practice to take you deeper than it could the first time. The first fast was the introduction. Subsequent fasts are the practice itself. The depth available is rare. Receive it.

Figure Guide

Every figure referenced in this book — the parasites and their eggs, the lifecycle diagrams, the clinical images — lives in an online figure guide. It is kept current and added to over time, which a printed page cannot be.

You will find it here:

eighthrs.com

The figure numbers in the chapters — Figure 4.1, Figure 10.3, and so on — match the guide. When you reach a figure and want to see the image, open the guide and find it by its number.

Quick Reference Charts

Practical tools, meant to be photocopied or photographed.

The charts that follow are stripped-down versions of the tracking tools and protocol references introduced throughout the book. Each one is meant to live with you during the work — clipped to a wall, tucked in a journal, or photographed on a phone for reference. Use them however serves you.

A 7-Day Signal Log

From Chapter 15 — Reading Your Body's Signals.

Day *Date*	**Energy** *1–10, when it dipped*	**Mental clarity** *1–10, fog or sharp?*	**Mood** *one or two words*	**Digestive** *gas, bloating, gurgling, nausea*	**Body odor & breath** *intensity; sweet, sour, metallic*	**Tongue** *coating: thick/thin, color*	**Skin** *breakouts, itching, clarity*	**Enema returns** *color, consistency, debris*	**Sleep** *hours, quality 1–10, dreams*	**Anything unusual** *anything that doesn't fit above*
Day 1										
Day 2										
Day 3										
Day 4										
Day 5										
Day 6										
Day 7										

The Daily Enema Chart

From Chapter 18 — Coffee Enemas & Liver Cleansing.

	AM — Coffee Enema	PM — Salt Water Enema
Timing	Morning, on rising	2 to 3 hours before sleep
Base liquid	48 oz water with ionic sulfated minerals	48 oz water with ionic sulfated minerals
Coffee *	3 tbsp organic light-roast, simmered 15 min, strained	—
Salt *	—	1 to 2 tsp Himalayan salt, fully dissolved
Clove oil *	2 to 3 drops, food-grade only	—
Black walnut hull tincture *	1 teaspoon	—
Milk thistle extract **	1 teaspoon	—
Aloe vera juice **	—	4 oz, inner leaf only
Magnesium chloride **	—	½ teaspoon
Pau d'arco tincture **	—	1 teaspoon
Temperature	Body temperature	Body temperature
Hold time	12 to 15 minutes, with position rotation	10 to 15 minutes
Replenish after	16 oz water, trace minerals, pinch salt, coconut water if available	16 oz water with trace minerals; magnesium glycinate before sleep
Purpose	Egg killer, adult parasite killer, liver protector	Soother, relaxer, antifungal sweep

* **Essential.** The minimum that makes this enema therapeutic.

** **Ideal.** The full protocol used in Weeks 2 onward.

*** **Situational.** Catalogued in Chapter 17.

The Herbal Antiparasitic Reference

Substance	Type	Tagline	Active Compounds	Primary Targets	Mechanism
Black walnut hull *	Whole-plant tincture (unripe green hull)	The adult killer	Juglone; tannins; naturally occurring iodine compounds	Adult tapeworms (especially); adult roundworms incl. hookworm and whipworm; adult intestinal flukes; Candida; various pathogenic bacteria	Direct toxicity
Wormwood *	Whole-plant tincture (*Artemisia absinthium*)	The larvae destroyer	Thujone (most active); artemisinin (in sweet wormwood); sesquiterpene lactones; bitter compounds	Parasite larvae across many species; juvenile parasites pre-reproduction; some adult roundworms; certain protozoa (incl. malaria parasites historically)	Reproductive interference; broad antimicrobial; moderate biofilm disruption
Clove *	Essential oil and tincture (*Syzygium aromaticum*)	The egg killer	Eugenol (primary)	Parasite eggs across species — the singular role nothing else fills; adult organisms; bacteria; fungi	Egg shell penetration; direct toxicity
Piperine *	Black pepper extract	The amplifier	Piperine (the active alkaloid of *Piper nigrum*)	Not antiparasitic itself — increases bioavailability of every other herb in the protocol	Inhibits drug-metabolizing enzymes; increases absorption up to 2000% for some compounds
Berberine **	Isolated alkaloid (from Oregon grape root, goldenseal, barberry)	The protozoa specialist	Berberine	Giardia (exceptionally effective); Cryptosporidium; broad-spectrum bacteria; Candida; some parasites	Membrane disruption; enzymatic disruption; significant biofilm activity
Oregano oil **	Essential oil (*Origanum vulgare*)	The membrane breaker	Carvacrol (primary); thymol (secondary)	Candida (exceptional); broad-spectrum bacteria; some protozoa	Membrane disruption; strong biofilm disruption

Substance	Type	Tagline	Active Compounds	Primary Targets	Mechanism
Mimosa pudica **	Seed	The mechanical scrubber	Mucilaginous compounds that gel in the gut	All worm species (mechanical removal); biofilm; heavy metals; toxins	Mechanical adsorption — physically grabs and removes
Chanca piedra **	Whole-plant tincture / capsule (*Phyllanthus niruri*)	The stone breaker	Phyllanthin and related lignans	Bile duct sludge and small biliary stones; supports liver during fluke clearing	Bile flow stimulation; anti-inflammatory in bile ducts
Milk thistle **	Standardized extract (*Silybum marianum*)	The liver protector	Silymarin (silibinin and related flavonolignans)	Not antiparasitic — protects liver cells during heavy detox phases	Hepatocyte membrane stabilization; supports liver regeneration
Dandelion root **	Whole-plant tincture / tea / capsule (*Taraxacum officinale*)	The bile mover	Sesquiterpene lactones; taraxasterol; inulin	Supports bile production and flow; mild laxative effect	Bile stimulation; supports liver in processing released toxins
Pau d'arco **	Inner bark tincture or tea (*Tabebuia* tree species)	The South American antifungal	Naphthoquinones (lapachol the most studied); beta-lapachone	Candida; certain protozoa incl. Cryptosporidium (as secondary); some bacteria	Direct toxicity to fungal cells; immune modulation
Pumpkin seed ***	Whole seed (*Cucurbita pepo*)	The paralyzer	Cucurbitacin	Tapeworms (particularly effective); roundworms; some flukes	Paralysis of parasite muscle tissue
Caprylic acid ***	Medium-chain fatty acid (from coconut oil)	The Candida disruptor	Caprylic acid (octanoic acid)	Candida albicans (primary); other yeasts	Membrane disruption — inserts into the fungal lipid bilayer

* **Essential.** The classic triad plus piperine. The minimum that makes the protocol work.

** **Ideal.** Broad-spectrum and liver-phase support. Used from the second week onward.

*** **Situational.** Used when specific conditions apply.

† **On taking capsules during the fast.** Several substances above are taken in capsule form. During a water fast, the preferred practice is to open the capsule and mix the powder into a small amount of water rather than swallow the capsule whole. Two reasons: digestive activity slows during fasting, so the capsule shell may not dissolve reliably; and gelatin capsules are an animal product some readers prefer to avoid during the fast. Vegetable cellulose capsules avoid the second concern but not the first. For powders too bitter to

mix with water (berberine, oregano-derived compounds), the capsule is acceptable as long as it is a vegetable-cellulose type.

The Full Timeline Comparison

The phases of the cleanse mapped against five common reader scenarios. Read the column that matches your situation. Day ranges are approximate. The order of phases is consistent.

Phase	No Herbs / First Time	Herbs / First Time	Herbs + Coffee Enema / First Time	Herbs / Second Time After 28-Day Fast	Herbs + Coffee Enema / Second Time After 28-Day Fast + Vegetarian Diet
Surface clearing	Days 1–5	Days 1–3	Days 1–2	Days 1–2	Day 1
Candida die-off begins	Days 10–14	Days 7–10	Days 5–7	Days 5–7	Days 3–5
First parasite cycle cleared	Days 14–21	Days 10–14	Days 8–12	Days 7–10	Days 5–8
Biofilm disruption	Days 15–21	Days 10–14	Days 8–11	Days 8–12	Days 5–8
Intestinal fluke die-off begins	Days 18–25	Days 12–16	Days 9–13	Days 9–13	Days 6–9
Liver fluke bile duct flushing	Unlikely without coffee enema	Partial	Days 10–15	Days 10–14	Days 7–11
Fluke eggs targeted by clove	Days 21–28	Days 14–18	Days 12–16	Days 10–14	Days 7–11
Second parasite cycle	Days 21–28	Days 14–18	Days 12–15	Days 11–15	Days 8–12
Deep layer release	Days 22–30	Days 16–22	Days 13–18	Days 13–18	Days 9–14
Third parasite cycle	Days 28–35	Days 20–24	Days 16–20	Days 16–20	Days 11–16
Liver fluke clearance	Rarely achieved	Days 22–28	Days 18–24	Days 16–22	Days 12–18
Intestinal lining regenerating	Days 25–35	Days 18–24	Days 15–20	Days 15–21	Days 11–17
Fluke egg second cycle cleared	Rarely achieved	Days 24–30	Days 20–25	Days 18–24	Days 13–18
Estimated full cleanse	28–40 days	22–30 days	18–25 days	18–25 days	15–22 days

What to Continue After the Fast

Reference for the post-fast continuation. Each element listed below has a specific role and a specific duration. Photograph or print this for reference during refeeding.

Element	Action After Breaking Fast
Trace minerals	Continue indefinitely
L-Glutamine	Continue 2-4 weeks for lining support
Clove tincture	Continue 3× daily until egg cycle complete (1-3 weeks)
Coffee enema	2-3× weekly initially; reduce to weekly, then monthly
Salt water enema	Reduce to as needed based on signals
Black walnut hull	Continue 2 weeks at reduced dose
Wormwood	Continue 1 week then discontinue
Berberine †	Continue 2-4 weeks as microbiome stabilizes
Mimosa pudica †	Continue 1-2 weeks
Milk thistle †	Continue 4-6 weeks for liver support
Probiotics	Begin and continue indefinitely
Fermented foods	Begin gradually and continue indefinitely
Coconut oil/MCT	Continue indefinitely as part of diet

† **On capsule preparation during refeeding.** Several substances above can be taken in capsule form. During the first 1-2 weeks of refeeding, the same guidance from Chapter 19 applies — open the capsule and mix the powder into a small amount of water rather than swallow whole. Digestion is still re-establishing, capsule shells may not dissolve reliably, and the liquid diet of early refeeding doesn't provide the digestive activation that capsules need. Once you're eating solid foods well (typically by week 2-3), capsules can be swallowed normally.

The Critical Two-Week Continuation

The two weeks immediately after breaking the fast. The protocol during this window determines whether the work consolidates or unravels.

The two weeks immediately after breaking the fast deserve specific attention. The protocol during this window is what determines whether the work of the previous month consolidates or unravels.

Element	Week 1 of Refeeding	Week 2 of Refeeding
Clove tincture	3× daily — non-negotiable	Continuing 3× daily
Black walnut hull	Once daily at half dose	Discontinued
Wormwood	Once daily for first 5 days, then discontinue	Discontinued
Mimosa pudica †	First 5 days	Discontinued
Milk thistle †	Daily	Continuing
Coffee enema	Every other day	Twice in the week
Probiotics	Begin Day 7 (single strain, low dose)	Increase gradually
Fermented foods	Day 5 onward (small amounts)	Wider variety; kefir if tolerated

† See the capsule note under the previous chart — capsule preparation guidance applies during early refeeding while digestion re-establishes.

Chart S — The Endocannabinoid System Across the Body

From Chapter 10. Six places in the body where the endocannabinoid system does its quiet work, in two columns: the way it shows up when the system is well, and the way it shows up when the system has thinned.

Body system	When the system is well	When the system is thinning
Sleep	The body softens toward sleep without being argued with. The mind quiets. Sleep is unfractured and the next morning is rested.	The day will not let go. Sleep takes longer to arrive, breaks across the night, and leaves the morning unfinished.
Mood	After a hard hour, the mood comes back to its own steady place the way water returns to its level after a stone is thrown.	Hard hours stay. The steadiness that should have returned by evening is still missing the next morning.
Pain	A small injury reports itself, the report is heard, and the pain takes its leave once the message has been received.	The pain that should have eased yesterday is still here today. A person begins to think of it as theirs to keep.
Hunger	Hunger arrives when the body has called for it and matches what the body has actually been doing.	Hunger arrives in the afternoon for reasons the afternoon did not produce. Appetite is something else wearing appetite's clothes.
Inflammation	When something has gone wrong, the alarm rises and then, the work being done, falls back to where it was before.	The alarm rises and stays risen. The joint, the skin, the gut keep simmering long after the original wrong has passed.
Gut motility	The slow ordered rhythm of the gut holds. Food enters, is taken in, is moved through at the steady pace the body has known for decades.	The rhythm falters. The gut speeds when it should slow, slows when it should move, forgets the timing it has known for years.

Chart T — The Arc of Repair After a Long Fast

From Chapter 25. A reference for what to expect across the months and years that follow a prolonged fast. The middle column tracks what is happening internally; the right column tracks what a person may experience and what is normal at each stage.

Time	What is happening inside	What a person may notice
First days	• Reintroduction begins with small amounts of simple food (broth, soft cooked vegetables). • Lining is reactivating digestion that has been paused for weeks. • Repair has not yet begun in earnest.	• Smaller appetite than expected; easily full. • Heightened sensitivity to flavor, salt, and sweetness. • Stools may be loose or irregular as digestion restarts.
First weeks	• Bacterial community begins to rebalance. • Immune cells beneath the lining come down off chronic alarm. • Body releases stored toxins and old undigested matter as eating resumes.	• Detox phase common in week one or two: looser stools, brief fatigue. • A heavier-than-usual evacuation event is possible. • Old food reactions begin to lessen.
First months	• Mucus layer rebuilds to full thickness. • Bacterial community completes most rebalancing. • New cells form on a clean substrate; each renewal cycle leaves the lining steadily improved.	• Reduced bloating after meals. • Foods that previously caused reactions may be tolerated. • Energy more stable; sleep quality often improves. • Skin may clear.
The years	• Lining renews every 3-5 days on a clean substrate. • Maintenance, not repair. • Capacity to absorb occasional insults (a poor meal, stressful week, needed medication) without reverting to chronic damage.	• Discomfort after a problem food is brief and clear, not dragging on for days. • Baseline digestion is reliable. • Rebuilding required only if life returns to chronic damage patterns.

Chart P — The Long-Arc Taper

The shape of the months that follow the first two weeks. Some elements taper toward absence; others continue indefinitely as part of how the practitioner now lives.

The protocol does not end when the first two weeks end. It thins. Some elements taper toward absence; others continue indefinitely as part of how the practitioner now lives. The shape of that thinning, set out below, is what distinguishes the practitioner whose results last from the one who was simply between fasts.

Element	Schedule
Clove tincture	3× daily through end of Week 7. Non-negotiable. The single most important continuation.
Black walnut hull	Once daily at half dose through end of Week 3. Then discontinue.
Wormwood	Once daily through end of Week 2. Then discontinue.

Element	Schedule
Mimosa pudica	Once daily through end of Week 4. Then discontinue.
Berberine	Once daily through end of Week 5. Then discontinue.
L-glutamine	Daily through end of Week 4. Optional continuation thereafter.
Milk thistle	Daily through end of Week 7. Optional continuation thereafter.
MCT or coconut oil	Continue indefinitely as part of the long-term diet.
Trace minerals	Continue indefinitely.
Coffee enema	Week 3: twice weekly. Weeks 4 to 8: once weekly. Beyond Week 8: monthly maintenance. Discontinue when energy is sustained and signals indicate no further need.
Probiotics — single strain	Day 7 onward through end of Week 2.
Probiotics — multi-strain	From Week 2 onward. Continue indefinitely.
Probiotics — spore-based	From Week 4 onward. Continue indefinitely.
Fermented foods	From Day 5 onward. Build to daily inclusion at most meals by Week 4. Continue indefinitely.
Bone broth	Weekly basis ideal. Continue as part of long-term diet.
Periodic resets	Quarterly: one-week antiparasitic maintenance. Annually: two-week intensive period. Every 3 to 5 years: consideration of another prolonged fast.

Chart Q — The Seven Pillars in Working Form. From Chapter 33 — The Long Partnership. The seven pillars paired with their practical specifics. The prose in the chapter is the why; this chart is the what.

Pillar	Practical specifics
1. Microbial community	Daily fermented food (kimchi, sauerkraut, yogurt, kefir). Plant variety across the week.
2. Gut wall	Bone broth weekly. L-glutamine in periodic short cycles. Olive oil, butter from grass-fed animals, occasional coconut oil.
3. Slowness of digestion	Sit-down meals. Adequate chewing. Several hours between meals.
4. Inflammation	Daily omega-3s. Polyphenol-rich foods (dark berries, green tea, turmeric, olive oil). Avoid industrial seed oils, refined sugars, processed foods.
5. Vagus nerve / nervous system	Adequate sleep. Daily walks. Breathing practice or meditation. Nourishing relationships kept; depleting ones thinned.
6. Toxin load	Water filter. Organic produce when feasible. Simple cleaning products. Periodic milk thistle. Regular sweating.
7. Longer rhythm	Quarterly: one-week antiparasitic maintenance. Annually: two-week intensification. Every 3-5 years: consideration of another prolonged fast.

Chart R — The Trace Minerals. From Chapter 3 — Trace Minerals, Bacteria & Enzymes. The seven trace minerals most often named in the chapter prose, with their roles and food sources. The body draws on as many as a hundred ionic sulfated trace minerals across its work; the chart below is a reference, not a complete catalog.

Trace mineral	Role and food sources
Zinc	Activates hundreds of digestive and immune enzymes. Found in oysters, grass-fed beef, pumpkin seeds, lentils, eggs.
Magnesium	Activates more enzymatic work than any other element; supports muscle relaxation and the energy work of the mitochondria. Found in dark leafy greens, pumpkin seeds, almonds, dark chocolate, avocado, fish.
Manganese	Protects the cells of the gut lining from oxidative damage. Found in pineapple, pecans, brown rice, leafy greens, whole grains.
Selenium	Activates immune defenses of the gut and supports the chemistry of detoxification, particularly during parasite die-off. Found in Brazil nuts (one or two a day is sufficient), seafood, eggs, organ meats.
Copper	Essential for the small fires of the mitochondria; supports connective tissue and iron metabolism. Found in shellfish, organ meats, dark chocolate, sesame seeds, cashews.
Chromium	Steadies the body's relationship with sugar; holds insulin's responsiveness across the day. Found in broccoli, grass-fed meats, whole grains, brewer's yeast.
Molybdenum	Activates the liver's deeper detoxification systems. Found in legumes, leafy greens, organ meats, whole grains.

The Coffee Enema Long-Arc Schedule

The arc of the months that follow. The role thins gradually as the body returns to its baseline.

The coffee enema does not end with the first two weeks. Its role thins. From a protocol practiced every other day or twice in the week, it steps down — first to a few times each week, then weekly, then monthly, then to as-needed only. The schedule below is the arc.

Period	Frequency
Week 3	Twice weekly.
Weeks 4 to 8	Once weekly.
Beyond Week 8	Monthly maintenance.
Solution	Standard solution — the additions like clove oil and black walnut tincture continue.
Discontinue	Once the practitioner has been eating normally for several weeks, energy is sustained at high baseline, no signals indicate continued need, and the body is integrated into post-fast equilibrium.

Chart U

The Liver-Gallbladder Flush Protocol

* * *

The liver-gallbladder flush is one of the oldest practices in this tradition and one of the most direct. It works by stimulating a sudden release of bile from the gallbladder and bile ducts, carrying out with that release the accumulated material — calcified bile components, hardened sludge, sometimes parasitic remnants — that has been stored over years. The flush is not subtle. The body knows what is being asked and, on the night of the flush, gives a clear report of having done it.

What follows is the full six-month protocol used in the year of preparation described in the chapter on preparing the body. For readers without a year of preparation time available, the minimum acceptable variation is given at the end. The full protocol — six monthly flushes followed by a six-month settle — serves the body better than a compressed version, because the body needs the time between flushes to integrate what each one has reached. The settle period at the end is not optional. It is the part of the protocol that has no ingredients.

Before each flush — five days of preparation

1. Begin five days before the flush night. For each of the five days, drink one gallon of water treated with ionic sulfated minerals and thirty-two ounces of organic apple cider (not vinegar — pressed apple cider, the cloudy unfiltered kind sold near the cold-pressed juices). Spread both across the day; do not drink either in one sitting.

2. The malic acid in the cider softens biliary deposits across the five days, preparing them to be released by the flush.

3. Continue eating normally during the five preparation days, with one shift: reduce or eliminate fats, especially heavy fats, in the last forty-eight hours. The gallbladder will be asked to expel a great deal of bile on the flush night, and a full reservoir gives the flush more to work with.

4. On the fifth day, eat a light lunch by two o'clock in the afternoon. After lunch, no further food until after the flush is complete the next morning.

The flush night itself

1. At six o'clock in the evening: dissolve four tablespoons of Epsom salt in three cups of filtered water. Drink three quarters of a cup. The taste is bitter and the body, especially after several previous flushes, will recognize and resist it. Drink it anyway.

2. At eight o'clock: drink another three quarters of a cup of the same Epsom salt solution.
3. At ten o'clock: in a glass jar, combine half a cup of cold-pressed organic olive oil with three quarters of a cup of fresh-squeezed pink grapefruit juice (or freshly squeezed lemon juice if grapefruit is unavailable or contraindicated by medications). Shake the jar until the mixture is uniformly cloudy. Stand near the bed. Drink the entire mixture as quickly as is possible without making the body reject it. Lie down on the right side immediately, knees drawn up toward the chest. Stay in this position for at least thirty minutes without moving.
4. The position matters. Lying on the right side, with the legs drawn up, opens the bile ducts most fully and allows the oil-and-juice mixture to do its work. Movement during this period interrupts the contraction the gallbladder is being asked to perform.
5. Sleep through the night in whatever position is comfortable. The work the flush is doing happens regardless of sleep position once the first thirty minutes have passed.

The morning after

1. On waking: drink three quarters of a cup of the remaining Epsom salt solution. This is the dose the body will most resist; it is also the dose that pushes the released material from the small bowel through and out. If the third dose does not go down, the night before will not finish.
2. Two hours after the third Epsom dose: drink a fourth and final three quarters of a cup of the Epsom solution.
3. Two hours after the fourth dose: the first food may be light — fresh fruit, a small smoothie, plain juice. Wait an additional two hours before introducing anything heavier.
4. What is released across the morning following a flush varies widely. Small green or dark-brown pebbles are the most common report. Larger objects, more substantial volume, or no visible objects at all are all within the range of normal first-flush experiences. See Chart V for what each category of released material is most likely to be.

The full protocol

One flush per month, for six months. The first flush typically produces the largest visible release. The second through fourth typically taper. The fifth often produces little. The sixth, in many practitioners, produces a renewed volume because deeper reservoirs that earlier flushes did not reach have finally opened.

After the sixth flush: stop. Do no further flushes for six months. The bile ducts and gallbladder need this time to find their own rhythm with what has been changed. Eat carefully, sleep carefully, and let the body hold the work without further intervention. The morning gut at the end of the six-month settle should be measurably different from the morning gut at the start of the six-month flush phase.

Total elapsed time from first flush to end of settle: twelve months. This is the full preparation pattern.

Minimum acceptable variation

Readers without twelve months of preparation time available may compress the flush phase, with proportional loss of effect. The minimum that retains meaningful preparation value: three monthly flushes over three months, followed by at least one month of settle before beginning the prolonged fast itself. Four monthly flushes followed by a two-month settle is preferable to three. Five flushes followed by three months of settle is closer to full. Six flushes plus six months of settle is the full version.

Compressing more aggressively than three flushes in three months — for example, attempting two or three flushes in a single month — is not recommended. The body needs the weeks between flushes to integrate what each one has reached. Flushes done too close together produce diminishing returns and ask the gallbladder to perform contractions it has not yet recovered from.

Contraindications and when to consult a physician

Do not perform a liver-gallbladder flush without first consulting a physician if any of the following apply: known gallstones large enough to potentially obstruct the bile duct (typically larger than half an inch on imaging); a history of pancreatitis; current bile duct or gallbladder infection; pregnancy or breastfeeding; current medications metabolized through the liver in ways that may interact with grapefruit (a non-exhaustive list includes statins, certain blood pressure medications, certain immunosuppressants, and some psychiatric medications); a history of significant cardiac arrhythmia (Epsom salt is magnesium sulfate and can affect cardiac rhythm in some bodies).

If during the flush night the body experiences sudden severe pain in the upper right abdomen radiating to the back or shoulder, persistent vomiting, fever, or yellowing of the skin or eyes, the flush should be stopped and emergency medical care sought. These signs may indicate a stone obstructing the bile duct, which is the principal serious adverse event possible with this protocol and which becomes proportionally more likely the larger the stones being released.

The protocol described here is for adults in reasonable general health. It is not appropriate for children, for the very elderly, or for any person whose condition has not been evaluated by a physician familiar with the specific contraindications above.

A final note

The flush is the most concrete preparation the body can do for a prolonged fast. Done across months, with the settle period that follows, it delivers to day one of the fast a body whose primary detoxification organ has been measurably opened, lightened, and restored to a working rhythm it had likely not held in years. The fast itself reaches further than any flush can. The flushes are how the body arrives at the threshold ready to receive what the fast does.

See the supplemental resources QR code at the back of this book for the recommended product list and printable version of this chart.

Chart V

What You May See and When

* * *

Across the prolonged fast, the body does its clearing work below the level a person can ordinarily see. The enema, by carrying the contents of the lower bowel out into a bowl, gives the practitioner the only direct view of the work the gut is doing. What appears in that bowl across forty days is varied, sometimes vivid, often unexpected, and not always identifiable to anyone who has not seen it before. This chart describes what the practitioner is most likely to encounter, what each category of material is most likely to be, and what the patterns across the arc of the fast suggest about the work's progress.

A note before the descriptions begin. The toilet bowl is not a microscope. Some of what appears in it can be identified with reasonable confidence — bile by its color and consistency, adult roundworms by their shape and size, tapeworm segments by their distinct rectangular form. Other material, especially the long rope-form structures the cleansing tradition has called mucoid plaque or rope worm, has not been settled in the medical literature. Conventional medicine reads these structures as compacted intestinal mucus expelled in larger pieces because the prolonged fast and daily enemas alter what the gut produces and how it moves. The cleansing tradition reads them as accumulated debris, biofilm, dead pathogens, or possibly an unidentified parasite. The honest position is that nobody has, to date, settled the question with the kind of evidence that closes it. What both readings agree on is that something has been in the gut long enough to have shape, and now is gone, and bodies that have been carrying these structures tend to feel different once they are no longer carrying them. The practitioner is not asked to resolve the disagreement. The practitioner is asked to look, and to read what their own body reports.

Bile

Bile is the fluid the liver makes to digest fats. It begins as a yellow-green secretion, and by the time it has done its work in the small intestine and traveled the length of the gut, bacterial action has converted it to the brown that ordinary stool carries. When transit is fast — or when a coffee enema dilates the bile ducts and stimulates a sudden release from the gallbladder — the bile arrives in the lower bowel still in its yellow-green or dark-green state, having had no time to convert. This is the green ooze the practitioner sees in the bowl after the morning enema, especially in the first weeks of the fast.

Clean bile, expelled by a body that has been clearing well, has the consistency of an ooze. It is fluid. It pours rather than holds shape. Its color is a yellow-green to deep green, sometimes shading toward olive or, when older bile has been stored a long time and is finally released, toward brown-black. What clean bile does not contain, when the gut beneath it has been cleared, is particulate matter. The practitioner whose enema is producing bile-only ooze, day after day, without distinct pieces suspended in it, is reading a body whose currently accessible reservoir of stored material has been exhausted.

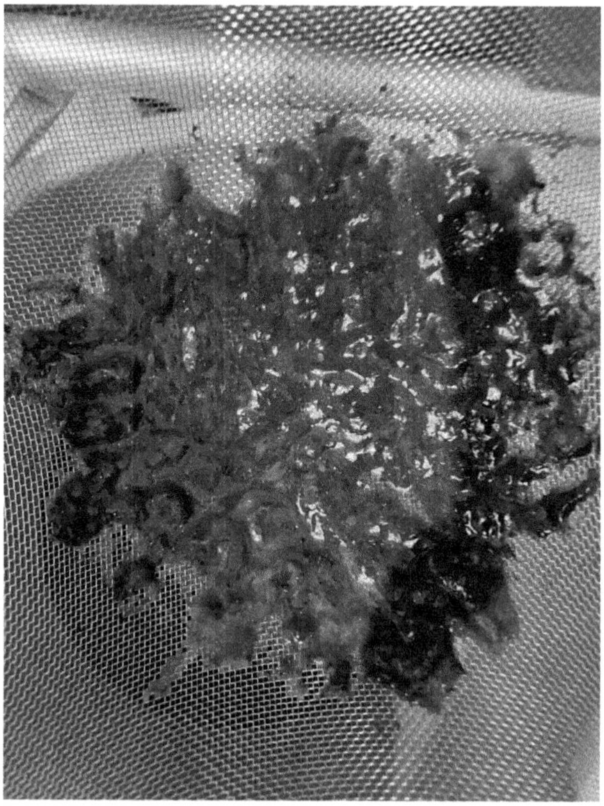

Bile on the screen — the green ooze the gut releases when the liver work begins.

Pebbles, stones, and small particulates

What appears in the bowl alongside the bile, especially in early and middle weeks, is most often a mix of materials. Small green or dark-brown pebbles, sometimes the size of grains of rice, sometimes larger, are the most consistently described. The cleansing tradition calls these gallstones, the same name used for the calcified deposits that form in the gallbladder and bile ducts and are visible on imaging in conventional medicine. The honest description of what these pebbles are, in a body undergoing prolonged fasting and enemas, is more layered. Some are calcified bile components — cholesterol crystals, bile salts, and bilirubin pigment that have hardened in the gallbladder and ducts over time, and have now been dislodged. Some, when the practitioner has performed liver-gallbladder flushes that include olive oil, are likely bile-soaked aggregations of the oil itself, formed by the interaction of the oil with the alkaline bile environment. Some are likely older biliary sludge that has compacted into pebble form across years.

What can be said with confidence is that the body has been holding them long enough for them to take form, and that they are no longer being held. What cannot reliably be distinguished, without laboratory analysis, is which of the pebbles in any given bowl are biliary stones, which are bile-soaked olive oil, and which are something else again. The practitioner is best served by noticing the trend over time — the volume reducing, the size diminishing, the pebbles eventually ceasing to appear — rather than attempting to classify each one.

Rope-form structures (mucoid plaque, rope worm)

Among the most striking things the practitioner is likely to encounter is the long rope-form structure that has come, in the cleansing tradition, to be called rope worm or mucoid plaque. These are stringy, sometimes rubbery, sometimes thick, sometimes flat and ribbon-like, ranging from a few inches to over a foot in length, occasionally longer. They have a recognizable structure — a starting point, an end point, and a kind of tensile integrity that holds until enough force is applied, at which point they break in a way that resembles the breaking of a long-dried worm or a length of weakened cord. Their color varies widely: brown, blackish-green, grey, yellow, sometimes with bile coloring throughout. Some have the appearance of a coiled or twisted structure, suggesting the shape of the gut they emerged from.

What these structures are has not been settled. The Russian researchers Volinsky and Gubarev proposed in 2013 that they are an unidentified parasite, calling them rope worms, and described five developmental stages. Their papers were not accepted by peer-reviewed journals. The cleansing tradition predating their work, going back to alternative-medicine practitioners in the early twentieth century, calls the same material mucoid plaque — accumulated mucus, biofilm, dead microbial material, and dietary residue, hardened over years into structured deposits. Conventional medicine reads them as ordinary intestinal mucus expelled in larger clumps because aggressive cleansing irritates the mucosal lining and the body produces more mucus in response. A 1930s Journal of the American Medical Association article described them, after colonics, as brown or blackish sheets, strings, and rolled-up wormlike masses of tough mucus with a rotten or dead-fish odor — and noted, regardless of what they were, that ill people who passed them reported relief of symptoms.

The practitioner who passes one of these structures sees what they see: a thing that had been in the gut, that had taken form, and that is no longer in the gut. The chart's recommendation is to let it be what it is, to note that it has come out, and to continue. The body that has been carrying this material tends to feel different on the day after one passes than on the day before. That difference, regardless of which name the structure is given, is the practical evidence the practitioner has to work with.

Parasite remnants

The parasites that have been the subject of the larger work of this book do, in some bodies, appear in the bowl during a prolonged fast with herbal antiparasitic protocol. They are distinguishable from the stones, the rope-forms, and the bile by their consistent and specific morphology.

Adult roundworms (Ascaris lumbricoides) are six to thirteen inches long, the thickness of a pencil, pink to white to off-white in color, and resemble in their general appearance a wet earthworm or a strand of cooked spaghetti. They are pointed at both ends and possess three small lips at the head end. The female is longer and straighter; the male is shorter and tends to have a curved or coiled tail end. When freshly passed they may still be moving, the way an earthworm moves on damp ground. When they have been dead longer, they have a shriveled, dried-out appearance and break under tension where a living worm would not.

Tapeworm segments (proglottids) are small, flat, rectangular pieces, typically a quarter-inch to an inch in length, white or pale yellow when freshly passed, drying to a yellowish or sesame-seed appearance when older. They may resemble grains of cooked white rice or cucumber seeds. Freshly passed segments may still be wriggling or moving; this movement is one of the strongest indicators that the object is a parasite segment rather than food residue or mucus. A tapeworm in the gut releases a continuous chain of segments, so the practitioner who finds one is likely to find more across the days that follow.

Adult pinworms (Enterobius vermicularis) are small white threads, about a third of an inch long, fine enough that they can be mistaken for cotton fiber or thread of fabric. They are most often visible at the anal opening rather than within the stool, since the female emerges to lay eggs in the perianal skin. The flat-rectangular forms the practitioner sees in the bowl that are smaller than tapeworm segments and longer-and-thinner than roundworms are most often pinworms or the smaller fluke worms. Distinguishing among them by sight alone is often not possible. What can be said is that something with parasite morphology has been passed, and the protocol that has been doing its work has reached it.

Hookworms, whipworms, and the larger flukes that occupy the bile ducts are less commonly seen in the stool, since they tend to remain attached to gut tissue and to die in place rather than detach and pass. The practitioner who has been carrying these may not see them at all, even after a successful clearing. This is one reason among several that visible material in the bowl is not the only measure of the work.

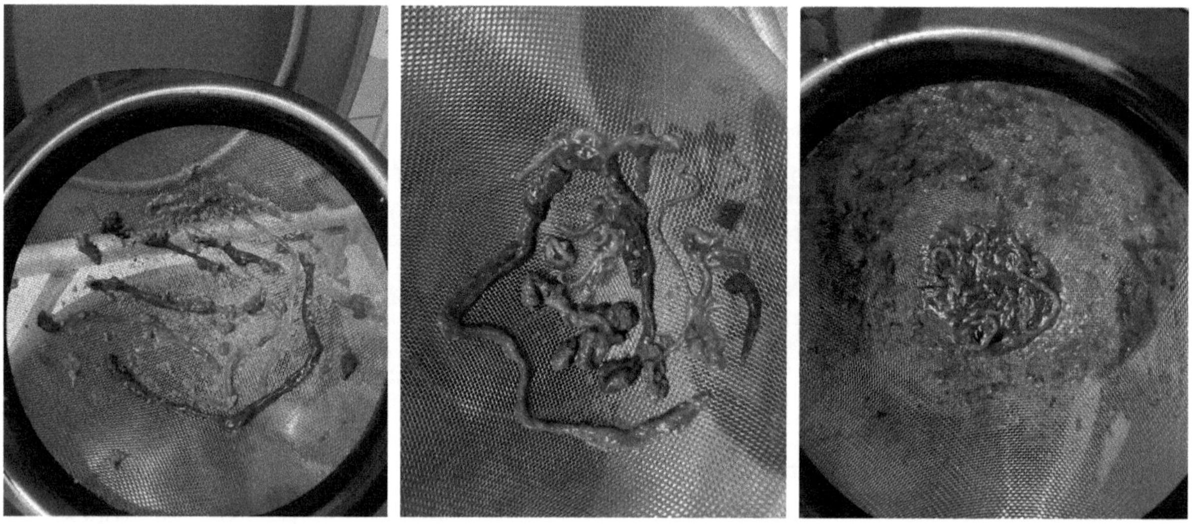

Rope-form material on the screen, released across the fast.

Patterns of completion

Across the arc of a forty-day fast, several patterns tend to emerge that, taken together, signal the work has reached its accessible layer. None of these patterns is a definitive stop signal on its own. The body that has been listening across the months of preparation and the weeks of the fast knows them collectively rather than individually.

The enema fluid quieting. In the first week, the water that comes out is heavily colored, full of particulate matter, and may be opaque with debris. By the second and third week, it carries less material and less color. By the fourth and fifth week, the fluid that comes out is closer to the fluid that went in, with intermittent bile staining and occasional small pieces. The water that comes back as it went in, day after day, is the gut reporting that the loose accumulated material has finished expelling.

The bile alone. As the gallbladder and accessible bile ducts release their stored material, the consistency of the bile-stained fluid changes. Early in the fast, the green ooze carries pebbles, fragments, and rope-forms within it. Later, the green ooze comes out as ooze alone — fluid only, without distinct pieces suspended within. Bile coming out as bile is one of the clearest signs the cleansing tradition reads as completion of the layer-clearing work.

The rope-forms ceasing. The long structured pieces, when they appear, do so on a schedule the body sets. They tend to appear most in the second through fourth week, and to taper off into the final weeks. When several days pass without a new structured piece, and when the days that follow continue to pass without one, the gut wall has finished expelling its loose accumulated material.

The body's own report. The morning gut, the energy on waking, the clarity through the day. A body that has cleared what was accessible begins to report a settled quietness that is recognizable from inside the experience even when difficult to describe from outside it. This report, which the prepared practitioner has been learning to read across the months of preparation, becomes the most reliable measure as the fast approaches its end.

On knowing when to stop

Two honest notes about completion. First, the layers of material the body holds extend deeper than any single fast can reach. The chapters on the layered gut and on the lining have already named that. What this fast clears is the currently accessible layer; what remains, in deeper reservoirs, will be the work of later fasts, of careful eating, of the slow long arc of the practice. The signs of completion in this chart are signs that this fast has done what this fast can do, not signs that the body has been cleared of all accumulated material across all layers. That work is longer.

Second, the risk of going too far is real and matters. Documented studies of prolonged water fasting show that the intestinal lining, while it renews, also undergoes measurable thinning and microvilli disruption during the fast itself. These changes revert with proper refeeding but are present while the fast is prolonged. The going has a stop signal. The coming back is where the lining either renews well or is asked to do too much before it has had time to thicken. The practitioner who reaches the signs of completion and continues fasting beyond them is asking a thinning lining to thin further, and the careful refeeding protocol described in the chapter on coming out of the fast becomes proportionally more important the longer the fast has gone. Listening at the end is what listening across the months of preparation has been preparing the practitioner to do.

A final note

The practitioner who has read this chart will recognize most of what appears in the bowl across the fast. What the chart has not done is replace the body's own knowledge of itself. The toilet bowl is a record of what has been released. The body that did the releasing is the only authority that can read what the release means for the work that remains.

For day-by-day visual confirmation across the arc of a prolonged fast, see the photo gallery referenced in the supplemental resources at the back of this book.

See the supplemental resources QR code at the back of this book for the recommended product list and printable version of this chart.

Chart Y

The Pre-Fast Checklist

* * *

By the time the close-in preparation arrives, the body has already been doing the work for months. The flush phase is finished or in its settle period. The dietary descent has been underway. The household has shifted. What remains, in the final two weeks, is a series of small specific tasks — confirming what is in the kitchen, confirming who has been told, confirming the body has what it will need — that protect the practitioner from arriving at day one and discovering something has been overlooked. This chart is the list. The reader is encouraged to print it (the QR code at the back gives access to a printable version) and physically check items off as they are completed.

One honest note before the list begins. The hardest task in the close-in preparation is not on this list. The hardest task is naming the day. The body has been ready for some time before the mind agrees, and the agreeing is not a step that can be checked off. A reader who finds themselves on the night before day one without the day actually being chosen yet should know this is a common experience and that the obstacle is not in the body. The list below cannot resolve the choosing. The list can ensure that, when the choosing happens, everything else is in place to receive it.

Two weeks before day one

The two-week mark is when close-in preparation begins. The dietary descent that has been underway should now arrive at one meal a day or close to it. Sleep should be the priority of the calendar. The household should know what is coming.

☐ Confirm the date you have chosen for day one. Write it down somewhere visible. If the date has not yet been chosen, choose it now.

- ☐ Inform the people in your life who will be affected by the fast: household members, employer if relevant, anyone who relies on you for care or work that will be reduced during the fast.
- ☐ Confirm any medical clearance you have sought. If you are on prescription medications and have not yet consulted a physician about the fast, do so this week, not in the final week.
- ☐ Take baseline measurements: body weight, waist circumference, blood pressure if you have a cuff at home, photographs from the front and side. These will matter later when you measure how far you have come.
- ☐ Confirm the kitchen is set up for the descent: ionic sulfated mineral concentrate, Himalayan sea salt, fresh organic produce for juicing, a working juicer, organic light-roast coffee for the morning enemas.
- ☐ Confirm the bathroom is set up: enema bag or bucket, the herbs you will be using during the fast, any topical or supportive items the protocol calls for.
- ☐ Confirm any travel or events on the calendar in the four weeks following day one. If something cannot be moved, factor it into the timing of the fast or move the fast itself.
- ☐ Begin reducing or eliminating alcohol if it has not already been eliminated. The body should not be processing alcohol in the final two weeks before a prolonged fast.
- ☐ Reduce social commitments that compete with rest. The fast will ask the body to do work that requires the body to not be stretched thin in the days leading up.

One week before day one

The final week is the closer-in window. The body should be on the descent it will continue into day one. The mind should be turning toward what is coming.

- ☐ Reduce solid food to one light evening meal. The body should be eating less than it is accustomed to in this final week.
- ☐ Begin the morning juice practice if it is not already underway. Fresh-pressed juices, low-sugar, predominantly green.
- ☐ Confirm hydration is consistent: water treated with ionic sulfated minerals, throughout the day, with Himalayan salt added in the proportion the chapter on hydration describes.
- ☐ Sleep eight hours where the body allows it. Rest more than usual.
- ☐ Reduce intense exercise. The body should be conserving rather than spending in this week.
- ☐ Conduct a final review of the household: are the people in it prepared for the days ahead, are the practical arrangements made, are there any commitments that have surfaced and need to be addressed before the fast begins.
- ☐ Re-read the chapters of this book that cover the early days of the fast (week one and the transition into ketosis). Knowing what is coming makes the experience cleaner.

- ☐ Write your intention for the fast. Put it in writing. Date it. Sign it. Keep it where you can find it during the difficult days.

Three days before day one

The three days before day one are the descent's last steady steps. For practitioners who have been doing the long descent across the prep year, these days may simply be the continuation of what has been ordinary. For practitioners who arrived at this list in compressed time, these days are the bridge from solid food into water.

- ☐ Eliminate solid food entirely. The diet for these three days is fresh-pressed juices, vegetable broth, herbal tea, and water treated with ionic sulfated minerals.
- ☐ Continue mineral hydration consistently. Twelve to sixteen glasses across the day.
- ☐ If you have been performing morning enemas as practice, continue. If not, the morning of day one is the natural point to begin.
- ☐ Sleep is the priority. Rest as the body asks.
- ☐ Speak with household members about the days ahead. Confirm anyone who will be supporting you knows what to look for and what not to worry about.
- ☐ Move any remaining tempting food out of the kitchen, or ask a household member to do so. Do not rely on willpower in the early days of the fast when temptation is at its strongest.
- ☐ Prepare a supply of the ingredients you will need for the morning juice and the morning coffee enema across day one and day two.

The day before day one

The day before is the threshold. The body has done the descent. The mind has, by now, named the day. What remains is one quiet day of completing the closing arrangements and resting.

- ☐ Final juice and broth day. Liquid only.
- ☐ Confirm everything on the previous lists has been completed.
- ☐ Bathe. Sleep clean linens. Set the bedroom up for restful sleep.
- ☐ Eliminate screens after sunset where possible. The mind should not be processing more inputs the night before than it must.
- ☐ Re-read your written intention.
- ☐ Sleep early. The morning of day one will arrive.

The morning of day one

Day one is the day the fast begins. Most practitioners find this morning unremarkable rather than dramatic; the body has been arriving at it for a long time, and the arrival itself is quiet.

☐ Wake at the time you intend to wake throughout the fast. Do not sleep in.

☐ Drink a glass of water treated with ionic sulfated minerals on waking. Add Himalayan salt to taste.

☐ Perform the first morning coffee enema if your protocol begins with day one (see Chart U for the liver-gallbladder flush protocol; see the chapters on coffee enemas for the daily fasting enema recipe).

☐ Take your morning herbs if your protocol calls for them.

☐ Eat nothing.

☐ Move into whatever the morning of day one is. The work has begun.

A final note

The list is done when the items are done. The fast is done when the body has finished doing what the fast asks. Between those two points is the work this book has been describing. Day one is the threshold. The body that crosses it has been preparing for a long time.

See the supplemental resources QR code at the back of this book for the recommended product list and printable version of this chart.

Supplement Timing Schedule

AM energy / PM recovery — fasting stack and post-refeed steady state

❦

How to read this

Two schedules. The first covers the fasting stack that supports the body through the final weeks of a prolonged fast. The second is the steady-state daily stack once refeeding is complete and the practitioner is eating a full whole-foods framework. The transition between them happens gradually across the fourteen-day refeed window — add dietary supplements (omega-3, creatine) back as food tolerance allows, and step thiamine down from 100 mg to 50 mg once whole grains return.

Color coding within each schedule: warm cream = morning energy block; pale green-gray = midday; cool blue-gray = evening calming/recovery block. The point is that the energy-supporting nutrients live in the first half of the day, and the calming/recovery nutrients live in the second half. The body has its own clock for what it needs when; the schedule respects it.

❦

Schedule A — The Late-Fast Stack

For the final weeks of a prolonged fast and the first three days of refeed. Schedule B phases in as food returns.

Notes on Schedule A

— The morning electrolyte mix should be diluted to roughly half-strength on a deeply fasted gut. Concentrated mixes are harder to absorb cleanly and can drive osmotic pull in the wrong direction. Sip over 30 to 60 minutes.

— Thiamine and B-complex spaced 30 minutes apart prevents the warm/buzzy crown sensation from stacking. The sensation itself is restoration noise, not warning noise — it represents B-vitamin metabolism coming back online in tissues that have been running depleted.

— D3 + K2 on the fast: ideally taken with a tablespoon of MCT or coconut oil if your protocol allows it. If not, hold until day 1 of refeed and take with the first dietary fat. Fat-soluble vitamins without fat are mostly excreted.

— Magnesium glycinate is non-negotiable at night. It is the molecule doing the most work for sleep onset, muscular calm, and the neuromuscular margin that prevents trigeminal signals from returning.

❦

Schedule B — The Post-Refeed Steady State

Once the fourteen-day staged refeed is complete and dietary intake is full, the daily stack shifts to this configuration. Thiamine drops from 100 mg to 50 mg as dietary thiamine returns. Omega-3 (algae oil) and creatine return as the fed-state stack. The magnesium evening dose increases.

Notes on Schedule B

— All fat-soluble vitamins (D3, K2, omega-3) live in the breakfast block because that is where dietary fat lives in the daily structure. Without fat present, the body absorbs roughly 30 percent of what is on the label. With fat, absorption climbs to 60–70 percent.

— B-complex with food, not on an empty stomach. The fasted-state empty-stomach dosing was a fasting-specific choice; once food is back, food is the better delivery vehicle.

— Calcium and magnesium continue to live on opposite ends of the day. They compete for the same absorption pathways, so giving them separate slots maximizes both.

— Creatine timing is flexible; what matters is consistency. The breakfast slot is the simplest place to land it so it does not get forgotten and does not crowd the evening calming stack.

— Glycine and L-glutamine are listed as "if using." Both are useful but optional; glycine for sleep, glutamine for gut-lining work in the first 4–6 weeks post-fast. Both can be dropped after the refeed window if they are not adding noticeable value.

❦

Quick reference — what goes when

Mornings are for the molecules that produce energy and restore cellular function: B-vitamins, thiamine, fat-soluble vitamins with breakfast fat, creatine for saturation, omega-3 with the meal.

Midday is for the splits: half the daily calcium, zinc-carnosine if using.

Evenings are for the molecules that calm, repair, and prepare the system for sleep: second calcium dose, glycine, glutamine, magnesium last.

The single most common timing mistake is taking magnesium in the morning. It will work, but it will pull the energy curve down through the middle of the day. Save it for the slot where its effect is what the body actually wants.

❦

Pre-Refeed Baseline Lab Requisition
A reference list of laboratory tests to draw on the final day of a prolonged fast, before refeeding begins.

CONTEXT FOR THE LAB / TECHNICIAN

The practitioner is on the final day of a medically-aware extended water fast and is requesting baseline labs BEFORE refeeding begins. This is a planned, supervised protocol — not a medical emergency, not an eating disorder.

Please note the following so reference-range flags are interpreted correctly:

• Insulin will be very low (expected, not pathological).

• Beta-hydroxybutyrate (BHB) will be very high (expected — deep ketosis).

• Thyroid will show conservation pattern (low T3, possibly elevated reverse T3) — expected, not pathological.

• Creatinine may be unreliable due to muscle mass changes — cystatin C is preferred.

• BUN may be elevated — protein catabolism, expected on extended fast.

- Uric acid may be elevated — purine turnover, expected.

Request a full copy of all raw results (not just summary) for personal documentation and the practitioner's own learning.

The practitioner is fasted. Provide the date of last food when scheduling.

TIER 1 — REFEEDING SAFETY (CRITICAL, before broth)

☐ Comprehensive Metabolic Panel (CMP)

☐ Phosphorus, serum

☐ Magnesium, RBC (NOT serum if possible — RBC is more accurate)

☐ Potassium (included in CMP — confirm reported)

☐ CBC with differential

☐ Thiamine (Vitamin B1), whole blood — refeeding safety

TIER 2 — NUTRIENT STATUS

☐ Vitamin B12 (active B12 / holoTC preferred; serum B12 if not available)

☐ Folate, serum (REPEAT — prior result <3.1 ng/mL = clinical deficiency)

☐ Vitamin D, 25-hydroxy

☐ Ferritin

☐ Iron + TIBC + transferrin saturation (full iron panel)

☐ Zinc, RBC

☐ Copper, serum

☐ Selenium

☐ Reticulocyte count

TIER 3 — METABOLIC SNAPSHOT (one-time, captures fasted state)

These values will change within hours of first food. Capturing the pre-refeed baseline is a one-time-only opportunity.

☐ Beta-hydroxybutyrate (BHB), serum

☐ Insulin, fasting

☐ Glucose, fasting (in CMP, confirm reported separately)

☐ Hemoglobin A1c

☐ Uric acid

TIER 4 — THYROID (conservation pattern expected)

☐ TSH

☐ Free T3

☐ Free T4

☐ Reverse T3

TIER 5 — INFLAMMATION / METHYLATION / LIPIDS

☐ hs-CRP (high-sensitivity C-reactive protein)

☐ Homocysteine

☐ Lipid panel (total cholesterol, LDL, HDL, triglycerides)

☐ GGT (gamma-glutamyl transferase)

☐ Bilirubin, direct and indirect (confirm both)

TIER 6 — HORMONES (recovery baseline)

☐ Cortisol, AM (morning draw)

☐ Testosterone, total and free

☐ DHEA-S

TIER 7 — KIDNEY (accurate function in low-muscle state)

☐ Cystatin C (preferred over creatinine in low muscle mass)

☐ Urinalysis (with protein, ketones, specific gravity, blood)

DELIVERY REQUESTS

- Please expedite results if possible (refeeding will begin shortly after the draw).
- Send full raw results via patient portal AND email (PDF).
- Flag any critical values to patient directly by phone.
- Indicate if no automatic supplement or medication recommendations are wanted — many practitioners doing this work interpret independently.

Thank you.

Reader Resources

Every figure, chart, and reference mentioned in this book — the parasite and bile photographs, the printable charts, and the recommended products — lives in a single online folder, kept current and added to over time. Scan the code, or type the address below into your browser.

eighthrs.com

www.ingramcontent.com/pod-product-compliance
Lightning Source LLC
LaVergne TN
LVHW070906210926
848482LV00017B/1008
* 9 7 8 0 9 9 9 8 9 9 0 4 5 *